Building ASL Interpreting and Translation Skills

Narratives for Practice (with DVD)

NANCI A. SCHEETZ

Valdosta State University

PEARSON

Boston ▪ New York ▪ San Francisco
Mexico City ▪ Montreal ▪ Toronto ▪ London ▪ Madrid ▪ Munich ▪ Paris
Hong Kong ▪ Singapore ▪ Tokyo ▪ Cape Town ▪ Sydney

To Richard
and
Melissa, Marie, Megghan and Chris, and Monique

Executive Editor and Publisher: Stephen D. Dragin
Editorial Assistant: Christina Certo
Marketing Manager: Kris Ellis-Levy
Production Editor: Gregory Erb
Editorial Production Service: Publishers' Design and Production Services, Inc.
Composition Buyer: Linda Cox
Manufacturing Buyer: Linda Morris
Electronic Composition: Publishers' Design and Production Services, Inc.
Interior Design: Publishers' Design and Production Services, Inc.
Cover Administrator: Elena Sidorova

For related titles and support materials, visit our online catalog at www.ablongman.com.

Between the time website information is gathered and then published, it is not unusual for
some sites to have closed. Also, the transcription of URLs can result in typographical errors.
The publisher would appreciate notification where these errors occur so that they may be
corrected in subsequent editions.

Cataloging-in-Publication data unavailable at press time.

ISBN-10: 0-205-47025-4
ISBN-13: 978-0-205-47025-9

Printed in the United States of America

10 9 8 7 6 5 4 3 2 1   EDW   11 10 09 08

Contents

Included on DVD

Included on DVD

⊙ Included on DVD

Included on DVD

Included on DVD

Included on DVD

Included on DVD

**PART IV Selections for Interpreting
          and Transliterating   271**

Included on DVD

Included on DVD

Preface

*B*uilding *ASL Interpreting and Translation Skills* has been designed for students taking courses in American Sign Language (ASL) as well as students and practitioners engaged in the field of interpreting who want to develop or enhance their skills. It has been developed to be used as a primary text in translation, consecutive, and simultaneous interpreting. This text will also find application in transliterating courses and as a secondary text in ASL courses. Designed as a workbook with an accompanying DVD, it has been divided into four parts.

Part I includes twenty-four chapters. Each chapter begins with a brief introduction to one of the specific grammatical features found in ASL. This provides students with essential background information before they translate the paragraphs found within each chapter. The discussion is followed by a sample paragraph that is glossed in ASL. Each chapter contains selections comprised of three- and four-sentence paragraphs. Presented in a workbook format, students have the opportunity to gloss each of the paragraphs and then practice their skills signing them. All of the examples contained in the first twenty-four chapters are signed on the accompanying DVD. At the end of each chapter, there is space allotted for students to write their own selection, gloss it, and practice signing it.

Part II, containing twenty-two chapters, is structured using the same basic format as Part I. Additional pedagogy pertaining to ASL principles is provided within the first twelve chapters. Throughout Part II the selections become increasingly longer. Chapters 13 through 22 do not include any specific pedagogy; rather, they are designed to let students draw from previous information and test their skills and their abilities by translating the narratives into ASL. Toward the end of Part II, the selections include more complex material in the form of practice paragraphs. This material is designed to segue into Part III.

Part III is divided into three sections: Multiple-Meaning Words, Idioms, and Vocabulary Building. These selections in Part III are longer and are designed to provide interpreters with source material that covers a wide variety of topics.

Within the first ten chapters of Part II, one multiple-meaning word is repeated several times within each of the selections. Generally, we do not hear these words used this way; however, by presenting them multiple times within a few short paragraphs, students are challenged to practice changing concepts quickly in order to express meaning accurately. Following each selection, five of the sentences have been pulled out, allowing students to focus on how they would gloss the individual sentences.

The second section within Part III, Chapters 11 through 15, focuses on English language idioms. Between five and seven idioms are presented in each of the narratives. The goal is not to model spoken language but rather to provide source material illustrating how these phrases are used and therefore, how they could be signed. At the end of each passage, individual sentences taken from the selection are provided for students to practice their translation skills.

The third part of Part III, Chapters 16 through 20, focuses on both enhancing and expanding vocabulary. Some of these selections have been taken from college texts, providing examples of varied and challenging source material. Within the field of interpreting, it is critical that practitioners acquire not only the mastery of both English and ASL but that they develop the skill of automaticity, so when they hear a word, they can immediately process what the word means, quickly retrieve the appropriate sign, and produce the message in a grammatically correct format. The exercises in Part III are designed to promote the development of these abilities.

Part IV contains selections of varying lengths. These can be used with students wanting to enhance both their consecutive and their simultaneous interpreting and transliterating skills. Part IV includes narratives, lectures, and passages from texts that might be read in a high school or college class.

Selected narratives from Part II through Part IV have been included on the DVD. Selections from the first twelve chapters in Part II are signed by Jeanne, with no voice added. Designated selections from Chapter 13 in Part II through the remaining chapters in Part IV are signed by a nationally certified interpreter. These narrations are presented in picture-in-picture format demonstrating simultaneous voice/sign interpretation. The symbol ⌾ indicates selections on DVD.

This workbook is designed as a teaching–learning vehicle. It has been developed to use in multiple classes starting with ASL I and continuing through simultaneous interpreting. It contains a wealth of source materials that vary in topic and in level of difficulty and complexity. Signers and interpreters are keenly aware of the importance of developing strong English and ASL skills. These exercises are designed to enhance those skills.

This text could not have been completed without the assistance of several individuals. The author wishes to extend thanks to Jeanne Ames and Amy Elton who diligently read through the examples, the transcription symbols, and the translations. Their insights were particularly helpful. The author also wants to extend special thanks to William Newell for his patience, perseverance, dedication, and the many hours he devoted to this project. His wealth of knowledge, his willingness to share his expertise, and his keen eye have been invaluable. This manuscript has certainly become stronger with his assistance. Special thanks are also extended to Chris McCuller for his technical assistance, the faculty in the Department of Special Education and Communication Disorders at Valdosta State University, and my family for their stories and words of support and encouragement throughout this project. The author also wants to thank all of the students who volunteered their time to record all of the narratives that are included in the text. Special thanks to Jeremy Williams, Megghan Brooks, and Chris McCuller for also volunteering their time to record some selections included on the DVD. The author also wants to express her gratitude to Jeanne Ames, Stephanie Fenton, Erin Salmon, and Christia Williams for the time they devoted to translating and signing/interpreting the selections for the DVD. Their expertise with the language and their willingness to invest hours to ensure the selections were signed/interpreted accurately will provide students with valuable models as they work toward mastering their own sign and interpreting skills. Heartfelt thanks are also extended to Mr. Bill Muntz who invested hours of his time recording all of the selections in the text, prepared the files for the DVD, and monitored the overall production of the speakers, signers, and interpreters. His expertise and attention to detail have resulted in producing quality examples for those who will use this text.

Thanks are also extended to the reviewers of this edition for their time and input: Jean F. Andrews, Lamar University; Lyes Bousseloub, California State University, Sacramento; Sue A. Cutler, Kalamazoo Valley Community College; J. Freeman King, Utah State University; William Newell, Valdosta State University; and Jean S. Plant, Georgia Perimeter College. And finally, thanks are extended to Steve Dragin and the staff at Allyn and Bacon for making this an enjoyable experience.

Transcription Symbols Representing American Sign Language with Written Transcription

Symbol	Example	Explanation
Capitalized English Words	MAN	Signs are illustrated and labeled with capitalized English words (these words are referred to as glosses).
- (hyphens)	NOT-YET	When words are joined together as in NOT-YET, the hyphen alerts the signer that the concept is presented with one sign.
fs-	fs-MARY	fs-hyphen is used to represent fingerspelling in ASL.
( ) Parentheses	(head nod, head moving from side to side)	Words represented in parentheses indicate an action or a movement, i.e., affirmative or negative responses. This can be done in conjunction with or independent of signs.
+	CLASS+ROOM	A plus sign between the word for sign glosses indicates a compound sign or a contraction.
++	WORK++	Plus signs following glosses indicate repetition of the sign.
# before the sign	# BANK	Fingerspelled Loan Signs.
IX	(IX)HE	Referential Indexing used for third-person pronouns (he, she, it, him her). When identifying a specific referent, it is included in quotes immediately after the gloss (i.e., 1X-"Mary").
IX-lf, IX-ctr, IX-rt	CAR IX-lf	Reference a pronoun by specific location. lf represents left; ctr, center; rt, right.
+AGENT	DANCE+AGENT	The Agent marker is used in ASL together with verbs such as DANCE, TEACH, PREACH to indicate the individual performing the action.
!	STAY!	An exclamation mark after the gloss indicates the sign is stressed; this is used for the emphatic form.
" "	"wave-right"	Quotation marks when placed around words written in lowercase indicate gesture-like signs.
IX-loc	TABLE-"there"	Information included in quotations immediately following a gloss can be used to specify the location of a place or an object.
-cont	SICK-cont	When -cont is placed after a gloss it indicates the verb is continuously inflected.
MOVE"right"	PUT "here"	Information about where something is located in space is shown in quotes, immediately after the gloss.
POSS	POSS "Joel"	POSS is used to indicate possessive pronouns. When necessary, the specific name of the referent is added in quotation marks immediately following the symbol (i.e., POSS "Joel" to indicate it is Joel's).
↔	DRIVE here and lf ↔	This indicates that the movement occurs between two different spatial locations.

Symbols for Non-Manual Behaviors

Symbol	Example	Explanation
y/s-q	<u>y/s-q</u> YOU HEARING YOU?	Yes/No Questions
whq	<u>wh-q</u> NAME YOU?	*Wh*-word questions
neg	<u>neg</u> NO, ME NOT STUDENT	Negation

(continued)

Symbol	Example	Explanation
t	_____t_____ SEE THERE MAN RED HAT, NICE HE.	Topic Marker. Indicates that eyebrows are raised while signing the topic and lowered for the comment.
-when-	-when- NEW HOUSE. UNLOAD. FINISH I TIRED.	Indicates when something happens.
cond	____cond____ WEATHER BAD, GAME CANCEL.	Conditional clause—this will always be the first part of the sentence when conditional clauses are used.
rs:	____rs:girl____ IX GIRL EXCITED	The "rs" indicates role shifting, signaling the person whose role the signer is assuming.
rhet-q	____rhet-q____ fs-SUE VP-TO-ME. WHY? CAR IX BREAKDOWN.	Rhetorical question.
nod	_____nod_____ ME FINISH READ, GIVE-YOU.	Assertions in ASL can be indicated by nod.
cs	__t___cs__ BOOK- THERE	The cs represents the cheek to the shoulder used to indicate close proximity in time or location.
oo	oo____ SMALL	Extremely small or thin.
Cha	__t__Cha__ MAN TALL	Extremely tall or large.

Symbols for Classifiers

Symbol	Example	Explanation
CL:C	MY GLASS ME CL:C PUT-THERE, GONE.	Represents a cylinder-like shape the size of a glass, cup, or bottle.
CL:CC	ME CL:CC CARRY TO OUTSIDE	Represents cylinder-like shape such as lamppost, coffee can, or flower pot.
CL:F	COINS CL:F IN A ROW	Small round, flat disk-like shape such as a coin or button.
CL:LL	PLATTER CL:LL BRING-TO KITCHEN	Large, round, flat disk-like shape such as a plate, larger platter, place mat, or frame.
CL:C˚	BOOK CL:C˚ GIVE-TO YOU	For objects such as a book, a flat box, a box of candy, or a stack of paper.
CL:O˚	NEWSPAPER CL:O˚ MOVE-TO COUNTER	For thin, flat objects such as a sheet of paper or a thin magazine.
CL:5	APPLES TWO CL:5-NEXT-TO-CL:5	For small round objects such as a baseball, an apple, or an orange.
CL:S>	MUGS CL:S> NEXT-TO-CL:S>THERE	For handle-like objects or objects with handles such as a broom, a pitcher, or a mug.
CL:5̈5̈	ME CL:5̈5̈-EYES-FALL-OUT	Used to represent small round objects.
CL:B	MAN HE CL:B "tall" DIRT CL:B-HANDFUL	Can vary to indicate smaller and larger sizes, piles, or amounts of something.
CL:A>	SHELF HAVE STATUES CL:A>	Objects that do not move, such as a house or other building, a statue.
CL:Λ	MAN CL:Λ STAND THERE, HE LOOK-AT-YOU	Person standing upright or an animal that stands upright such as an ape.
CL:Y	TWO AIRPLANE CL:Y- NEXT-TO CL:Y	Aircraft with wings (not helicopters or rockets).
CL:V	SEE MY DOG CL:V -THERE	A crouched or sitting person or animal.
CL:1	MAN HE CL:1 WALKED DOWN STREET	An upright person or animal such as a bear walking on its hind legs.
CL:11	PICTURE BIG CL:11-SQUARE-SHAPE	To indicate the outline of a shape such as a window.
CL:CC	CHAIR CL:CC LONG-THERE	To describe thickish objects such as a sofa, counter, low hedge, or a thick border or edge.
CL:B	SHE FORGET LEFT MAGAZINE CL:B-THERE	To describe a flat surface or object such as a tabletop, countertop, or small rug.
CL:G	SHELF HAVE DIRT CL:G-THIN-LAYER-ON-CL:B	CL:G is used to show various thicknesses, widths, or depths.
CL:BB	I NEED PAPER CL:BB-THICK STACK, FOR-FOR RESEARCH PAPER	CL:BB is used to show greater thickness, width or depth.

Based on transcription symbols found in: Lentz, E.M., Mikos, K., & Smith, C. (1989). *Signing naturally: Teacher's curriculum guide.* Berkeley, CA: Dawn Sign Press. Baker, C., & Cokely, D. (1980). *American Sign Language: A teacher's resource text on grammar and culture.* Silver Spring, MD: T.J. Publishers. Humphries, T., & Padden, C. (2004). *Learning American Sign Language* (2nd ed.). Boston: Allyn and Bacon. Humphries, T., Padden, C., & O'Rourke, T.J. (1994). *A basic course in American Sign Language* (2nd ed.). Silver Spring, MD: T.J. Publishers.

PART I

Selections for Beginning ASL Students

Pronouns, Locations, and Use of Sign Space

American Sign Language (ASL) is a rich language used within and among members of the Deaf community. Like other languages, it provides a systematic means for communicating thoughts, ideas, and feelings through the use of conventional symbols (Schein, 1984). ASL uses the visual representations of concepts utilizing three-dimensional space to transmit information (Borden, 1996).

The articulatory system of ASL uses "images made by fingers, hands, and arms—images that are linguistically shaped by movements of the eyebrows, lips and cheeks, by the hunching and thrusting of the shoulders, by the signer's posture" to communicate with those who share a common language (Schein & Stewart, 1995).

While spoken languages follow a linear order, sound by sound, word by word, ASL is produced visually with signs simultaneously communicating additional information, i.e., number, adverbials, questions versus statements, and other grammatical information. This simultaneous additional information is conveyed through the signs, spatial relationships, and sign movements and non-manual signals. As a result, signed messages require a two-part process on the part of signers. First, signers initiating a message must possess the ability to construct mentally a visual image of what they want to convey. Second, they must be able to accurately present concepts visually to ensure that recipients of the message are provided with the information that is intended. From the onset, if novice signers can begin to create in their minds a mental image of what they want the receiver to understand, they start to develop insights into the construction of ASL. However, if they fail to grasp this concept and instead produce signed messages that are structured to represent English words and English word order, the visual concept is frequently lost. This can, and frequently does, lead to misunderstandings and communication breakdowns.

Signed messages are produced in the signing space. Signers/interpreters produce signs in an area that includes the space from the waist to the top of the head. The majority of signs are made within a space referred to as the normal or general signing space. This provides the viewer with the opportunity to maintain eye contact while at the same time observing the speaker's hands and upper torso to read/understand aspects of the signs and non-manual signals being presented. Although the signing space extends approximately six to eight inches above the head and out from the shoulders, the area reserved for fingerspelling is much smaller (Scheetz, 1998). Figure 1.1 provides an illustration of the space used to communicate using signs and fingerspelling.

Sign space plays an integral role in ASL. It provides the backdrop for thoughts, ideas, and concepts to be expressed. It also affords the signer/interpreter the opportunity to describe relationships, incorporate directional verbs, and utilize time indicators.

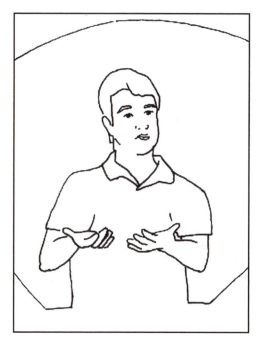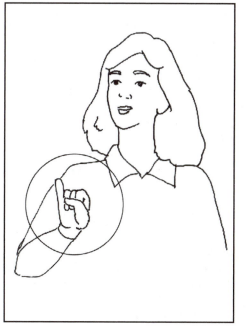

FIGURE 1.1 Use of Sign and Fingerspelling Space
Source: Courtesy of Marie A. Scheetz

According to Borden (1996) there are four basic reality principles that must be followed to promote the correct use of space within ASL. First, information must be conveyed from the **general to the specific**. Once the background and the big picture are established, details can be added. Second, ASL communicates **concrete information before abstract** information. In essence, objects must be in place within the signing space before any actions can occur. Third, **spatial relationships** must be established that reflect how these concepts are related to one another in the "real world." Fourth, ASL adheres to **chronological order**, creating scenes in space that represent the events in the actual order that they occurred. In essence, the concepts that are produced in sign space should be as much a reflection of the real world as possible (Borden, 1966, p. 18).

Through ASL, nouns (people, places, and things) can be identified and established within the signer's sign space. This is accomplished by first identifying the individuals, events, or objects that are being discussed and then establishing their locations within the general sign space. Once identified, signers/interpreters can use these locations to refer back to these individuals, places, or events.

In ASL this process is called *pronominalization*. When incorporating pronouns in ASL, the noun is produced first, followed by spatial indexing that is frequently accompanied with eye gaze to a space that becomes designated as the person, place, or thing (Kelly, 2001).

Signers can refer to people or things whether they are physically present or not, by pointing, using one of several handshapes, or by shifting their eyes to a specific point in space. Furthermore, multiple locations can be established in space and remain for the duration of the conversation. Several strategies are employed by signers when establishing the locations of people or things. In instances when describing events that occurred in the past, the signer will reference them in the order that they occurred, thus following the reality principle (Borden, 1966). In situations in which individuals are being referenced, they will be arranged in space around the signer's body so that they may be referred to later in the discourse.

Sometimes pronouns in English can be ambiguous—for example, as in "Tony insulted Jorge and then he hit him." In this example, we aren't certain who hit whom. In ASL there is no ambiguity when expressing the equivalent sentence (Markowicz, 1980): JORGE IX-lf, TONY IX-rt. IX-rt-Tony INSULT IX-lf-Jorge. IX-lf-Jorge PUNCH IX-rt-Tony.

When referencing is used appropriately to refer to a noun or nouns that have been previously established in the designated sign space, the signer/interpreter is effectively using pronouns in ASL.

Practice selections are included below to provide you with the opportunity to practice translating English into ASL. When translating these sentences, gloss them in ASL the way that you would sign them. Transcription symbols have been included at the beginning of this text to assist you with your translations. Once you have translated the paragraphs, practice signing them. Pay particular attention to your use of sign space and your placement of nouns and use of pronominal references.

Throughout Part I of the text, examples of how to gloss English sentences have been provided. Please note that these are only examples of one way these can be glossed. The examples are not intended to be viewed as the only way these sentences can be signed. As with any language, ASL can express the same ideas using different signs and structures.

You will find each of the examples signed on the DVD. Additional selections, indicated by an asterisk, are also signed or interpreted on the DVD.

 EXAMPLE 1.0
....

Marti lives here in New York. Karla lives in California. They are both university teachers. Marti is deaf and has one brother and no sisters. Karla is hearing and has two sisters.

fs-MARTI IX-rt LIVE NEW-YORK, fs-KARLA IX-lf LIVE CALIFORNIA. TWO-OF-THEM TEACH UNIVERSITY. IX-rt-Marti DEAF. HAVE BROTHER ONE, SISTER NONE. IX-lf-Karla HEARING. HAVE SISTER TWO.

Selection 1.1: Mary Lives in New York

Mary lives in New York. She has one brother and one sister. Her parents are deaf, just like Mary. Her brother and sister are both hearing.

_____

_____

_____

_____

Selection 1.2: Tom's Learning ASL

Tom's taking a class at the university. He's learning to be a sign language teacher and is taking an ASL I class. When he doesn't understand, he asks the teacher to explain again. He's the only man in his class.

_____

_____

_____

_____

Selection 1.3: Fingerspell That Again

Please fingerspell your name again. I didn't understand what you spelled. Oh, I see, you're from California. Do you go to school there? What's the name of the college?

5

CHAPTER 1
....
Pronouns,
Locations, and Use
of Sign Space

PART I

PART II

PART III

PART IV

_____

_____

_____

_____

Selection 1.4: Susan Attends School

Susan's hard of hearing. She goes to a mainstreamed school. When she doesn't understand, she writes her questions on paper. Then the teacher explains more to her.

_____

_____

_____

_____

Selection 1.5: A Teacher at the Residential School

Who's the man teaching at the residential school? Where's he from? Is he hearing, hard of hearing, or deaf? Which class does he teach? Where did he attend college?

_____

_____

_____

_____

Selection 1.6: My Father

Your teacher's my father. He's a nice man. His name's Michael Worth, but he's called M.J. He writes books, teaches classes, and has a deaf father and a hearing mother.

_____

_____

_____

_____

Selection 1.7: The French Teacher

Do you know the name of the high school French teacher sitting by the door? She knows English and is now learning Spanish and sign language. Then she will know four languages. I can't remember her name. I knew it before but now I've forgotten it.

_____

_____

_____

_____

Selection 1.8: The Elementary School

I know the high school is over there and the college is over here. But where's the elementary school? Is it over there by the high school or over here by the college? I don't remember where my father said it was. If you explain to me again where it is, I know I can get there.

_____
_____
_____
_____

Selection 1.9: Learning Sign Language

Excuse me, what's your name and where are you learning sign language? I'm learning it too. Do you take classes from the deaf man at the university or are you a student at the high school? Why do you want to learn ASL? Do you have a deaf sister or brother? My friend's deaf and I want to sign to her.

_____
_____
_____
_____

Selection 1.10: What Does It Mean?

Do you know what the girl standing by the window signed? Does she want a pen, paper, or a book? I didn't understand her. I need to have her explain it again. I'm just now taking a sign language class and I need to learn more. She's a student at the residential school in New York; she isn't hearing.

_____
_____
_____
_____

Free Expressive Practice: Introduce yourself, demonstrating your ability to locate nouns and pronouns within your sign space.

Hi, my name is _____ and I live _____. (Provide additional information.) _____

_____
_____
_____

CHAPTER 2

Directional Verbs

Verbs play a significant role in all languages. They function as the main elements in predicates, providing a mechanism for expressing actions, states of being, or relationships between two or more objects. They may be inflected to indicate tense, aspect, voice, and mood. Unlike nouns that name people, places, and things, verbs convey information by describing what these people, places, and things are doing, what is being done to them, as well as actions that occur between them.

In American Sign Language (ASL) verbs are expressed in a variety of ways. According to Padden (1983), as cited in Smith, Lentz, and Mikos (1988), verbs in ASL can be placed in either of two primary categories: plain, inflecting, also referred to as directional verbs, or spatial verbs. **Plain verbs or nondirectional verbs** are referred to as those that require the signer to specify the subject and the object. These verbs can only name an action and can't be modified in their movement to provide any other information (Borden, 1996, p. 61). When using plain/nondirectional verbs, it is critical that signers explicitly mention who is initiating the action and who is the recipient of the action. Because these verbs are always signed in the same manner, they do not convey subject or object specific information (Smith, Lentz, & Mikos, 1988, p. 108). Some examples of plain/nondirectional verbs in ASL include EAT, DRINK, PLAY, LIKE, NEED, THINK, and WANT.

Directional verbs utilize directionality of movement to indicate who is the initiator and who is the recipient in the interaction. In these instances both the subject and the object are identified by changing the direction, location, and the movement of the sign. Some examples of directional verbs in ASL include GIVE, CHOOSE, PAY, and LOOK AT. When signers want to indicate that they are giving someone something, the sign moves away from the body in the direction of the recipient. This hand movement and direction often replaces the function served by word order in English (Schein & Stewart, 1995, p. 36). In essence, the subject is easily identifiable based on the direction of the sign movement (Smith, Lentz, & Mikos, p. 108).

When employing the use of directional verbs, it is critical that signers begin the sign in the appropriate location in sign space and move the sign in the direction of the recipient of the action. In these instances, the spatial location of the signer designates the first person, the individual with whom the signer is communicating becomes the second person, and any other individuals or things become the third person (Cokely & Baker-Shenk, 1991, p. 67). It is essential that all parties involved in the communication exchange are aware of the spatial locations that are designated through the use of directional verbs. In the event that these identifications are not made and the appropriate use of sign space is not followed, breakdowns in communication can occur.

There are several categories of directional verbs. Borden (1996) categorizes three different types of directional verbs. The three types consist of one-directional: travel verbs, nontravel verbs, and object verbs. One-directional verbs are so designated because they are used to depict the act of traveling from one location to another while at the same time creating a location for the individual/object to go. Inflecting/one-directional travel verbs include GO, COME, FLY, and RUN.

One-directional nontravel verbs allow the signer to identify the object of the verb. In these instances the signer is able to convey the specific initiator of the action and the object or individual who is the recipient of the action. Inflecting/one-directional nontravel verbs include, but are not limited to, ADVISE, ASK, PAY, SEE, and TELL.

One-directional object verbs share all of the characteristics of the two previous groups. However, verbs functioning in this group are designed to act on a third object within the sentence. Some of the one-directional object verbs include BRING/CARRY, BUY, and SEND (Borden, 1996, p. 95). See Figure 2.1 for an example of a one-directional object verb.

Cokely and Baker-Shenk (1991) further describe another category of directional verbs as being reciprocal in nature. In these instances, the signer can indicate that two people or two groups of people are engaged in the same activity at the same time by using both hands to produce like signs. When this occurs, each hand represents the action of one person or group. Based on the location of the hands, their direction of movement, and the palm orientation, the signer can indicate which person(s) or group(s) are involved in the action (p. 73). When using the reciprocal directional verbs communication technique, two individuals can look at each other at the same time, groups can exchange information or trade places, and people can stay in constant contact with each other.

Spatial verbs require the identification of the subject and the object; however, because spatial verbs allow for changes in directionality, they function in the same manner as inflecting verbs. Spatial verbs allow the signer to indicate if he or she is placing an object above or below, or if the individual is retrieving an object from a designated area. Within this context the signer must indicate who is initiating the activity before demonstrating where the object is located. Examples of spatial verbs include PUT-UP, BRING-DOWN, GET-FROM-ABOVE, PUT-DOWN-BELOW, and so forth.

In the selections that follow several of them contain directional verbs. First, change the English text into ASL; second, practice signing the sentences demonstrating your command of directional verbs. Example 2.0 is signed on the DVD.

 EXAMPLE 2.0

Yesterday Bill told me he would help me find the sign language class. He said he knew where it was. I asked him when he could help me. He said he would show me today.

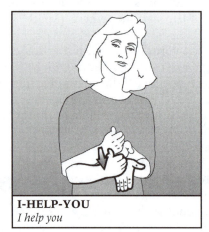 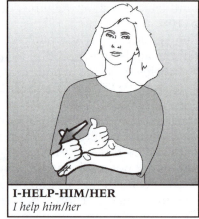

I-HELP-YOU
I help you

I-HELP-HIM/HER
I help him/her

FIGURE 2.1 Example of a Directional Verb

Source: From Humphries, Tom, & Carol Padden, *Learning American Sign Language*, 2/e. Published by Allyn and Bacon, Boston, MA. Copyright © 2004 by Pearson Education. Reprinted by permission of the publisher.

_____ t _____ nod _____
YESTERDAY fs-BILL TELL-me, SIGN LANGUAGE CLASS he-HELP-me FIND.

_____ rs ___ whq _____
IX-rt-he SAY KNOW WHERE CLASS. me-ASK-TO-he, "HELP-me WHEN"? IX-rt-he SAY TODAY SHOW-me.

Selection 2.1: The Teacher Helps Out

I told the teacher I didn't understand what she meant. She told me she'd help me. She explained again and told me to bring her the book. She looked at the lesson, explained more, and then I understood.

_____
_____
_____

Selection 2.2: Please Help Me

Please hurry and go to the library and bring me the box of books. I need them to teach my class. I want to show the students the signs they need to learn today. Thanks for helping me.

_____
_____
_____

Selection 2.3: Sending a Box to California

Did you watch TV today? The man was demonstrating how to send chairs and tables to California from Georgia. You need a box for the two items. Go to the post office, pay the woman, and she'll help you send them to California.

_____
_____
_____

Selection 2.4: Finding the Restroom

Excuse me, is the restroom by the bookstore or the cafeteria? Can you help me? Please tell me where it is. I asked the woman at the desk in the library but she didn't know. She told me you could show me where it is.

_____
_____
_____

Selection 2.5: Bring Chairs to the Table

The teacher told the students to bring their chairs and books to the table. She gave them pens and paper and told them to explain what they learned in sign language class.

_____
_____
_____

Selection 2.6: Locating the Gold Paper

Hi, where's the gold paper? I need it to take to the library. The woman there will send it to the bookstore. I'll go with you to get it. Can we go now?

_____

_____

_____

Selection 2.7: Meet Monique

Come on! Please hurry! I want you to meet Monique. Can you come? She's over there sitting at the table in the cafeteria by the window. She's really a nice woman. She helped me move when I came here to college.

_____

_____

_____

Selection 2.8: Where Is the Office?

Do you remember where the office is? Is it down the hall by the classroom or is it across from the elevator? I want to give my paper to the teacher. Then I want to go to the cafeteria and get a drink.

_____

_____

_____

Selection 2.9: The Lady in the Cafeteria

I'm going to the cafeteria. Do you want to come? I need some coffee and candy. Do you know the woman who works there? She's also in my French class. We went to elementary and high school together. Now we're learning French together.

_____

_____

_____

Selection 2.10: Jason's Sign Language Class

I don't know where Jason's learning sign language. I know he has classes at a university but I don't know the name of the college. His teacher's deaf and Jason told me that he enjoys teaching. Jason said the teacher comes in, blinks the lights, says "good morning," and he's ready to begin.

_____

_____

_____

Free Expressive Practice: Create your own selection here demonstrating your command of directional verbs.

_____

_____

_____

_____

Descriptive Adjectives

merican Sign Language like other languages provides many ways for describing people, places, and things through the use of adjectives. However, unlike in English, adjectives may appear before or after the noun. When describing an individual to someone for the first time, the gender of the person is always mentioned first. This is followed by describing the individual's most unique or distinguishing characteristic.

In ASL, once the gender and the unique features of the individual have been established, a description of the person tends to follow a particular order. Height tends to be mentioned first followed by the person's body type, the color of the person's hair, and his or her hairstyle (Smith, Lentz, & Mikos, 1988, p. 90). Adjectives used to describe the person's hair, eyes, and other physical characteristics can occur either before or after the nouns they are modifying.

Therefore, when describing a tall man with red curly hair in ASL it could be signed either MAN TALL HAIR RED CURLY or as TALL MAN RED CURLY HAIR. In English, the same description would be presented as, "the tall man with red curly hair," placing the descriptive adjectives before the noun or within the prepositional phrase.

Descriptive adjectives are also used to describe clothing, including patterns found on fabrics and objects as well as the length and style of fashions. Plaids, polka dots, and stripes can be portrayed through sign. When describing sizes and shapes, signers frequently represent these patterns through the use of classifiers.

Classifiers, although not unique to American Sign Language, serve an important role when communicating using the language. Some classifiers are used to represent nouns, indicate noun location, demonstrate noun movement, and describe the functionality of objects. In these instances, they frequently function as predicate phrases (Newell et al., in press).

Other classifiers function as descriptive adjectives. This category of classifiers is referred to as Size and Shape Specifiers (SASSes). Size and Shape Specifiers are used to describe objects. Differentiated by handshape, these classifiers can show the particular size, shape, and texture of objects, and distinguish between shallow objects and objects having depth (Baker & Cokley, 1980, p. 308). In these instances, the noun is identified first followed by the descriptive adjective that can be represented with a classifier.

Classifiers are represented with the abbreviation CL. There are numerous classifiers used to describe size and shape. Two examples of SASSes are the CL:F and the CL:G. The CL:F handshape represents small round flat objects, such as coins, polka dots, small flowers located on a particular piece of fabric, small pieces of candy, or buttons.

When describing buttons on a shirt, dress, or blouse, the signer would begin by signing SHIRT, DRESS, or BLOUSE. This would be followed by fingerspelling the noun, button (fs-BUTTON), and then signing the classifier, in this instance CL:F indicating the size, location, and the relationships to previously identified objects. This provides the signer with a visual representation of buttons, thus indicating if they appear vertically, horizontally, diagonally, or randomly on an object.

The CL:G classifier is used to describe the width or thickness of an object. By using this descriptive adjective, the signer can describe how thick a book is, how much rain was collected in a bucket after a torrential thunderstorm, and so forth. Examples of the CL:F and the CL:G handshapes are represented in Figure 3.1.

In the selections that follow, translate the English into ASL. Then practice signing these sentences while incorporating descriptive adjectives.

 EXAMPLE 3.0
....

Julie is a short, thin woman who has cute clothes. Have you seen her blue and grey striped sweater with the three buttons on the outside of each sleeve? She looks good in it.

<u>   t   </u>

WOMAN NAME fs-JULIE IX-rt-she SHORT-STATURE THIN, CLOTHES CUTE.

<u>   y/n-q   </u>

FINISH SEE IX-rt-Julie SWEATER BLUE HAVE GREY CL:4-stripe-on-chest,

SLEEVE fs-BUTTON THREE CL:F-on-outside-wrist? IX-rt-she APPEARANCE GOOD.

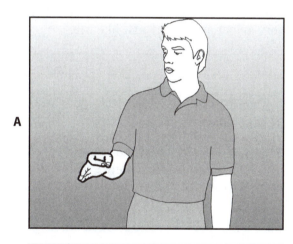

A

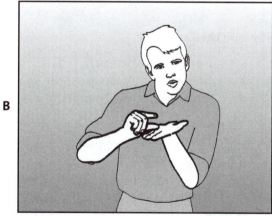

B

FIGURE 3.1 **(A)** Example of the Classifier CL:F Used as a Descriptor to Represent Small, Flat Objects; **(B)** Example of the Classifier CL:G Used as a Descriptor to Represent Width or Thickness

Source: From Humphries, Tom, & Carol Padden, *Learning American Sign Language,* 2/e. Published by Allyn and Bacon, Boston, MA. Copyright © 2004 by Pearson Education. Reprinted by permission of the publisher.

Selection 3.1: The Woman in the Library

Did you see the woman sitting at the table in the library? She's tall, medium build, curly brown hair, and blue eyes. She was wearing a red dress with white stripes. She's my sign language teacher.

_____

_____

_____

Selection 3.2: The Man in the Cafeteria

Who's the man in the cafeteria? He's short, has black hair, a beard, brown eyes, and is really, really thin! He had on a blue coat today. He's so arrogant. He ordered me to go to the library and bring him a book.

_____

_____

_____

Selection 3.3: Woman with the Gray Hair

See the woman with the gray hair. She has on a hat, a short-sleeve orange V-necked shirt, and a brown skirt. She's tall, a little chubby, and she looks like my mother. She's very sweet and smart just like me.

_____

_____

_____

Selection 3.4: Who Is That Snob?

Who's that snob? What's her name? She's not smart; she's not pretty. She's not friendly. She has black hair that's cut close. She's from New York. Why do you think she moved here? Maybe her dad got a job teaching at the university.

_____

_____

_____

Selection 3.5: The Boy with the Curly Hair

Do you know that boy, that one with the curly red hair and the blue eyes? When the teacher asks him questions, he's always right. He hasn't made a mistake yet. He's just like the little girl with the blonde hair. She's smart too.

_____

_____

_____

Selection 3.6: Ricky's Always Late

Ricky's always late for class. He's tall and usually wears shirts with snaps down the front. He's hard of hearing and he doesn't understand the teacher. He prefers to go to the library and look at thick books. He doesn't know sign language, but he can understand fingerspelling.

15

CHAPTER 3

Descriptive
Adjectives

PART I

PART II

PART III

PART IV

_____

_____

_____

Selection 3.7: Who Is Twyla?

Who's Twyla? Is she tall or short? Does she have good sign skills? Is she the one by the man with the black hair, beard, and the striped shirt? I don't know what she looks like. Please describe her again.

_____

_____

_____

Selection 3.8: Writing My Paper

I can't go on and write my paper because I haven't read the book. I've got to go to the library and read today. They keep the windows open in the library and it's cool. I'll have to wear my long sleeve red shirt with the white dots when I go so I can stay warm.

_____

_____

_____

Selection 3.9: Motorcycle Man

See the grey house over there with the red car in the front and the motorcycle in the driveway? What's the man's name who owns the motorcycle? You know he's medium height and build, has black curly hair, and one gold tooth. Who is he?

_____

_____

_____

Selection 3.10   The Bus Driver

The bus driver lives in an apartment over there. He drives his car to work and then gets on the bus. He always wears a blue and white striped shirt and blue pants. The students like him. He's nice and friendly.

_____

_____

_____

Free Expressive Practice: Using the lines below, write your own selection. Include in your selection a description that can be signed using Size and Shape Specifiers.

_____

_____

_____

_____

CHAPTER 4

Noun/Verb Pairs

There are a variety of ways that verbs are expressed in ASL. While some are anchored to the body, as in TO-HAVE and TO-LIKE, others change directions to indicate the initiator and the recipient of the action (see Chapter 2), while others are related in form to a noun in what are called noun/verb pairs.

In these types of ASL verbs, each noun/verb pair share handshape, location, and orientation parameters of the sign formation and are distinguished by regular changes to the movement parameter. In these instances, nouns and verbs that are related to each other in meaning are differentiated by **movement frequency**, the **movement direction** (one direction or bidirectional), and the **manner of movement** (continuous or quick abrupt movements) (Supalla & Newport, 1978). Research conducted by Supalla and Newport (1978) showed that in most noun/verb pairs, the nouns are produced with repeated, small, quick movements while their related verbs are signed with repeated or continuous movement delivered in either a one-directional or bidirectional manner. An example of a bidirectional noun/verb pair is BABY and ROCK-BABY (Baker & Cokely, 1980, p. 107).

An example of a noun/verb pair is CHAIR and TO-SIT. In this noun/verb pair, the noun has a short, repeated movement, and the verb is produced with a single continuous movement. This is shown in Figure 4.1.

There are several noun/verb pairs, including signs such as DOOR and OPEN/CLOSE-DOOR, BOOK and OPEN/CLOSE-BOOK, WINDOW and OPEN/CLOSE-WINDOW, in which the verbs are signed with single one-directional movements and the nouns are signed with smaller repeated movements.

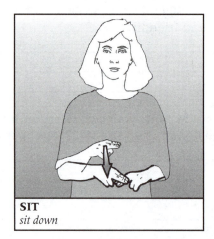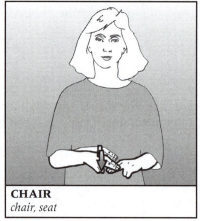

| SIT | CHAIR |
| *sit down* | *chair, seat* |

FIGURE 4.1   Example of a Noun/Verb Pair SIT/CHAIR

Source: From Humphries, Tom, & Carol Padden, *Learning American Sign Language,* 2/e. Published by Allyn and Bacon, Boston, MA. Copyright © 2004 by Pearson Education. Reprinted by permission of the publisher.

Below you will find several selections that include noun/verb pairs. Translate the English sentences into ASL and then practice signing them.

EXAMPLE 4.0
....

When Chris gets up in the morning, he finds his green comb, combs his hair, brushes his teeth, gets dressed, closes all of the windows, and drives to work. He is a fitness instructor.

<u>   when clause   </u>

EVERY-MORNING fs-CHRIS WAKE-UP DO++ GET-UP, IX LOOK-FOR COMB GREEN, COMB-HAIR, BRUSH-TEETH, GET-DRESS, #ALL WINDOW CLOSE-WINDOW, FINISH DRIVE-TO WORK. HIMSELF TEACH EXERCISE fs-FITNESS.

Selection 4.1: Four Things for Mom

Mom asked me to do four things for her. She asked me to close all of the windows, throw out the garbage, turn off the lights, and close the door when I went to school. I told her I'd do it.

_____

_____

_____

Selection 4.2: The Science Teacher

That science teacher's so friendly and so smart. She really wants us to learn and she doesn't mind when we make mistakes. She wants us to open our books, read, think for ourselves, and answer questions. In her class, we sit in our seats and write papers about how we feel and about things we prefer.

_____

_____

_____

_____

Selection 4.3: Megghan's House

Megghan lives over there by the university. Her address is 1617 Oak Street. She likes to ride her bike to the campus and visit her friends who live in the dorm. Her friends like to exercise. They walk around the campus, and they ride their bikes. They all enjoy having fun outdoors.

_____

_____

_____

_____

Selection 4.4: Tamika and Her Clothes

Tamika has lots of clothes. All of her blouses are in the top drawer. All of her skirts are in the second drawer, and all of her jackets are in the third drawer.

She gets up in the morning, turns on the light, turns on the TV, opens the top drawer, takes out her clothes, and gets dressed. Then she drives to school.

RS TAMIKA HAVE MANY CLOTHES. #ALL BLOUSES DRAWER TOP, #ALL SKIRTS DRAWER TWO. #ALL JACKET DRAWER THREE. EVERY MORNING SHE WAKE-UP DO++ LIGHT-ON, TV-ON, TOP DRAWER-OPEN, CLOTHES TAKE, GET-DRESS. FINISH DRIVE-TO-SCHOOL.

Selection 4.5: Can You Help Me?

Can you help me? Please help me find my comb. I need to comb my hair. I left it on the chair last night. Did you sit on it? If you find it, please bring it to me.

_____

_____

Selection 4.6: Looking for Candy

I need some chocolate. Can you help me find the candy machine? I thought it was down the hall on the left by the door by the elevator. I saw a girl eating a Snickers so I know there must be a machine. Do you think someone opened the door and that's why I can't find the machine?

_____

_____

_____

Selection 4.7: The Bookstore

The bookstore's on your left on the corner. The bookstore has books, paper, pencils, water, soda, and food. It's ok to eat in there. You see students opening and closing used books looking for the nicest one.

BOOKSTORE WHERE? CORNER YOUR LEFT. HAVE WHAT? BOOKS, PAPER PENCIL, WATER, SODA, FOOD. IN THERE YOU CAN EAT. YOU SEE STUDENTS #DO ++ OPEN-BOOK CLOSE-BOOK WHY? SEARCH FOR BEST ONE.

Selection 4.8: I Need Some Coffee

I need some coffee. The cafeteria has good coffee. They keep their cups warm. Then when you go to drink the coffee, it is always hot. I'm going there now. Do you want me to bring you some?

_____

_____

_____

Selection 4.9: A New Phone

I'm buying a new phone. When I went to call my friend, all I could hear was noise. It's just not working. I need one that I can depend on.

_____

_____

_____

Selection 4.10: Casey Loves to Fly

Casey loves airplanes. He's a pilot and he loves to fly. He has flown from California to New York in a small plane. I like to look at his plane when it's on the ground.

_____
_____
_____

Free Expressive Practice: Write your own selection here incorporating noun/verb pairs.

_____
_____
_____

PART I

PART II

PART III

PART IV

Topic/Comment

Frequently in American Sign Language (ASL) the topic is signed first, followed by a comment. When this occurs in ASL, it is referred to as topic/comment structure or topicalization. Signers indicate topics by raising their brows, tilting their heads, and maintaining eye gaze on the person being addressed or the object that is being referenced (Baker & Cokely, 1980). In these instances, the signer can set the stage for the information that will follow. By identifying the focus of the narrative, the signer is then free to add comments that can be in the form of statements or questions.

When using topicalization, the signer determines if he or she wants to introduce the subject or the object of a sentence first. This is influenced in part by the context of the discussion and by the focus of the communication.

In the selections that follow, change the English text into ASL and practice signing the sentences.

 EXAMPLE 5.0

Have you been to the airport lately? Yesterday I went there to pick up my mom and I was surprised to see how much it has changed. It isn't small any more and it has become very busy with planes flying in and out every five minutes.

<pre>
    t   y/n-q
_____ _____
AIRPORT, YOU FINISH TOUCH RECENTLY? YESTERDAY ME GO-1f PICK-UP MOM.
          rhet-q
        _____
 ME SURPRISE, WHY, AIRPORT CHANGE. PAST AIRPORT SMALL, NOW BIG. IX-1f-
there BUSY++ EACH 5-MINUTE++ MANY AIRPLANE FLY-TO-LAND, FLY-TO-TAKE-
OFF. WOW #BUSY.
</pre>

Selection 5.1: John's Exciting Day

John's mom showed up at his apartment this morning and told him she had a surprise for him. He looked out the window and there was a black and grey motorcycle. It was really cool! John was so excited. He thanked his mom and told her he'd ride it to class.

_____

_____

_____

_____

21

CHAPTER 5
Topic/Comment

PART I

PART II

PART III

PART IV

Selection 5.2: The Hungry Student

Sissy had to hurry to get to the university so this morning she didn't eat. Today she has a test in English and she's nervous; she wants to pass it. She's very good at Spanish but not English. She couldn't eat because she was upset. Now she's tired, hungry, and cranky.

_____

_____

_____

Selection 5.3: Jose's Apartment

Jose has a really cool apartment. It's over there by the university. It's near the dorms and the library. There's a bus that goes from his apartment to the college so Jose doesn't have to drive. He doesn't really like the bus but he doesn't have a car or a motorcycle.

APARTMENT JOSE'S POOL. CLOSE - TO UNIVERSITY, DORM, LIBRARY.
JOSE NOT HAVE CAR OR MOTORCYCLE. HE TAKE BUS
FROM APARTMENT TO COLLEGE.

_____

Selection 5.4: Driving Test

See the woman over there, the tall, thin one with the blonde hair in the pink dress? She has to take her driving test. She's very nervous. I told her to calm down and stop worrying. She must pass the test so she can drive to her office. I told her that she will pass the test.

WOMAN, TALL, THIN HAIR BLONDE DRESS PINK YOU SEE HER?
DRIVE TEST SHE HAVE. SHE NERVOUS I TELL CALM
DOWN WORRY STOP. TEST SHE MUST PASS DRIVE TO
HER OFFICE. I TELL HER SHE WILL

Selection 5.5: Marci

Marci's not feeling good today. She's hot and then she feels cold. She looks very pale and she said she feels sick. All night she tossed and turned. Now she's very tired. She doesn't like to feel sick. She'll have to skip class today and take her test when she feels good again.

_____

_____

_____

_____

Selection 5.6: A Request

Do you mind helping me today? I need some books from the library but I can't go over there. Will you please go to the library for me get my books and bring them here? I'll be in the classroom down the hall next to the elevator. If you don't mind, it would really help me. Thank you.

Selection 5.7: The Garbage

I don't know what I smell but something stinks. It could be the garbage. Would you mind throwing it out? I'll open the doors and the windows. Wow! It doesn't smell good. I have to leave for class, and when I come back I'll clean the apartment. My mom and dad will come today, and we don't want it to smell in here.

STINK I DON'T-KNOW WHAT I SMELL. MAYBE GARBAGE.
THROW-IT CAN YOU? DOOR WINDOW I OPEN. WOW
SMELL BAD. I HAVE CLASS NOW WHEN I ARRIVE
I WILL CLEAN. MY PARENTS SHOW UP WE DON'T-WANT SMELL.

Selection 5.8: Televisions and Lights Are Different Today

Televisions are different today. How we turn them on and off is different. We don't use a knob-type switch to turn them on and off. We use a pushbutton switch. Lights are the same way. We can use a lever-type switch to turn lights on or off. We can use a pushbutton switch. Car lights use a knob-type switch to turn them on and off.

TODAY TV DIFFERENT. TURN-ON OFF HOW DIFFERENT
KNOB SWITCH NOT USE. WE USE PUSHBUTTON. LIGHTS
SAME-AS. TURN ON OFF LEVER-TYPE WE CAN OR
PUSHBUTTON. CAR LIGHTS HAVE KNOB TURN ON OFF

Selection 5.9: The Irritated Teacher

Mr. Smith teaches at the high school. Wow! Was he mad today! Fourteen of his students skipped class. He didn't like that at all. He went ahead and gave a test to the ten students sitting in class. The ones who skipped will flunk. They'll be sad when they come to class.

Selection 5.10: Reading a Good Book

Today I didn't have class so I spent all day reading a good book. It was an interesting book about a boy who lives far away from here. His parents are both teachers, the same as mine, so I could sympathize with what he wrote about. He explained that his parents rode bikes to school and that he walked to his class. It was interesting.

_____

_____

_____

_____

Free Expressive Practice: Using the lines below write your own selection. Include in your selection sentences that lend themselves to topic/comment.

_____

_____

_____

_____

PART I

PART II

PART III

PART IV

Negation, Negative Incorporation, and Modals

When forming negative statements in ASL, the sign NOT can be used to express negation or respond to others' questions. In these instances, the sign NOT can be placed either before or after the noun it is describing. Therefore, when responding to the question "Do you think it will rain tomorrow?" the signer can express a negative view in ASL by signing TOMORROW RAIN NOT or TOMORROW NOT RAIN.

Negative statements can also be expressed through negative incorporation. In these instances, the signs LIKE, WANT, and KNOW can be produced by twisting the sign so the palm faces downward thus indicating the positive intent has been changed and is negative in nature. For example, the sentence, "I don't like ice cream," can be

<u>   t   </u>

signed ME NOT-LIKE ICE CREAM or ICE CREAM NOT-LIKE ME.

Signers can also convey intent by use of modals in sentences. Signs such as WILL, CAN, SHOULD, and MUST can be signed one of three ways, either before the verb, after the verb, or before the verb and again at the end of the sentences. Therefore, the English sentence, "I must study for the test" can be expressed in ASL one of three ways: first, ME MUST STUDY FOR TEST; second, ME STUDY MUST FOR TEST; or third, ME MUST STUDY FOR TEST MUST.

Change the following selections, written in English, into ASL, then practice signing the sentences.

 EXAMPLE 6.0

Mark doesn't have any money. Yesterday he really needed to buy gas for his car, and he didn't know what to do. He didn't want to borrow money from his friend again. He decided he had to find a job so he could drive his car.

fs-MARK BROKE. YESTERDAY IX-rt-Mark CAR, GAS NEED BUT IX-rt-he STUCK,

<u>   t   </u>

MONEY NONE. MONEY IX-rt-he BORROW POSS-"Mark" FRIEND AGAIN,

<u>   neg   </u>

IX-rt-he NOT-WANT. KNOW WHAT-DO. IX-rt-he DECIDE #JOB MUST FIND

<u> rhq </u>

WHY? DRIVE AROUND CAN.

25

CHAPTER 6
....
Negation, Negative
Incorporation,
and Models

PART I

PART II

PART III

PART IV

Selection 6.1: The New Teacher

Do you know who the new ASL teacher is? Is she hearing or deaf? I don't know who'll be teaching. Sue told me that the new teacher gets mad if students show up late for class and will flunk you if you can't tell her the answers.

_____

_____

_____

Selection 6.2: The School Year Starts Soon

School will start again soon. Moms and dads will drive their children to school. Some will be nervous, some excited, and some happy. Some will go to mainstreamed schools and some to residential schools. When the first day is finished, all of the students should calm down and be eager to learn.

_____

_____

_____

_____

Selection 6.3: Straight Hair

Sheila doesn't like curly hair. She thinks it looks like a Brillo pad. She prefers hair that is straight with a little wave in the front. She said curly hair makes her look ugly and makes her nose and ears look big. Stan told her she should be happy that she isn't bald.

_____

_____

_____

Selection 6.4: Library Fine

Today I have got to go to the library and pay my fine. It really makes me mad. My sister took my book to read and didn't give it back to me. Now it's late. Mom told me to calm down that she would take it back to the library for me. I don't like it when my sister takes my books.

_____

_____

_____

Selection 6.5: Coffee

I can't drink coffee at night. When I do, I toss and turn all night and am tired all the next day. When I want to drink coffee, I drink it either in the morning or at lunch. My parents can drink five or six cups of coffee at night and they're fine. It doesn't make them nervous or excited. I can't do it.

_____

_____

_____

_____

Selection 6.6: Jamia's New Bicycle

Jamia doesn't like to exercise. She would rather ride in the car than walk. So I was really surprised when she got a new black bicycle. It has ten speeds, and she rides it to class in the morning and again in the afternoon. She wants to join the bike club at the college. They ride five to ten miles a week. Wow!

_____

_____

_____

_____

Selection 6.7: Marnie

Have you seen Marnie? She's so excited. Tonight she is going out with Bill. She met him in her sign language class. He's tall, medium build, has black hair and blue eyes. He really seems friendly. They should have a really good time.

_____

_____

_____

Selection 6.8: Todd

Todd asked me to go with him to meet his brother tonight but I told him I was sorry that I couldn't go. I have more reading to do and I've got to write an essay on the book to give to the teacher. I would rather go with him than read and write but I want to pass the class. He said he understood.

_____

_____

_____

_____

Free Expressive Practice: Write your own selection here. Be sure to include sentences that include negation, negative incorporation, and/or modals.

_____

_____

_____

_____

Classifiers: Describing Location and Movement

There are several types of classifiers. Although some function as descriptive adjectives (see Chapter 3 for a discussion of how classifiers can be used as descriptive adjectives [Size and Shape Specifiers]), classifiers can also represent nouns in predicate phrases (Valli & Lucas, 2000). In these instances, the noun must be identified first. Once the noun is clearly understood, the classifier handshape that represents the noun is signed to identify or refer to the person, object, or location in three-dimensional space.

In essence, these classifiers serve a similar function as the pronouns *he, she, or it* serve in English. For example, in ASL the index finger is used to refer to the individual object, person, or location and is represented as CL:1 when writing about ASL.

Classifiers can also be used in predicate phrases to describe movement. For example, when a signer wants to represent that a vehicle is moving from one space to another, the specific vehicle would be identified, e.g., car, truck, bus, and so forth. This would be followed by the CL:3 handshape. After placing the classifier at the point where the vehicle is located, it can then be moved to indicate the direction that it traveled. Further discussion of how classifiers are used to represent nouns, movement from one location to another, and group activities will be described in subsequent chapters. Examples of the CL:1 classifier and how it can be used to indicate movement are included in Figure 7.1. An example of the CL:3 classifier is included in Figure 7.2.

In the selections that follow, change the following paragraphs into ASL and practice signing them.

EXAMPLE 7.0

Before I went to class I put my glass next to the sink. It was dirty. When I came back, the kitchen table had three stacks of plates and glasses all over it. Someone must have done the dishes. Now I need to put the plates and glasses in the cupboard.

BEFORE ME GO-TO CLASS, KITCHEN fs-SINK ME CUP CL:C-"put-next-to-sink."

<u>   t   </u>

HAPPEN ARRIVE HOME, IX-there KITCHEN TABLE, SEE PLATES CL:LL THREE-"stack-of-plates," GLASSES CL:C-"all-over." SOMEONE WASH-DISH FINISH. NOW CUPBOARD CL:LL-"plates" CL:C-"glasses"PUT-AWAY MUST

Selection 7.1: Sue's Kitchen

Sue's kitchen is so nice. When you open her cupboard, you see all of her glasses in neat rows on the bottom shelf. Her small plates are next to her large plates

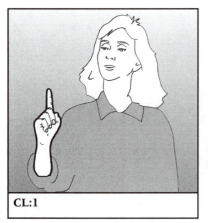
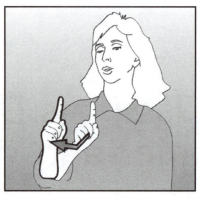
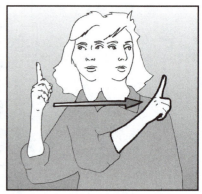

Person going by quickly

FIGURE 7.1 CL:1 and CL:1 Movement

Source: From Humphries, Tom, & Carol Padden, *Learning American Sign Language,* 2/e. Published by Allyn and Bacon, Boston, MA. Copyright © 2004 by Pearson Education. Reprinted by permission of the publisher.

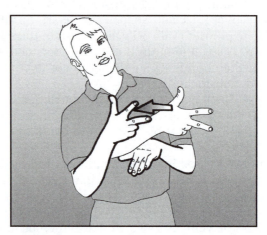

FIGURE 7.2 Example of Classifier CL:3 Used to Represent Vehicles and Vehicle Movement

Source: From Humphries, Tom, & Carol Padden, *Learning American Sign Language,* 2/e. Published by Allyn and Bacon, Boston, MA. Copyright © 2004 by Pearson Education. Reprinted by permission of the publisher.

on the second shelf, and her platters and bowls are on the top shelf. Sue's plates are white with red and blue dots all over them. They look very patriotic.

_____

_____

_____

_____

Selection 7.2: Renee's Shoes

Renee likes to shop. She enjoys going in and out of stores. She likes to buy clothes but she really enjoys shopping for shoes. She has several pairs of shoes—I don't know how many shoes she has but I think she has more than fifty pairs. She has black shoes, brown shoes, white, and red. Her favorite ones are black. She has ten pairs of black shoes that all look different.

_____

_____

_____

_____

29

CHAPTER 7
....
Classifiers:
Describing Location
and Movement

PART I

PART II

PART III

PART IV

Selection 7.3: The Missing Grapes

This morning I left a bowl of grapes on the table and went to class. Four hours later I came back and they were gone. I don't know who moved them. I asked my brother if he knew where they were and he said "No." I asked him if he'd look for them while I threw out the trash. He said he'd be happy to help me.

_____

_____

_____

_____

Selection 7.4: Dirty Dishes

All week I have been busy going to class and taking tests. Now it looks like I haven't done dishes in a month. Plates, glasses, cups, and silverware have been left all over the table. Tonight I'll clean the kitchen. I don't like a mess but I didn't have time to clean. I'll have more time next week.

_____

_____

_____

_____

Selection 7.5: Where's My Candy?

Who hid the candy? You know, the candy that was in the bowl in the kitchen? This afternoon it was here and now it's gone. I told you not to touch it. I'm hungry, and I want it. I don't mind if you took some, but I want it back. Where did you put it? Please give it to me.

_____

_____

_____

_____

Selection 7.6: Candles

Do you like candles? I do. I like the big thick ones and those that are tall and thin, the size around of a silver dollar. Steve has several candles in his living room and in his bathroom. The ones in the living room are blue and white and are rather large. The ones in his bathroom are small and white and sit all around his tub.

_____

_____

_____

_____

Selection 7.7: Paul's Cars

Paul has six cars. Two are white, two are black, one is blue, and one is green. He drives the green one back and forth to class three days a week. He drives the blue car to take the garbage to the landfill. The blue car doesn't smell good. His dad gave him one of the white cars, and he bought the black ones. In six months he'll sell two of them.

_____

_____

_____

_____

Selection 7.8: The Canister Set

I need to buy a canister set. I saw one in Tampa that I like. The set has four containers. One's large, one's a little smaller, one's medium size, and one is small. All of them are white with apples, oranges, peaches, and grapes on them. They look better than the white ones without any fruit. I'll buy them next week.

_____

_____

_____

_____

Free Expressive Practice: Write your own selection here. Be sure to incorporate at least two classifiers that describe either size and shape or nouns in conjunction with their locations.

_____

_____

_____

_____

Establishing Tense in ASL

To establish tense in ASL, time adverbial signs are used. Since ASL does not inflect verbs for tense—for example, ASL does not add "ed" to verbs to indicate past tense—the tense must be clear through the use of time adverbials. Time adverbial signs include words such as NOW, TODAY, YESTERDAY, RECENTLY, PAST, FUTURE, TOMORROW, LATER, and are usually stated at the beginning of a sentence. When these signs are produced, they follow an imaginary time line that runs through the signer's body and into the areas in front of and in back of the body (Baker & Cokely, 1980). In general, present tense signs are made in the immediate sign space in front of the signer's body, while those indicating future tense extend in front of the signer's body, and those representing past tense are move toward the signer's back. See Figure 8.1 for an example of the time line.

Time adverbials are produced along the "time line" relative to when actual events occurred or will occur. Therefore, when something happened centuries ago or will not happen until some time in the distant future, the time adverbial sign will be modified to show the relative length of time. When indicating that events took place a long time ago or will not happen for many years, signers frequently use facial expressions to further modify the time frame. In these instances the puffed cheeks facial expression accompanies the signs, thus emphasizing the time frame.

It is important to note that the direction of movement of the time signs is always signed in relation to present time (Baker & Cokely, 1980, p. 176). Also, keep in mind that once the tense has been established, it remains constant until the signer changes it.

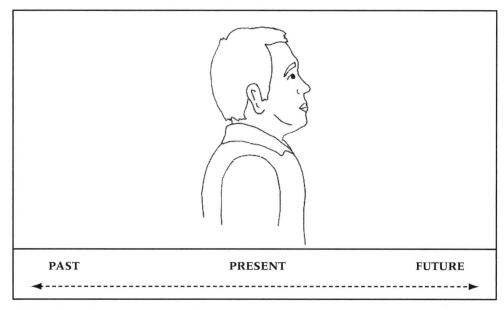

| PAST | PRESENT | FUTURE |

FIGURE 8.1   Time Line Used in ASL to Denote Present, Future, and Past Tense
Courtesy of Marie A. Scheetz

In addition to utilizing the above time adverbial signs in sentences, the sign FINISH can also be incorporated into sentences to indicate that an action has been completed. In these instances one can indicate that one has finished eating, is through reading a book, or has completed his or her classes. In this regard, the sign can also be used as a conjunction to indicate when one event ended and another event began. This is illustrated in sentences that describe multiple activities. For example, "After I went to the store, I drove home, and then I cooked dinner." ME GO-TO STORE FINISH DRIVE-TO HOME COOK DINNER. Although used as a time sign, FINISH can also be used to indicate the extent or limit of something as in "We're just co-workers," US-TWO WORK SAME #JOB FINISH, or to express that you want someone to stop an activity that he or she is engaged in doing. In this instance, FINISH is signed with a single sharp movement as in "Stop teasing me!" TEASE-ME FINISH! (Humphries & Padden, 2004).

In the selections that follow change the following English text into ASL and practice signing.

 EXAMPLE 8.0

Years ago I taught at a residential school for the deaf in Colorado. I really enjoyed my students. Later I got married and moved to Pennsylvania where I began teaching English to deaf students. Today I train teachers to work with deaf students.

                                                                               t

MANY YEAR PAST, ME TEACH DEAF-SCHOOL fs-COLORADO. MY STUDENT IX-they, ME ENJOY TEACH IX-they. LATER, ME MARRY FINISH, MOVE-TO fs-PA, TEACH ENGLISH IX. DEAF STUDENT IX-they. NOW, ME TEACH FUTURE TEACHER GROUP IX-plural circular-ref. back HOW THEY TEACH DEAF STUDENT.

Selection 8.1: Peter's Family

Peter's family lives in New York. His family moved there from Russia. His parents divorced when he was 2, and he has lived with his mom ever since. He has two sisters and one brother. When he grows up, he's planning to take classes at the university. He wants to take classes in Russian history.

_____

_____

_____

_____

_____

Selection 8.2: My Roommate

Recently I got a new roommate. She's short, thin, has brown hair and brown eyes. Her name's Kyla, she's deaf, and she grew up in California. She moved in yesterday and I got to meet her. The two of us share the same birthday—it's really interesting. I think we'll enjoy being roommates—she has good sign skills.

_____

_____

_____

_____

33

CHAPTER 8
Establishing
Tense in ASL

PART I

PART II

PART III

PART IV

Selection 8.3: My Aunt Betty

Do you know my Aunt Betty? She's a teacher at the residential school. She went to school with your mom. She's been married for twenty-seven years now and has three children. They're all grown up and have moved out. Her roommate introduced her to my uncle Bob. They went together through college. She told me she'd like to meet you.

_____

_____

_____

_____

Selection 8.4: Tami's Family

Tami and her boyfriend got married when they were 17. They separated when they were 18 and got a divorce one year later. Then they started dating again and got married again last year. They want to have several children. Tami will finish college in six months. When she's through, they'll start their family.

_____

_____

_____

_____

Selection 8.5: The Ideal Husband

How do you know if your boyfriend will be the ideal husband? First, he should be your best friend. He should like you and love you. He should be friendly and not arrogant. He should tell you how he feels and admit when he's wrong. The two of you should like some of the same things and prefer to do things together.

_____

_____

_____

_____

Selection 8.6: The Surprise Party

Grandpa will be 70 this year. He loves birthdays and since he was a little boy has wanted a surprise party. This year for his birthday we'll surprise him. We've invited all of our aunts, uncles, and cousins to come for the party. We also invited many of his good friends. I'm so excited—I can't wait to surprise grandpa.

_____

_____

_____

_____

Selection 8.7: Tim's Girlfriend

Tim's girlfriend's name is Jessica. She's my daughter's roommate and a real cutie. She and my daughter are both college students and live in an apartment about fifteen miles from the campus. The two girls are about the same height, and both of them have short hair. Jessica and Tim will get married next year, and my daughter will have to find a new roommate.

_____

_____

_____

_____

Selection 8.8: Teresa's Family

Teresa's Deaf and lives in Denver. She has two brothers but no sisters. Both of her brothers are hearing as are her parents. One of her brothers is married and has three children, two boys and a girl. Teresa's nephews and her niece know how to sign. They like to stay with their Aunt Teresa in Denver.

_____

_____

_____

_____

Free Expressive Practice: Create your own selection here. Demonstrate your use of time indicators and/or the use of the sign FINISH.

_____

_____

_____

_____

Age, Time, and Counting Numbers

ASL follows specific rules when the signer wants to indicate a person's age or the time of day. In these instances, the sign OLD and the sign TIME are produced first followed by a number sign. In both instances, the numbers 1 through 5 are produced with the palm turned outward. However, when one wants to identify a specific number of objects in ASL, the number can be signed before or after the noun it is referring to as in TREE THREE or THREE TREE and for the numbers 1 through 5 the palm faces inward.

In ASL signs for days of the week can change their movement to indicate regularity. The handshape for the sign remains the same, only the movement changes. The signer can express that an event occurred on a specific day or illustrate that it takes place regularly on that same day by modifying the movement. For example, the sign SATURDAY can be changed to express EVERY-SATURDAY by vertically moving the sign down in front of the signer's body. In this respect, days of the week can be presented in a downward, vertical movement signifying that the activity occurred each or every Sunday or Monday, rather than happening on only one Sunday or Monday.

Times of the day (e.g., morning, afternoon, evening) can also be modified to indicate the frequency of an activity. For example, when the signer wants to explain that an event occurs every morning as opposed to happening on only one morning, the sign MORNING is produced in a continuous horizontal movement across the signer's body thus expressing the meaning EVERY-MORNING. Figure 9.1 illustrates time repetition, indicating each and every and time regularity indicating number of days.

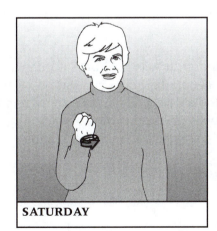
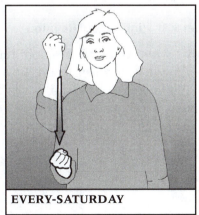

SATURDAY   **EVERY-SATURDAY**

FIGURE 9.1   Time Repetition: Changing Saturday to Every Saturday

Source: From Humphries, Tom, & Carol Padden, *Learning American Sign Language,* 2/e. Published by Allyn and Bacon, Boston, MA. Copyright © 2004 by Pearson Education. Reprinted by permission of the publisher.

Modification of signs is not limited to the times of the day or the days of the week. It can be used to indicate events that occur on a weekly, monthly, or yearly basis. In this respect, the regular movement of the sign for ONE-WEEK or ONE-MONTH can be signed repeatedly while moving the sign horizontally to indicate EVERY-WEEK or downwards to indicate EVERY-MONTH (Baker & Cokely, 1980, p. 186). By repeating the movement of the sign, and signing the appropriate time adverbial (e.g., PAST, FUTURE), the listener is alerted to the fact that the activity being discussed has or will take place on a regular basis.

The following selections are written in English. Change these sentences into ASL and then practice signing them.

 ### EXAMPLE 9.0

At 10 o'clock I've got to go to the school for the deaf. I promised I'd read a story to the children in Ms. Abby's room. She has twenty-one children in her class, fifteen girls and six boys. They love to have stories signed in ASL. I will read a story about Mrs. Wishey Washey. It will be fun!

                                                               <u>rhet-q</u>

TIME-TEN, GO-TO DEAF-SCHOOL ME MUST. ME FINISH PROMISE CHILDREN WHAT?

                                     <u>   t   </u>

STORY ME READ IX-there fs-MS fs-ABBY-poss ROOM. POSS "Ms. Abby" CLASS HAVE CHILDREN: TWENTY-ONE, GIRLS FIFTEEN, BOYS SIX. IX-rt-they LOVE-IT STORY USE-ASL. STORY TITLE fs-MRS, fs-WISHEY fs-WASHEY ME READ. WILL #FUN!

Selection 9.1: Grandma Needs a Hearing Aid

Grandma is very hard of hearing—really she's almost deaf and she needs a hearing aid. She's very stubborn and refuses to get one. Every Friday I go and see her. When you talk to her, she doesn't understand, and you tell her the same thing again and again. Then she answers with "I know that." I wish she would change her thinking and buy one.

_____

_____

_____

_____

Selection 9.2: High School Reunion

Recently I went to my high school reunion. It was held on Saturday at eight o'clock. Wow! It was fun to see how people had changed. Some of my old friends still looked young and others looked very old. While some remained good looking, others had become chubby. I could remember some of their names but forgot others. It felt strange going back to my high school.

_____

_____

_____

Selection 9.3: Dirty Laundry

Can you meet me at 3:30? I want you to go with me to the laundromat. I have a pile of dirty clothes that I need to wash. Please come to my house and we can

37

CHAPTER 9
....
Age, Time, and
Counting Numbers

PART I

PART II

PART III

PART IV

go together. I want to finish it so I can go away this weekend. If I don't get it done, I'll have to stay here this weekend.

_____
_____
_____

Selection 9.4: Anyone Know Josh?

Do you know Josh? He's medium height and build, has a mustache and a pot-belly, and is full of mischief. He was in my French class last year. He knew all the answers and was a little crazy. Some people thought he was odd, but he was very nice. He helped me pass that class.

_____
_____
_____

Selection 9.5: Watching TV

How many hours a night do you watch TV? Do you watch the news? What's your favorite program? I watch about one hour of TV a night. I like *Entertainment Tonight*. I can watch it for thirty minutes and know what is happening. Sometimes I watch a movie or sports. I don't like game shows and refuse to watch them.

_____
_____
_____
_____

Selection 9.6: The Neighborhood

Do you remember who used to live in the gray house across the street from my parents? I can't remember their names. They lived there for twenty years. She stayed at home and he taught at the elementary school. They were so friendly and many weekends had parties. Their names have slipped my mind.

_____
_____
_____
_____

Selection 9.7: The Smith Family

The Smiths have been married for eleven years. They have three children. Ron's 8, and the twins, Char and Chris, are 6 years old. Tomorrow afternoon they're having a birthday party for all three children. They were all born on the fourteenth of May. How would you like to share your birthday with your brother and sister? I think I'd prefer my own day.

_____
_____
_____
_____
_____

Selection 9.8: Autumn and Amber

Autumn and Amber are sisters. Autumn's almost 30 and her sister is about 25. They both went to the Florida School for the Deaf. Autumn's married and has three children, two boys and a girl. The boys are 7 and 5, and the little girl is 3. She works as a teacher of the deaf in California. Amber's still in college. She'll graduate in a few months. She hopes she can find a job after she graduates.

_____

_____

_____

_____

_____

Free Expressive Practice: Create your own selection here. Demonstrate your command of incorporating age, time, and counting numbers.

_____

_____

_____

_____

Additional Work with Classifiers

In previous chapters information has been provided regarding how classifiers are used as descriptive adjectives and how they can function as referents for nouns and pronouns. In this chapter classifiers are examined with regard to how specific classifier handshapes are used to represent categories of objects and how they function to indicate the action of the predicate.

In Chapter 7, classifiers that can be used to represent a particular group of nouns were discussed. You will recall that because the handshape represents all of the members of a particular group, it is essential that the noun be identified first followed by the appropriate classifier. When representing the category of vehicles, for example, the car, boat, truck, train, or other form of ground transportation, it is followed by the CL:3 classifier. Thus, when conversing, the signer can identify where the vehicle is located and demonstrate how and where it changes locations or moves.

Classifiers can be used to reflect objects that are stationary or are moving; for example, aircraft, individuals, or animals in upright positions and individuals or animals in crouched or sitting positions (Humphries & Padden, 2004). Examples of classifier handshapes that are used to represent various groups of nouns are included in Figure 10.1.

Classifiers can be used to further demonstrate individual, animal, or object movement. In classifier predicates, the palm orientation, location, and/or movement of the classifier can change to depict the way an individual or animal walks, turns, or the direction he or she is approaching from. When using classifier predicates, the signer produces the classifier in a specific location in three-dimensional space. For example, the signer can sign DOG followed by the CL:V to indicate where a dog is located. Then by moving the CL:V to another location in space, it becomes clear that the dog moved from one place to another (Valli & Lucas, 2000, p. 83).

The following selections have been written in English. Translate them into ASL and then practice signing them.

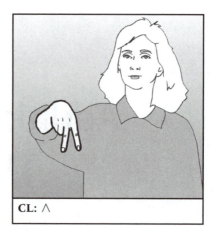

PART IV

CL: ∧

Person standing upright or an animal that stands upright such as an ape.

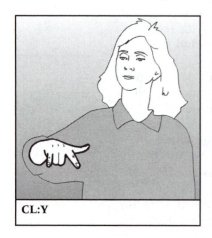

CL:Y

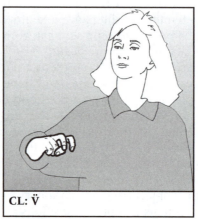

CL: V̈

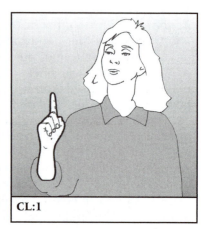

CL:1

Aircraft with wings (not helicopters or rockets).

A crouched or sitting person or animal.

An upright person or animal such as a bear walking on its hind legs.

FIGURE 10.1 Classifiers Representing CL:∧, CL:Y, CL:V̈, and CL:1
Source: From Humphries, Tom, & Carol Padden, *Learning American Sign Language,* 2/e. Published by Allyn and Bacon, Boston, MA. Copyright © 2004 by Pearson Education. Reprinted by permission of the publisher.

EXAMPLE 10.0
....

Jane started walking toward her car when she realized she forgot her key. She turned to go back to the house when she spotted her neighbor coming toward her. The two of them chatted for a few minutes, and then he walked in the house with her to get his jacket. He had forgotten it the night before when he and his wife had been over for dinner.

$$\overline{t}$$

fs-JANE IX-rt CL:∧ CAR, IX-rt REALIZE KEY FORGET. IX-rt CL:∧ HOUSE HAPPEN SEE

$$\overline{when}$$

NEIGHBOR MAN IX-lf CL:1 walk toward Jane. TWO-OF-THEM CHAT SHORT, FINISH, TWO-OF-THEM ENTER HOUSE. PAST NIGHT MAN POSS "his wife" # ALL-us EAT TOGETHER. IX-rt-he FORGET LEFT COAT IX-rt-he LOOK-FOR FIND.

41

CHAPTER 10
....
Additional Work
with Classifiers

PART I

PART II

PART III

PART IV

Selection 10.1: Jake's New House

Jake bought a two-story house in New York. It has a basement and an attic. The living room, dining room, kitchen, and bathroom are all on the first floor. There are three bedrooms, a family room, and another bathroom on the second floor. The family room has big windows on two sides. He lives in the house with his two dogs that love to sit in the family room by the windows.

_____

_____

_____

_____

Selection 10.2: Busy Saturday

Saturday was a busy day. I got up at 5:00 A.M. I went for my morning jog around the lake. Then I came back, and I cleaned house until 1:00. When I was finished, I went to the grocery store, walked up and down every aisle, came home, and baked a cake. Then it was time to cook dinner.

_____

_____

_____

_____

Selection 10.3: The Man in the Library

Monday I was sitting in the library reading. Every time I looked up I saw a man with blonde hair and blue eyes staring at me. I started to stare back. After about an hour the man and his friend walked over to me. "I'm sorry I was staring, but I thought you were an old flame." With that they turned and sauntered out.

_____

_____

_____

_____

Selection 10.4: The Airport

I love to go to the airport and see all of the planes on the runway. They're in such a nice straight line. I also like to sit and watch the people walk by. Some walk quickly, some just meander, and sometimes you see someone who staggers. Sometimes you see girls in short shirts, and frequently you see men in ties and jackets.

_____

_____

_____

Selection 10.5: Juanita's Kitchen

Juanita has a beautiful house. Her kitchen's my favorite. She has a breakfast bar that is "L" shaped. People love to sit around her breakfast bar because it faces a huge window. When you look out the window, you can see a wide border of pink flowers that she's planted. On the other side of the flowers is a round swimming pool. I can just sit there and take it easy.

_____

_____

_____

_____

Selection 10.6: Sam's Schedule

Every morning Sam gets up at 6:00. She has breakfast, reads the newspaper, and drives to the residential school. Sometimes she gets stuck in traffic and has to wait for 30 minutes before the cars start to move. She teaches from 8:00 to 3:00. Every Monday she walks three miles with her friends. Every Wednesday she goes to church. This Friday she'll drive to her parent's house and spend the weekend with them.

_____

_____

_____

_____

Selection 10.7: Retirement Home

When I retire, I want a small house. Right now I have a big house, and I get tired keeping it clean. When I retire, I want to take it easy, rest, do some swimming, watch TV, read books, and fly to see my grandchildren. I don't want to clean house every week. If it's a small house, I can clean it in half a day.

_____

_____

_____

_____

Selection 10.8: Coffee Drinker

Are you a coffee drinker, or do you like tea? Sometimes I like coffee with my breakfast. My friend drinks coffee all day long. She drinks about fifteen cups a day. I asked her if she can sleep at night, and she said yes. I think if I drank that much coffee I couldn't sleep and would end up walking back and forth to the bathroom all night.

_____

_____

_____

_____

Free Expressive Practice: Create your own selection here. Demonstrate your command of using classifiers.

_____

_____

_____

_____

_____

CHAPTER 11

Expressing Negatives Using None

In Chapter 6, various ways of making negative statements in ASL were discussed, in particular how to use the sign NOT and negative incorporation in sentences. As you will recall, the sign NOT can be signed either before or after the noun or the verb to express negative feelings or describe adjectives. In addition, negative statements can also be expressed through negative incorporation as in NOT-KNOW and NOT-WANT.

This chapter focuses on how to express negatives using the sign NONE. In ASL, the sign NONE can be used in a variety of ways. It can be used in conjunction with verbs to indicate that you didn't see or hear anything by signing SEE NONE or HEAR NONE. It can also be used in sentences to indicate zero quantity as in HAVE NONE MONEY ME, meaning I don't have any money, or HER ANSWER UNDERSTAND-NONE ME, meaning I didn't understand her answer.

When using signs that demonstrate negation, it is important that a negative headshake accompany the signs. Appropriate facial expressions should also be produced simultaneously, thus conveying the negative intent of the message.

The following sentences are written in English. Change them into ASL and practice signing the sentences.

 EXAMPLE 11.0

I must go to the store. I opened the refrigerator today and realized I have no milk, no eggs, and no bread. I went to the cupboard hoping to find something to eat and realized that I was out of soup, crackers, and cereal. I am so hungry. I've got to go now.

<u>   rhet-q </u>
ME GO-TO STORE MUST, WHY TODAY fs-REF CL:S-pull-open-door, REALIZE HAVE MILK, EGGS, NONE. ME GO-TO CUPBOARD CL:S-pull-open-door HOPE FIND FOOD,

<u>cond</u>
LOOK FRUSTRATE: SOUP, CRACKER, CEREAL, RUN-OUT. HUNGRY ME! NOW ME GO-TO STORE.

Selection 11.1: Miss Audra's Cakes

Miss Audra makes cakes that are twelve layers high; none of them are any smaller. Each layer's about one-half of an inch high. She starts with eggs and butter and adds flour and sugar. She goes to the store every week to buy what she needs. Sometimes she makes twenty-five cakes a day. She sells each cake for $20.00 but they're worth it. There are no other cakes like Miss Audra's.

_____

_____

_____

_____

Selection 11.2: Missi's Diet

Last week Missi started a diet. Every morning she eats cereal. For lunch she eats chicken and salad, and for dinner she has soup. She can't eat any potatoes, bread, or cheese on her diet and no ice cream. She can drink all of the coffee or tea she wants but no soda. I don't think I would like her diet.

_____

_____

_____

_____

Selection 11.3: Shopping in France

Alex was shocked to find out how much everything costs in France. He went shopping for food and found that steak cost $18.00 a pound. A carton of milk was $6.50 something, and apples were $1.00 each. Nothing was under a dollar. He was afraid he would run out of money if he stayed there a long time. Nothing was cheap. Wow!

_____

_____

_____

_____

Selection 11.4: The Earthquake

Did you hear about the earthquake in Peru? I didn't hear anything about it. My dad told me there was an earthquake on Monday and several people were hurt. It was awful. Now the people don't have any water, and many of their homes are gone. What do people do when that happens?

_____

_____

_____

_____

Selection 11.5: The Cabinets

Would you mind straightening the cabinets up for me? They're such a mess, and I have no room to put my groceries. I went shopping and bought a lot of food on sale. Now my cans of vegetables and soup are all mixed up. My boxes of cereal, popcorn, and tea are in the wrong places, and there's no room for my chips. Thanks for helping me.

_____

_____

_____

_____

Selection 11.6: The Budget

Zoe's on a budget. When she goes to the store, she can't spend more than $45.00. She looks for cheap meat and refuses to buy expensive cereal. She never buys soda and drinks water instead. She buys a lot of spaghetti because it's cheap, and she can't afford salad. It's hard when you don't have much money.

_____

_____

_____

_____

Selection 11.7: The Vegetarian

Tiffany's a vegetarian. She doesn't eat red meat or chicken. She'll eat eggs, vegetables, and fruit. She eats soup if it doesn't have meat in it. She prefers potato soup. Every day she eats salad, and occasionally she'll eat eggs for dinner. She's been a vegetarian for thirteen years.

_____

_____

_____

_____

Selection 11.8: Who Has Time to Cook?

Who has time to cook today? So many people have very busy jobs, and they have no time to cook. They go to work in the morning and come home at night tired from being so busy at work. When you're tired and hungry, you just want to eat—not cook. Do you like to cook? I like to cook on Sunday when I don't have to go to work.

_____

_____

_____

_____

Free Expressive Practice: Create your own selection here demonstrating your ability to incorporate negating statements.

_____

_____

_____

_____

_____

Additional Work with Noun/Verb Pairs

In Chapter 4 noun/verb pairs were discussed and practiced. As you will recall, in ASL in most noun/verb pairs the nouns are produced with repeated, small, quick movements, while their related verbs are signed with repeated or continuous movement. In noun/verb pairs such as AIRPLANE, FLY-TO; COMB, COMB-HAIR; BICYCLE, RIDE-BICYCLE; TYPEWRITER, TYPE; and, BROOM, USE-BROOM (SWEEP), the noun is signed with a smaller movement while the verbs are produced with a larger repeated movement.

Supalla and Newport (1978) analyzed the movement of numerous nouns and verbs in noun/verb pairs. Their analysis focused on three "dimensions": first, the frequency of the movement and whether it was a single movement or a repeated movement; second, the directionality of the movement, if the sign moved in only one direction (unidirectional) or if it moved in two directions (bidirectional); and third, if the sign was produced with a smooth movement or if it ended abruptly.

Although it is not the purpose of this text to provide an in-depth look at the linguistics of ASL, it is interesting to note that when these noun/verb pairs were analyzed, the researchers found the movement of the nouns in each of the pairs was almost always signed with a small, quick movement, even though the verbs might be signed with a repeated bidirectional or unidirectional movement (Baker & Cokely, 1980, p. 105).

Another mechanism in ASL for deriving nouns from verbs is through affixation. In these instances a compound sign is produced whereby the agent marker used in ASL is combined with the verb to indicate the individual performing the action. Some examples of this variation include TEACH, TEACH+AGENT; DANCE, DANCE+AGENT; and PREACH, PREACH+AGENT. However, it is important to note that ASL tends to be verb dominant, so the sign PREACH+AGENT is generally restricted to a more formal register. In less formal signing, ASL tends to favor verbs over nouns. Thus, in informal conversation when responding to the questions, "What do you do?" the signer would respond TEACH ME rather than signing ME TEACH+AGENT (Newell, 2006). See Figure 12.1 for an illustration of affixation.

Below you will find several selections that include noun/verb pairs. Translate the English sentences into ASL and then practice signing them.

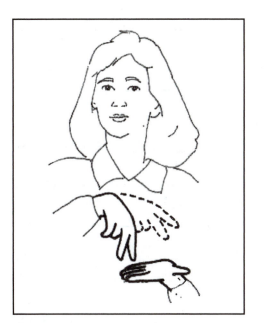
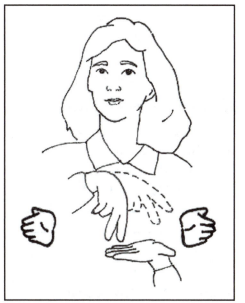

FIGURE 12.1 Example of a Noun/Verb Pair Changing DANCE to DANCE+Agent Suffix
Courtesy of Marie A. Scheetz

 EXAMPLE 12.0
....

I've got to remember to get some gas tomorrow. I have to drive to the airport and pick up my sister. She flies in at noon tomorrow. It would be awful if my car ran out of gas on the way to pick her up. She would not be happy.

TOMORROW MUST REMEMBER fs-GAS PUT-GASOLINE-IN. TOMORROW NOON. MY SISTER. IX-sister FLY-TO-here ME MUST DRIVE-TO AIRPORT PICK-UP.
<u>   cond   </u>
SUPPOSE TOMORROW ME DRIVE-TO AIRPORT HAPPEN fs-GAS TRUE-
<u>   cond   </u>   <u> neg </u>
BUSINESS RUN-OUT. SISTER HAPPY NOT.

Selection 12.1: Sharon's Party

Sharon invited me to her party. A lot of the teachers we used to teach with were also invited. She's having it next Friday but I can't go. I'm really stuck. I've got to work until 11:30, and she said the party would be over by 10:00. I called her and told her I couldn't come, that I'd be typing away for hours. Maybe I can go to her next one.

_____

_____

_____

_____

Selection 12.2: Shawn's Car

There's something wrong with Shawn's car. It broke down on Wednesday, and he thinks there's something wrong with the engine. He used my phone and called his friend and asked if he could drive him to work. His friend's car's broken too. I guess he'll have to borrow a bicycle and ride the bicycle to work.

_____

_____

_____

_____

Selection 12.3: Sue and Jerry

Last week Sue and Jerry worked late. They cleaned cabinets, got in the car, drove to the mall and went shopping, visited friends, and helped some of the movers at the church. They're in the process of moving offices. Now they're worn out. On Saturday they plan to stay home, watch TV, and relax.

_____

_____

_____

Selection 12.4: New Computer

Wow! You have a new computer. It's nice. When did you buy it? Where did you get it? Is it a Dell or a Gateway? Can I use it next week to type my paper? The teacher told me all sixteen pages have to be typed, and I don't want to use my old typewriter.

_____

_____

_____

Selection 12.5: The Party

We need to buy some food and drinks for the party. The whole dance line will be coming. We need some Coke, Pepsi, and bottled water. We also need to get some popcorn and peanuts. We have meat and bread for the sandwiches. I don't want to run out of food. I know a lot of the dancers will be hungry and they'll eat a lot.

_____

_____

_____

Selection 12.6: The Hairdryer

Can I use your hairdryer to dry my hair? Mine's broken. I tried to call Pat on the TTY and ask her if I could borrow hers, but she's not home. I'll have to go to the store tomorrow and buy a new one.

_____

_____

_____

Selection 12.7: The Airport

I really like to go to the airport and look at all of the planes lined up on the runway. They take off one after another and fly in all different directions.

Some fly toward California; others fly toward New York. It's just fun to sit and watch them.

_____

_____

_____

_____

49

CHAPTER 12
....
Additional Work
with Noun/
Verb Pairs

PART I

PART II

PART III

PART IV

Selection 12.8: My Grandparents

My grandparents are both deaf. Last week grandpa bought two hearing aids but he hasn't put them on yet. Grandma refused to buy an aid. She said her hearing is ok. Now when she watches TV she turns it way up. It hurts my ears.

_____

_____

_____

Selection 12.9: Bad Week

I've had a bad week. First I hurt my leg at dance class, and one of the other dancers had to take my place. Then my car got a flat tire. I went to call my friend for a ride and discovered her car was broken. Then, when I finally got home and opened the cabinets to get something to eat, I noticed that we were all out of food.

_____

_____

_____

Selection 12.10: Broken Computer

My computer won't start. I've tried everything, and I give up. I'll call Bobby later and ask him to come over here and see what's wrong with it. I don't think it's the battery, because I just bought a new one. What do you think's wrong with it?

_____

_____

_____

Free Expressive Practice: Create your own selection here to demonstrate your command of noun/verb pairs or your use of the agent marker.

_____

_____

_____

_____

Conditionals

We use conditional sentences in English to alert those around us to the conditions under which we will embark on an activity and the result or consequence that we anticipate will happen if and when the conditional expectations are met. Frequently in English we begin conditional sentences with the word "if." In English the condition and result may be expressed condition first or result first.

In ASL sentences can be structured to include a condition and a result. In essence, these sentences are comprised of two parts: a condition, which is stated first, followed by the result or the consequence. When indicating the condition, the eyebrows are raised and the head is tilted up and back, the eyebrows are then lowered, and the head assumes a neutral position during the consequence. When structuring sentences in this manner, the sign SUPPOSE or #IF sometimes precedes the condition. However, conditional sentences may also be expressed using facial grammar (raised and then lowered eyebrows, thus indicating the condition and the consequence) without adding the signs SUPPOSE or #IF. When translating conditional sentences, the transcription symbol <u>cond</u> is used when the conditional portion of the sentence is signed.

Below you will find several selections that include conditionals. Translate the English sentences into ASL, and then practice signing them.

 EXAMPLE 13.0

The man from the relay services company is coming tomorrow to talk about what they do. I want to hear what he has to say. If I can get out of class on time, I'll come to the meeting. If I can't, I'll have to miss it. Please get the information for me if I don't show up. Thanks.

TOMORROW MAN FROM VIDEO RELAY COMPANY COME-HERE LECTURE ABOUT fs-VRS. ME WANT GO-TO.

<u>   cond   </u>   <u>   cond   </u>
FINISH ON-TIME, NOT POSTPONE, SHOW-UP CAN ME. #IF CLASS

                            <u>   cond   </u>   <u> neg </u>
EXAGGERATE, MISS MUST. IF ME SHOW-UP, PLEASE FOR ME GET MAGAZINE-pamphlet, PAPER HAND-OUT SO-FORTH GET. THANK-YOU.

Selection 13.1: Feeling Sick

Yesterday I was sick all day. Last night I tossed and turned all night. First, I was hot, then cold. If I don't feel better in the morning, I'll go to the doctor. I've got a lot to do, and if I stay sick I won't be able to study and pass the test.

51

CHAPTER 13
....
Conditionals

PART I

PART II

PART III

PART IV

Selection 13.2: Working with John

I don't like to work with John because he's so hard to satisfy. He wants every-thing perfect. If you're not exact with your work, he won't accept it. He tells you to go back, sit down, and do it again. Then he wants to look at it to make sure it's right.

Selection 13.3: Car Problems

My car has had many problems lately. First I had two flat tires, and then I had problems with the engine. If I don't show up for class, please tell the teacher the reason why. I don't want her to think that I don't like her class—I do—my car is just old, and it breaks down frequently.

Selection 13.4: Lots of Money

All of us would like to have lots of money. Suppose someone gave me a lot of money. I would buy you a new house and a new car. I'd give some money to my parents and grandparents. I'd pay all of my bills. What would you do if I gave you a lot of money?

Selection 13.5: The Teacher

The teacher told us we had to come to class tomorrow or we'd flunk the test. I think I can stay home and pass the test. I really disagree with her. Why? Well, that teacher always reads exactly from the book. I can stay home and read the book myself, and then study, and I'm sure I'll pass.

Selection 13.6: Moving

Are you ok today? Someone told me that you have to move in month. Is that true? Wow! You'll have to leave all your friends. Your roommate will have to find someone to live with. If he can't find someone, will he have to move to a new apartment? I'm sorry you have to move.

Selection 13.7: My Boyfriend

Yesterday I found out my boyfriend likes another girl. She's egotistical and a snob. She's short, chubby, and not cute. She isn't even friendly. Last week I asked him if he wanted to go with another girl, and he said "No." Now, I'm hurt. If your boyfriend told you that, wouldn't you feel the same way?

_____

_____

_____

Selection 13.8: Buying Books

I need to register for class tomorrow. Then I need to go to the bookstore and buy my books. Sometimes it's hard to find a parking place. If I can't find one, will you drive me and I'll get out and buy them while you drive around? That would help me so much.

_____

_____

_____

Selection 13.9: Moe's

Do you know where the new restaurant is? You know—Moe's? I think it's across the street from Target, next to the gym. They make Mexican food, and it tastes good. If it's not raining tomorrow, I'll meet you there at noon, and we can have lunch together. I'll ask Minnie if she wants to go with us.

_____

_____

_____

Selection 13.10: Hungry Girl

Yesterday I was so hungry! My boyfriend and I went to the restaurant near the university for lunch. I ordered two chicken sandwiches, a large Coke, and six cookies. Then I ate some chocolate candy. My boyfriend ate one sandwich and had a small Coke. This is the first time I've eaten more than he has. If I keep eating like this, I'll weigh more than he does.

_____

_____

_____

_____

Free Expressive Practice: Create your own selection here. Demonstrate your command of how to incorporate conditionals into your sentences.

_____

_____

_____

_____

Using Conjunctions in ASL

Within Chapter 8 there is a brief discussion regarding the sign FINISH. You will recall that in ASL FINISH can be used in multiple ways to express information. When placed before or after a verb, it indicates that an action has been completed. The English sentence "I have already eaten dinner" can be represented in ASL as "ME FINISH EAT DINNER" or "ME EAT FINISH DINNER."

Furthermore, FINISH can be used as a conjunction to join one or more activities together. In these instances, the sign FINISH is used with the same meaning and function as "then" in English. Used in this manner several activities can be linked together. When joining the following thoughts together—"I flew to Boston; I stayed for two weeks with my brother; then, I flew home"—the sign for FINISH can be utilized as a conjunction and is illustrated as follows: "ME FLY-TO BOSTON STAY TWO-WEEKS FINISH FLY-TO HOME."

Other words used as conjunctions in ASL include HAPPEN, FIND, WRONG, FRUSTRATE, and HIT. HAPPEN is used to indicate unexpected events; FIND conveys unexpected discoveries. WRONG is signed for unexpected events happening without warning, FRUSTRATE is signed as a conjunction for unexpected obstacles, and HIT is signed to express unexpectedly positive circumstances (Humphries & Padden, 2004, p. 191).

When signing the selections that follow, translate the English text into ASL and practice signing the sentences. Several of these selections contain opportunities to use conjunctions.

 EXAMPLE 14.0

Last week I went to the store to buy a new Sidekick, but they were all out of them. I called my friend and found out that they had some at the store on Park Street. I was so excited. I drove right over and bought one.

LAST-WEEK ME GO-TO-there STORE BUY SIDEKICK NEW, FRUSTRATE SIDEKICK RUN-OUT. ME TTY-to MY FRIEND, I-X TELL-ME STORE HAVE SIDEKICK. STORE fs-

<u>when clause</u>

PARK fs-ST. I-X-loc HAVE. THRILLED ME! TTY FINISH DRIVE-TO STORE BUY FINISH.

Selection 14.1: Going to a Movie

Yesterday Ross and I went to see a popular movie that was playing at the theater. There was a long line of people. We inched our way to the ticket window.

When we arrived at the window, the woman told us that they'd run out of tickets. We were headed back to the car when all of a sudden I fell.

_____

_____

_____

_____

Selection 14.2: The Trip

Two years ago my brother and his wife went on a trip. They flew from Atlanta to Philadelphia and stayed with his wife's grandparents for one week. Then they drove to Baltimore and stayed for two days before driving on to Boston. After three more days, they flew back to Atlanta and came home.

_____

_____

_____

_____

Selection 14.3: My Favorite Sport

I love softball, and I'm very skilled at it. Before, when I was in high school, I played soccer, tennis, and hockey. I was so-so at them. When I finished high school, I played softball in college. We got to travel to several other colleges to play. Scads of people used to come and watch us; our team was very successful.

_____

_____

_____

_____

Selection 14.4: Baryshnikov

Baryshnikov's a brilliant dancer; he's so talented. He has toured England and all over the United States, including Chicago, Philadelphia, Boston, Detroit, and Atlanta. People line up to buy tickets and go in and see him. He's been dancing for fifteen years. Five years ago he hurt his knee and was unable to dance for several months. Now he's dancing again.

_____

_____

_____

_____

Selection 14.5: The Car Accident

Three years while I was driving I had an accident. A car hit me broadside, and I was hurt. I called my dad and let him know I was in the hospital. He hurried over to see me. The doctor said I'd be ok and that if I rested, I could go home in six days. When I could finally go home, I was so happy.

_____

_____

_____

_____

55

CHAPTER 14
....
Using
Conjunctions
in ASL

PART I

PART II

PART III

PART IV

Selection 14.6: Math Class

Sabrina's very good in math but Todd isn't. He's so inept; he struggles with math and always has to ask the teacher for help. Every night he studies for two hours, but he still struggles. Sabrina's planning to become a math teacher in the future. Todd wants to become a carpenter. He's talented with woodwork, but he must get better with math to be successful.

_____

_____

_____

_____

Selection 14.7: Looking at Art

People buy tickets and enter museums to look at all of the artwork. Some of the paintings are strange, some make you feel depressed, and some are wonderful. While some of the artists appear very skilled, others are so-so. In three months, I'll go to an art show in Chicago.

_____

_____

_____

Selection 14.8: Megghan's Dog

Six months ago Megghan got a new dog named Taz. Taz weighs about 55 pounds, is black and white, and has long straight fur. A year ago he was hit by a car and now he can't use his left front leg. For a year he's been walking with a limp. He's a very sweet dog. He likes to ride in the car, sit by people, and eat ice cream.

_____

_____

_____

_____

Selection 14.9: Damon Plays Baseball

Damon's a baseball player. He plays for UGA. Yesterday he was playing and was up to bat. A ball came and hit him in the eye. They had to take him to the hospital. The doctor said he couldn't play for two weeks. Now he must sit and watch the other players. He's so bored and is eager to play again.

_____

_____

_____

_____

Selection 14.10: The South

Ten years ago Dan moved from Washington to the South. Now he misses the snow. He'd like to trade places with someone who lives in Baltimore and move to a colder area. His mom disagrees with him. She likes the warmth. She told him he could decide if he wants to move back. If he moves, she'll put off visiting him until it gets warm.

_____

_____

_____

_____

_____

Free Expressive Practice: Create your own selection here. Incorporate the use of at least one conjunction in your selection.

_____

_____

_____

_____

Additional Work with Verbs and Classifiers

There are several types of verb forms in ASL. Some verbs are body anchored, meaning that they contact the body when they are signed, as in HAVE, ENJOY, KNOW, and TIRED. This body contact tends to limit the amount of movement of the verb (Baker & Cokely, 1980, p. 268). Others incorporate movement to change nouns into verbs, as in SIT/CHAIR, BOOK/OPEN-BOOK. Still others alter their direction to indicate the initiator and the recipient of the activity as in HELP-me/HELP-you, GIVE-me/GIVE-you and so forth.

Classifiers are used in predicates in many ways. See Chapters 7 and 10 for a discussion of how they are used to describe location and movement. After identifying the person, place, or thing, the movement of a classifier, for example, can indicate how someone gets in and out of vehicles and on and off animals. In these instances, the individual or object must be identified first before the movement can be described. When demonstrating an individual standing by and then getting in and out of a car, the signer represents the individual standing by using the CL:Λ classifier. This can be changed to the bent-V classifier handshape to indicate that the person is seated. Likewise, when exiting the vehicle, the CL:V̈ classifier handshape is used to show the person exiting the car and changing to the CL:Λ once the individual is again standing in an upright position. Figure 15.1 provides examples of these classifiers.

The following selections include a variety of verb forms. Translate the English sentences into ASL and then practice signing them.

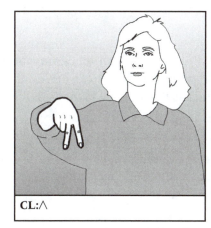 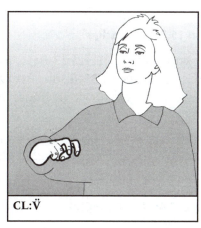

FIGURE 15.1 Examples of the Classifiers CL:Λ and CL:V̈ (Bent-V) Used to Represent Persons Standing and Persons or Animals in a Crouched Position

Source: From Humphries, Tom, & Carol Padden, *Learning American Sign Language,* 2/e. Published by Allyn and Bacon, Boston, MA. Copyright © 2004 by Pearson Education. Reprinted by permission of the publisher.

EXAMPLE 15.0

Can you help me tomorrow? I need to send letters out about the Miss Deaf Ohio Pageant. I think if we send out fifty letters to sponsors we will be okay. Can you come over around nine o'clock in the morning to help?

<u>   y/n-q   </u>   <u>   t   </u>

TOMORROW HELP-me CAN YOU? ME LETTER SEND-TO MANY ANNOUNCE

                <u>   cond   </u>

fs-MISS DEAF fs-OHIO PAGEANT. SUPPOSE CAN DISTRIBUTE-TO FIFTY SUPPORT+++ WE FINE FEEL.

                  <u>   y/n-q   </u>

DON'T-MIND TOMORROW TIME-NINE YOU COME HELP-me?

Selection 15.1: Shannon Was a No Show

Yesterday Shannon told me she'd meet me at 7:30 at the restaurant. I went in and waited. Now it's 8:30, and she still hasn't shown up. I guess I'll just get in my car and go home. If she had car problems, she couldn't call me because she doesn't have a cell phone.

_____

_____

_____

Selection 15.2: Smoking Regulation

Did you know that you can't smoke in restaurants in Florida any more? They passed a law saying where food's served you can't smoke. Now many people have to go outside and stand around if they want a cigarette. It's great for people who don't smoke, but I'm sure people who smoke don't like it.

_____

_____

_____

Selection 15.3: The Judge

Do you know Wetzel Brown? He is a tall, big man with black hair and blue eyes. He's the judge in Madison. Every day he gets in his car drives about six miles to work, goes in the court house, and sits there while lawyers defend their clients.

_____

_____

_____

Selection 15.4: The Deaf Club

Back in 1974 many Deaf people went to Deaf clubs. Every Friday the clubs would serve food and show captioned movies. Today many Deaf people watch captioned movies on their TVs at home. I miss going to the Deaf club. It was a good way to meet many nice people.

59

CHAPTER 15
....
Additional Work
with Verbs
and Classifiers

PART I

PART II

PART III

PART IV

_____

_____

_____

Selection 15.5: When Valerie Arrives

I promised my friend Valerie that I'd show up at the airport and meet her when her plane landed. Once she gets off the plane, we'll walk to the car and drive to the country. My house is about forty-five miles from the airport. When we get there, we'll ride horses.

_____

_____

_____

Selection 15.6: Tons of Homework

Every night that teacher gives her students a huge pile of homework. Her plan is that they'll master the course work. All of the students feel so much pressure to finish the work. They'll be excited when the semester ends.

_____

_____

_____

Selection 15.7: The Waitress

Ashley works as a waitress at Red Lobster. She's very skilled at writing the orders but very inept at serving people their right food. She gave one man steak instead of chicken, and she gave another man water who had ordered beer. She says there's nothing to being a waitress, but I think she needs help.

_____

_____

_____

Selection 15.8: Where Do You Want to Go?

Do you want to go biking, swimming, flying, or to the club tomorrow? You're the one graduating, so you decide. I'll be happy to pick you up after graduation, and we can go together. Just tell me what time to come and where to meet you. We have all day so we can do whatever you want.

_____

_____

_____

Selection 15.9: Inside the Lawyer's Office

When you go inside the front door at the lawyer's office, you follow the hall around to the left, and you'll find the waiting area. Sit down and be patient. The lawyer who'll help you knows law and is skilled at defending criminals.

_____

_____

_____

Selection 15.10: Movies on Airplanes

Many times when you have to fly for several hours, they'll show you a movie. Once the plane takes off, the movie will appear on a small screen that comes down from the ceiling. The movies are great for hearing people but not for deaf people because they don't have any captions.

_____

_____

_____

_____

Free Expressive Practice: Create your own selection here. Be sure to include classifiers and directional verbs in your selection.

_____

_____

_____

_____

Giving Directions in ASL

When giving directions to locations in ASL, the general location is given prior to giving specific information. The general location is signed first, followed by a starting point, and then directions are given from that point. The person giving directions will normally attempt to establish a known reference point close to the destination or location by using the sign KNOW and a typically well-known landmark that is close to the final location. This will become the starting point from which specific directions are given (Newell, 2006). Eye gaze is a very important feature of ASL. While giving directions, it is important to visually follow the path the directions are taking.

When describing how buildings or geographic locations are located in relationship to each other, classifier handshapes can be used for clarification. In these instances, the building or location can be identified, followed by the classifier CL:A or CL:5̈ (see Figure 16.1). Once established, the location of additional buildings or geographic areas can be established. Keep in mind that it may be appropriate to produce classifiers on both hands to indicate there is more than one building. After all of the locations have been identified, the relationship of the first building/area to those subsequent buildings/areas can be established by referencing. As with other classifiers, it is important to note that the building/area must be identified first before a classifier can be used. Signs such as CLOSE-TO, ACROSS-FROM, and MIDDLE-OF are used when giving directions. Often the destination location will be repeated near the end of the directions with the sign THERE as the final sign (Newell, 2006).

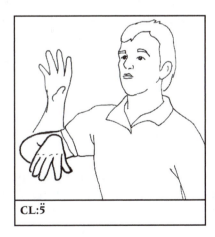
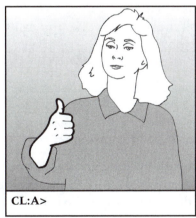

CL:5̈

CL:A>

Objects that do not move such as a house or other building, a statue.

FIGURE 16.1 CL:5̈ and CL:A Classifier Representing Cities, Heaps of Items, and Buildings
Source: From Humphries, Tom, & Carol Padden, *Learning American Sign Language,* 2/e. Published by Allyn and Bacon, Boston, MA. Copyright © 2004 by Pearson Education. Reprinted by permission of the publisher.

Below you will find several selections that focus on giving directions. Translate the English sentences into ASL and then practice signing them.

EXAMPLE 16.0

I like to eat at The Hut near the college. It only takes about five minutes to get there. Drive four blocks down Oak Street and turn left on Meeker Street. Drive another three blocks and you'll see a Shell station in the middle of the block on the right-hand side. The Hut is right next to it.

                                                    _____rhet-q_____

ME LIKE EAT fs-THE fs-HUT NEAR COLLEGE. DRIVE HOW LONG TO fs-THE fs-HUT, APPROXIMATELY FIVE-MINUTE. KNOW fs-OAK fs-STREET, DRIVE STRAIGHT-on-Oak-Street FOUR fs-BLOCK SEE, fs-MEEKER fs-ST INTERSECTION, CL:3-vehicle-turn-left. DRIVE THREE fs-BLOCK, MIDDLE LOOK-to-right SEE fs-SHELL fs-STATION IX-there fs-THE fs-HUT NEXT-TO IX-there.

Selection 16.1: The Mall

I like to shop at the mall in Tampa. It's close to my house. All I have to do is go straight down my street for three blocks. At the third light I turn left and go north for about half a mile. It's right there on the corner at the intersection of Pine and Oak. The police drive around the lot all day so it's safe to shop there at night.

_____

_____

_____

_____

_____

Selection 16.2: Fat Daddy's

Have you been to Fat Daddy's Restaurant? It just opened recently. It has a big sign in front with the name on it and a picture of a sandwich. It makes different kinds of sandwiches. It's located across from the gym next to the building where all the doctors work. You can't miss it—the roof is hot pink!

_____

_____

_____

_____

Selection 16.3: TV Repair Shop

Will you please unplug the big-screen TV for me? I have to take it to the repair shop. Yesterday it just shut down. I don't know why. I was watching it, and all of a sudden it just stopped working. If you'll put it in my car, I'll drive downtown and park and ask the man to get it out of my car for me.

_____

_____

_____

_____

63

CHAPTER 16
....
Giving
Directions
in ASL

PART I

PART II

PART III

PART IV

Selection 16.4: Shalonda's Apartment

Shalonda recently moved into a new apartment. When you leave the library, you go straight down Main Street for about ten miles. It's quite a ways. You cross over the bridge and turn right at the corner where the gas station is. You'll be going west. Continue until you see the sign on your right that says Melrose Place. Her apartment's behind the first building on your left.

_____

_____

_____

_____

Selection 16.5: Take the Box to the Post Office

Please close the box on the table, tape it up, and take it to the post office for me. I need to get it sent to your cousin. Be careful with it. It's full of glasses, and I don't want them to break. When you go into the post office, tell the woman to please insure it for $200 because the glasses are very expensive.

_____

_____

_____

_____

Selection 16.6: The New Coke and Snack Machines

Did you know that they've added two new machines in our building? If you take the elevator to the second floor, they're located down the hall around the corner by the water fountain. The drink machine has both Coke and Pepsi in it—how strange. The snack machine has popcorn, candy, and other things to eat.

_____

_____

_____

_____

Selection 16.7: The Hospital

To get to the hospital, you go left at the corner and then go straight ahead through two intersections. At the corner of Smith and Jones, you will see Moe's restaurant on one corner and Dalton Books on the other corner. Turn right there—continue to go straight through four more lights, and the hospital will be on your right.

_____

_____

_____

_____

Selection 16.8: Cindy's Mountain Home

Cindy lives in the mountains. She has a beautiful home. When you go in the front door, you're in a big living room. The kitchen's next to the living room, and there's one bathroom behind it. There are windows all around the house.

The bedrooms are all located on the second floor, and there's one more bathroom up there too.

_____

_____

_____

_____

Selection 16.9: Marie's Restaurant

Marie's restaurant's across from the church. Every Sunday people go to church from 9:00 to 10:00 and then go to Marie's for breakfast. The restaurant's located close to Don's house. Sometimes after breakfast we go to Don's and go bike riding. It makes for a nice Sunday.

_____

_____

_____

Selection 16.10: Looking for an Outlet

Sometimes it's hard to find an outlet. The TV and VCR and lights are all plugged into the wall in the living room. The computer and the printer are plugged into the wall in the bedroom. The hairdryer's plugged into the wall in the bathroom. I need to unplug something so I can plug in my telephone.

_____

_____

_____

_____

Free Expressive Practice: Create your own selection here. In your selection, include a minimum of two locations and then describe either how you would get from one location to the other, or where something is located within a building.

_____

_____

_____

_____

CHAPTER 17

Working with Time: Describing Plurals and Regularity

Chapter 9 described how to incorporate time to convey the various days of the week as well as how to indicate weeks, months, and years. Information has also been presented that explains how signs can change one of their parameters to change one day to all day, one Sunday to every Sunday, and so forth.

Weeks, months, and years can be modified to express the difference between one week and weekly, one month and monthly, and one year and yearly. The sign for WEEK is produced with a repeated, circular movement to indicate an event or activity occurs more than one time. Likewise the sign for MONTH is made in a circular manner, thus indicating the event or activity occurs once each month. See Figure 17.1 for an example of the differences between MONTH and MONTHLY.

Numbers can also be incorporated when indicating the various times of the year to specify the exact number of weeks, months, and years. The numbers 1 through 9 can be incorporated into the signs as in 3-WEEK, 6-MONTH, and so forth. However, for numbers larger than 9, the number is usually signed before the week, month, or year.

When the number being described is an approximation rather than an exact number, the sign APPROXIMATELY can be signed prior to or immediately following the number. The sign APPROXIMATELY conveys that the time in question is "about" or "around" a specific time as in "APPROXIMATELY TIME-11." In these instances the signer is clarifying that the time frame is not an exact number. Also,

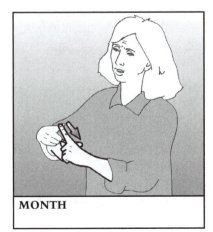 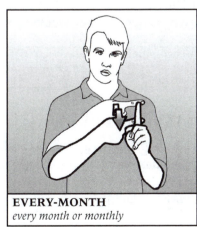

MONTH

EVERY-MONTH
every month or monthly

FIGURE 17.1   Example of Month and Every Month

Source: From Humphries, Tom, & Carol Padden, *Learning American Sign Language,* 2/e. Published by Allyn and Bacon, Boston, MA. Copyright © 2004 by Pearson Education. Reprinted by permission of the publisher.

the number handshape may be shaken slightly to indicate "around or about" a certain time (Newell, 2006). The sign APPROXIMATELY can also be used in conjunction when describing age or monitory amounts to indicate an individual is "about 50" or the vase is worth "about $75.00."

Below you will find several selections that include time indicators. Translate the English sentences into ASL and then practice signing them.

 EXAMPLE 17.0

Tomorrow I will start my new diet. I will exercise every day and eat healthy food. I will get up tomorrow morning at 4:45 and go to the gym. Do you want to go with me? I only plan to stay for about an hour. Then I'll go home and shower.

TOMORROW NEW fs-DIET START ME. EVERYDAY EXERCISE, EAT RECOVER

$$\underline{\hspace{4em}\text{when}\hspace{4em}}$$
FOOD WILL ME. TOMORROW MORNING ME GET-UP TIME 4:45 GO-TO GYM.

$$\underline{\hspace{2em}\text{y/n-q}\hspace{2em}}\qquad\qquad\underline{\hspace{2em}\text{mm}\hspace{2em}}\qquad\underline{\text{when}}$$
YOU WANT JOIN ME? ME PLAN STAY APPROXIMATELY ONE-HOUR. FINISH GO-TO HOME SHOWER.

Selection 17.1: Summer Vacation

Every year my family flies to Colorado to visit my husband's parents. This year we'll go in July. We'll stay for two weeks and then fly to California to visit my sister. I haven't seen her in three years, and I can't wait to see her. We'll stay for four days and then fly home.

_____

_____

_____

Selection 17.2: Summer Classes

Last summer I started taking classes at the university. For ten weeks we went to class every Monday, Wednesday, and Friday from 9:00 to 12:00. On Tuesday and Thursday I had class from 8:00 until 4:00. Next summer I'll only have to take two classes for four weeks. I am so glad.

_____

_____

_____

Selection 17.3: Winter Retreat

In two years a group of my friends and I are going to get together in the mountains in Canada. We plan to ski, ice skate, and play ice hockey. All of us enjoy cold weather. Every month the five of us talk on the phone and plan our vacation. We've been taking vacations together every two years for the past ten years.

_____

_____

_____

Selection 17.4: Shopping for a New Car

Please meet me tomorrow around 10:00 so we can go and look for a new car. I need something cheap that won't be expensive to drive. I don't want to pay more than $7,000. I'd prefer a four-door car but will take a two-door. I'll plan to meet you at the Nissan dealership where they have the used cars.

_____

_____

_____

Selection 17.5: Missi's Busy Schedule

Missi is one busy woman. Every Monday she goes to dance class. Every Wednesday she has Spanish class. Weekly she does volunteer work at the hospital, and when she's not there, she's at her regular job. On Saturday mornings she meets her jogging friend on the corner near your house at 7:30, and they run for three miles.

_____

_____

_____

_____

Selection 17.6: The Cheater

I don't like people who lie and cheat. Sometimes you see students cheating in class. They're too lazy to study and show up for class without their work. You can see them looking at other people's papers and copying their work. Even though you see it, no one wants to squeal on them.

_____

_____

_____

Selection 17.7: Outdoor Activities

Do you like to do things outside? Do you prefer doing things outside when it's hot or cold? Some people really like to surf and go fishing. Other people like ice skating and skiing. If you like cold weather and mountains, skiing is the perfect sport. If you like to be outside when it is hot, surfing or fishing can be fun.

_____

_____

_____

_____

Selection 17.8: Bad Habits

That man has some really bad habits. He goes to bed late, oversleeps in the morning, and is always late for work. When he gets there, he takes forty-minute coffee breaks. He's just lazy. I told him he needs to go to bed earlier, arrive at work on time, or he'll be fired. Then who will hire him?

_____

_____

_____

_____

Free Expressive Practice: Create your own selection here. Be sure to incorporate at least two time indicators.

_____

_____

_____

_____

CHAPTER 18

Quantifiers

Quantifiers such as MANY, A-FEW, SOME, and SEVERAL can be signed either before or after a noun. These quantifiers may be combined with nouns that can be counted, such as plants, apples, bicycles, desks, teachers, and so forth, indicating how many of these nouns there are. Quantifiers such as A-LITTLE, PLENTY, and SOME can be signed together with noncount nouns such as COKE, COOKIE, and CHICKEN, which can be counted indicating how much or how many of these nouns there are. In ASL, to sign ME HAVE COKE SOME REMAIN-ING or ME HAVE SOME COKE REMAINING would both be appropriate, likewise, BICYCLE SEVERAL JOHN HAVE or JOHN HAVE SEVERAL BICYCLE would also be acceptable.

Below are several selections that include quantifiers. Translate the English sentences into ASL and then practice signing them.

 EXAMPLE 18.0

Bronwyn has been a teacher for several years. During that time she has collected many children's books. She has so many she can fill ten tall bookshelves. Some of her books are for young children, 3- and 4-year-olds, while others are for kindergartners and older children. She has plenty of books.

<u>   t   </u>   <u>   when   </u>

fs-BRONWYN TEACH SCHOOL SEVERAL YEAR. SINCE START TEACH, IX-rt-she

<u>   mm   </u>

COLLECT CHILDREN BOOK MANY. BOOK MANY. ME LOOK, FEEL POSSIBLE

<u> nod </u>   <u> t </u>

TEN BOOKSHELF (2h CL:B-loc "floor to ceiling"++)" FULL CAN. BOOK HAVE VARIETY DIFFERENT++ AGE. SOME FOR CHILDREN YOUNG CHILDREN AGE-3, AGE-4. OTHER BOOK FOR CHILDREN GO-TO KINDERGARTEN. SOME FOR OLD+ER CHILDREN. IX-rt-she HAVE BOOK PLENTY IX-rt-she.

Selection 18.1: Winter Sky

Have you ever been up north in the winter and looked up at the sky on a cold evening? If it's clear, you can see the moon and many, many stars. There's a big difference between looking at the sky in the city and in the mountains. The lights from the city make it hard to see the stars. There are no lights in the mountains.

_____
_____
_____
_____

Selection 18.2: Summer Theater

Did you see the article in the newspaper yesterday about the summer theater on Jeckyll Island? It said there'd be several plays this summer and 10 percent of them would be signed. A few of them will take place outside. We should go this summer and support the theater group.

_____
_____
_____

Selection 18.3: Soccer Game

Next year the world soccer games will be held in France. I've heard that England has a strong team. They'll be playing against the United States. I imagine many people will go to the games. If we want to go, we should buy our tickets now. If we wait, I don't think we'll be able to get any.

_____
_____
_____
_____

Selection 18.4: Bar-B-Q

Next Saturday we're having a barbeque. It will start around 5:00 and continue until late in the evening. I want to invite all of you to come. We'll have plenty of food and drinks. Wear some comfortable clothes and bring your suit because we're going to play tennis and go swimming. If it's too hot outside, we'll go in and watch movies.

_____
_____
_____
_____

Selection 18.5: Mountain Driving

You have to pay attention to the road when you're driving in the mountains. It curves back and forth as you drive up toward the top. From your car window you can look down, and many times you can see rivers winding along the roads. When you get close to the top, the air is cool and you can feel the sun on your face.

_____
_____
_____
_____

Selection 18.6: Emily's Children

Emily's been married for ten years and would like to have several children. If she can't have children, she'd like to adopt. She and her husband have talked about adopting children from Russia. They would like to have five boys and five girls. Do you think that's a lot of children?

_____

_____

_____

_____

Selection 18.7: The President

The president of the United States lives in the White House in Washington, DC. He has a huge job and stays very busy. He's always in meetings and travels all over the world. People either support the president and believe in his ideas or they dislike him and are against his ideas. Are you for or against the president?

_____

_____

_____

_____

Selection 18.8: Classes

Marie has eight classes this semester. Each of them requires several papers. Some of them will only need to be a few pages long, while one or two of them will demand a lot of writing. She has a major paper due for her Deaf Heritage class. She'll need to go to the library, research several articles, and start writing. She must have a minimum of ten sources, and the paper must be at least twenty pages in length.

_____

_____

_____

_____

_____

Free Expressive Practice: Create your own selection here. In your selection, include a variety of quantifiers.

_____

_____

_____

_____

_____

CHAPTER 19

Repeatedly, Continually, and Reduplication

There are a number of action verbs in ASL that repeat their movement to indicate that an action occurs frequently. As you recall, verbs such as GO-TO, SHOW-TO, and PAY-TO are directional verbs. Based on the direction they are signed, they indicate who initiates the action and who receives the action. These signs can also be repeated to alert the signer that the action occurs numerous times. In this way the sentence "I went to the Deaf Club" can be changed into "I went frequently to the Deaf Club" by repeating the sign GO-TO. Figure 19.1 provides an example of a repeated verb movement.

When indicating frequency, facial grammar may be altered, thus alerting the listener to the fact that the activity takes place with a great deal of difficulty (clenched teeth), easily without any effort (mm), or in a lazy manner (th) (Newell, 2006). The non-manual signal written th can be expressed on the mouth to indicate the activity is completed in a lazy manner or without paying attention to the task at hand. When a task requires a lot of effort, pursed lips accompany the sign, signifying the amount of effort required to complete the task. For an in-depth discussion on facial grammar, consult Baker and Cokely, *American Sign Language: A Teacher's Resource Text on Grammar and Culture* (1980). Figure 19.2 provides examples of facial grammar related to the amount of effort associated with an activity.

Verbs can also be produced in a circular motion to indicate the action occurs continuously. A circular repeated motion indicates an activity that is continuous/ongoing. For example, waiting for a long time is indicated in ASL by modifying the movement of the sign WAIT and signing it in a circular motion.

There are a few nouns that can be repeated to indicate that they are plural. Examples of some of these signs include SENTENCE, RULE, and SPECIALITY-FIELD (Baker & Cokely, 1980, p. 377). Other signs are repeated in multiple locations in space with a horizontal or vertical sweeping motion, which makes them plural. Some examples of signs that change from singular to plural when reduplicated are WINDOW, WINDOW++, DOOR, DOOR++, TREE, TREE++, and BOOK, BOOK++.

In Chapter 18, quantifiers were discussed, explaining how they can be combined with nouns to indicate plurality. Classifiers in their plural forms can also be used to make nouns plural. For example, the sign CAR represented by the CL:3 classifier can be repeated CL:3-in-a-row to indicate that there is a row of cars rather than just one.

Change the following selections from English to ASL and practice signing them.

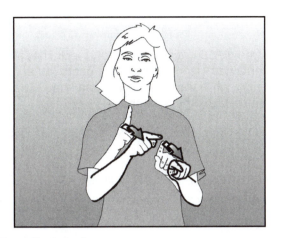

FIGURE 19.1 Go-There-Repeatedly

Source: From Humphries, Tom, & Carol Padden, *Learning American Sign Language,* 2/e. Published by Allyn and Bacon, Boston, MA. Copyright © 2004 by Pearson Education. Reprinted by permission of the publisher.

Lips pursed to show lack of intensity or effort, ease:

Mouth opening and closing, to show intensity or effort:

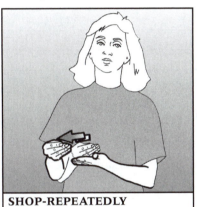

SHOP-REPEATEDLY
to shop easily

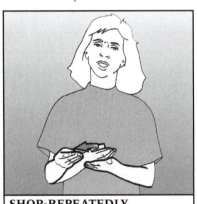

SHOP-REPEATEDLY
to spend a lot of time and effort shopping

Tongue slightly protruding through pursed lips to show carelessness or lack of deliberation:

Lips pursed together and eyebrows squeezed together to show diligence, care, or deliberation:

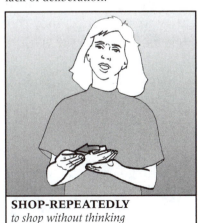

SHOP-REPEATEDLY
to shop without thinking

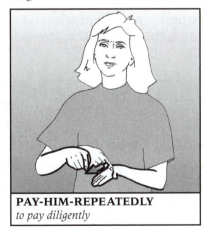

PAY-HIM-REPEATEDLY
to pay diligently

FIGURE 19.2 Examples of Facial Grammar

Source: From Humphries, Tom, & Carol Padden, *Learning American Sign Language,* 2/e. Published by Allyn and Bacon, Boston, MA. Copyright © 2004 by Pearson Education. Reprinted by permission of the publisher.

EXAMPLE 19.0

Mom and her friends from AASD get together every week. They all graduated at the same time and have remained friends. Weekly they get together for lunch and sit around and visit. Once in a while they go bowling. Sometimes they plan trips, but most of the time they just enjoy each other's company.

EVERY-WEEK MOM, POSS-mom FRIEND FROM fs-AASD GATHER-TOGETHER.

$$\overline{\ \ t\ \ }$$

FRIEND #ALL GRADUATE TIME SAME, STILL FRIEND SINCE. EVERY-WEEK LUNCH SIT CL:V CHAT++, ONCE-IN-WHILE, GO-TO fs-BOWLING. SOMETIMES PLAN TRAVEL,

$$\underline{\ \ rhet-q\ \ }$$

BUT MOST THEY ENJOY WHAT CHAT++.

Selection 19.1: Winter in Pennsylvania

In Pittsburgh in the wintertime it's too cold to go outside. Many days it snows and snows and a foot stays on the ground. When this happens, many people stay in and read lots of books, watch movies, and cook lots of soup. Then when spring comes and it's warm, they go outside again.

_____

_____

_____

Selection 19.2: Paying Bills

Every month I sit down and pay bills diligently. Then when I'm through, if I have money left, I go shopping. I like to buy clothes, but I really like to shop for shoes. Do you like to go from store to store shopping? Some people don't enjoy that. For me it's a lot of fun.

_____

_____

_____

Selection 19.3: Volleyball Game

Last Saturday Mike and his friends and John and his friends played volleyball for three hours. Mike's team won. When they were finished, they cooked hot dogs and hamburgers and sat around and talked. It was a perfect day to be out-side—warm, but not too hot.

_____

_____

_____

Selection 19.4: Camping

Do you like to go camping in the woods? I like to go in the fall when the trees change color. It's fun to hike in the mountains, fish, and cook over a campfire. When it gets dark, you can lie down and see all of the stars. I wish I could go every week but I can't.

_____

_____

_____

Selection 19.5: Summer Fun

Summer is my favorite time of the year. I don't like winter because it gets too cold, and it rains or snows a lot. Fall is so-so but in the summer there's no school —you can ride bikes, skate, or play football all day and stay up late. You can also go swimming and play basketball or volleyball. If I could change anything, I'd make it summer all year.

_____

_____

_____

_____

Selection 19.6: The Buffet

Alan loves going to Ken's on Thursday night. He goes every Thursday because they have all-you-can-eat chicken. The waitress brings you a plate of chicken, French fries, and salad. Then when you run out of chicken she brings you as much as you can eat. Alan eats and eats. He always leaves feeling full.

_____

_____

_____

_____

Selection 19.7: The Complain Game

Have you ever played the "Complain Game"? Last Saturday was my first time. Everyone sits around in a circle and complains. Some complain about work, others about restaurants, some complain about their family. I didn't think it was much fun. I won't play again.

_____

_____

_____

Selection 19.8: Movies

Big J loves to go to the movies. It doesn't matter what's playing, he'll go. Usually he goes every Saturday at three o'clock. He likes to go in the afternoons because it's cheaper. Sometimes he has to wait in line for a long time if it's a popular movie. Other times he's the only one in the theater. I don't know if I could go every week, could you?

_____

_____

_____

_____

Free Expressive Practice: Create your own selection here. Try to incorporate nouns or verbs that can be signed repeatedly, continually, or reduplicated.

_____

_____

_____

_____

Using Predicate Adjectives to Indicate Repetition

In ASL nouns and verbs can repeat their movements to indicate plurality or that an activity happens repeatedly. For example, the signer can repeat the sign for CHILD with a sweeping movement in space to create the plural CHILDREN. Likewise, verbs can be repeated as in GO-TO to illustrate that the signer regularly goes to a specific location or event or goes to several different places. Adjectives can also be repeated to express that a condition exists or happens repeatedly over a period of time. For example, one can describe that there are several different church denominations located within a one-mile radius by signing CHURCH APPROXIMATE ONE fs-MILE HAVE CHURCH DIFFERENT++ IX-there++.

Predicate adjectives can be produced in a circular fashion indicating that the condition continues for an extended period of time. In these instances, the signer can indicate that an activity is ongoing. An example of a predicate adjective that can be signed continuously is when a student wants to express that the teacher gives her the same type of math problems every night and that they never change. In this sentence the sign for SAME would be repeated in a circular manner. EVERY-NIGHT TEACHER GIVE-TO ME MATH PROBLEM SAME-circular++.

Change the following selections from English to ASL and practice signing them.

 EXAMPLE 20.0

My daughter seems to be frustrated all the time lately. She's taking a class for the third time and still can't seem to pass the tests. She worries continuously about what she'll do if she fails the class again. I hope all of this worry doesn't make her sick.

SINCE MY DAUGHTER IX-rt-she SEEM FRUSTRATED-circular. IX NOW TAKE-UP CLASS THIRD TIME, STILL PASS TEST CAN'T. IX-rt-she DWELL-ON-circular.

<u>   t   </u>

WHAT-TO-DO #IF FAIL AGAIN. DAUGHTER DWELL-ON-circular, HOPE NOT BECOME SICK IX-rt-she. CAUSE IX-rt-she SICK CAN.

Selection 20.1: Sophie's Trip

Sophie has been worrying about her trip for weeks. She's flying from California to Europe and will then travel around by train. She's worried that her plane

77

CHAPTER 20
Using Predicate
Adjectives to
Indicate Repetition

PART I

PART II

PART III

PART IV

will be late landing and that she'll miss her train. If that happens, she'll have to rent a car and she doesn't like to drive. I hope she'll have fun.

_____
_____
_____
_____

Selection 20.2: Quiet House

My house is so quiet now. All of our children have moved out and are living in different places. Some parents are relieved when their children grow up and leave—they look forward to doing things alone. I feel a little depressed. I miss cooking for a lot of people and talking for hours.

_____
_____
_____
_____

Selection 20.3: The Hotel

Have you been to the new hotel in Chicago? It's absolutely beautiful! There are fireplaces and green plants in every room. The shops in the lobby have everything from clothes to jewelry. I shop there regularly. And the three restaurants are wonderful. The chef is skilled at cooking chicken and fish.

_____
_____
_____
_____

Selection 20.4: Ed

Ed's the supervisor where I work, and none of us likes him. He's very strict and argues with all of the workers. He complains all the time and is never satisfied with anyone's work. I wish he'd find a new job with a different company. He might be happier and complain less.

_____
_____
_____
_____

Selection 20.5: Internet Resources

There are so many resources on the Internet today. It doesn't seem to matter what you're looking for, you can find it. I needed to find some information on Deaf culture for my ASL class. Wow! I was amazed to see how much information is out there on Deaf people.

_____
_____
_____

Selection 20.6: Hurricane Season

Don't you hate it when hurricane season starts? For people in the South and the Southeast the destruction can be horrific! When a Category 3 or higher hurricane hits, there is damage everywhere. Between the continuous rain and the wind it seems like everything within a fifty-mile radius is affected. I feel so sorry for people whose homes are destroyed because of bad weather.

_____

_____

_____

_____

_____

Selection 20.7: Music

There are so many different kinds of music to choose from today. Country, Heavy Metal, Jazz, and Classical music are just a few. If you turn on your radio, you can find almost anything you want to listen to. When Ross is driving for a long periods of time, he likes to set his radio to the country station and sing along with the music.

_____

_____

_____

_____

Selection 20.8: Maintaining Your Proper Weight

Almost all diet and exercise programs say the same thing. If you want to lose weight, you must diet and exercise. Most programs recommend that you exercise at least thirty minutes every day and limit your intake of high-fat food, sugar, and starches. Research shows if you even walk thirty minutes every day, you can lose ten pounds in a year.

_____

_____

_____

_____

Selection 20.9: Visiting James

James has been sick for months. He goes to the doctor regularly and owes him a lot of money. The doctor gave him a lot of pills, and he takes them weekly. I wish I could help him; he can't drive and doesn't get out much. I live so far away, and I can only come and visit on the weekends.

_____

_____

_____

_____

Selection 20.10: Shy Sheila

Sheila used to be very shy. She stayed at home all the time because she would get embarrassed easily. Then she met Joe. He helped her feel confident. From then on she started to go out and meet people and have fun. It's nice that the two of them are going together now.

_____

_____

_____

_____

Selection 20.11: The Botanist

A friend of my father's is a botanist. He has lived next door to my parents for years and is leaving next week on a trip. He'll travel all around collecting plants from everywhere. I think he's starting in New York and will then travel from place to place in Europe. Altogether he'll be gone six months. He does some exciting research.

_____

_____

_____

_____

Free Expressive Practice: Create your own selection here. Include in your selection nouns, verbs, or adjectives that can be reduplicated.

_____

_____

_____

_____

_____

CHAPTER 21

Rhetorical Questions

Rhetorical questions are another form of questions found both in English and American Sign Language. They are generally not intended to be answered by the person being addressed; rather, they are designed to be answered by the individual speaking or signing the question. Rhetorical questions are used to introduce information or to draw attention to the information that will follow. When expressed in ASL, the eyebrows are raised, and the head is tilted forward as in yes/no questions. Question signs such as WHY, HOW, WHERE, WHAT, and WHO may be used when signing rhetorical questions. Oftentimes when HOW and WHY are signed, the word "because" is frequently voiced for the rhetorical.

For example, the sentence "I've got to go to the store and by some food because I don't have any" can be signed in ASL,

        <u>rhet-q</u>

ME GO-TO STORE MUST, WHY HAVE FOOD NONE.

Likewise, in the sentence "I passed the test because I studied hard" can be signed in ASL,

        <u>rhet-q</u>

TEST ME SUCCEED HOW-wg STUDY-long time.

Several of the following statements can be signed using rhetorical questions. Change these selections into ASL and practice signing them.

 EXAMPLE 21.0

Todd wants to move from Colorado to Texas because he hates cold weather. He's been looking for a job for six months now, and once he finds one he'll be on his way. He has so many things to move but I think he'll get a U-Haul and pack it up when he's ready to move. I hope he finds a new job soon.

    <u>t</u>   <u>affirmation</u>   <u>rhet-q</u>

KNOW TODD, NOW LIVE COLOR fs-ADO, WANT MOVE-TO TEXAS. WHY? IX-rt-he VOMIT-IT WEATHER COLD. SINCE 6-MONTH IX-rt SEARCH++ FOR GOOD #JOB.

    <u>cond</u>   <u>PAH</u>

HAPPEN FIND #JOB   SUCCESS, FOR SURE IX-rt-he MOVE WILL. HE HAVE

        <u>cond</u>

THING MANY++. READY MOVE-AWAY, IX-rt GET fs-UHAUL fs-TRUCK, PUT-IN POSS-Todd THING++. HOPE IX-rt-he FIND NEW #JOB SOON, "cross fingers."

Selection 21.1: The Dancer

Katrina majored in dance for three years. She attended two different universities and studied under the best instructors. Then she changed her major to nursing because she thought she'd have a hard time finding a job as a dancer. Today she works full time as a nurse and continues to dance for enjoyment.

_____

_____

_____

_____

Selection 21.2: Smith's Poultry Shuts Down

Tom has worked at Smith's Poultry for fourteen years. Last year the company closed, and he was laid off. He looked and looked for another job, but many other people were looking, too, so he didn't find one. Now he's drawing unemployment. He doesn't like it because he feels embarrassed but his family has to eat.

_____

_____

_____

_____

Selection 21.3: Change in Careers

Paul has worked for the state for twelve years. Now he's making plans to go back to school. He either wants to be a carpenter or a welder. He doesn't want to go to school for four years because he wants to hurry and earn money again. When he finishes, he wants a job with good benefits, in which he can get annual raises.

_____

_____

_____

_____

Selection 21.4: The Interpreter

Zoe went to school for four years to become an interpreter. She took about sixty hours in her field and now feels prepared to accept many different assignments. While in school she completed an internship in which she got to observe interpreters working in schools, doctor's offices, and churches. Now that she's finished she wants to interpret at the high school.

_____

_____

_____

_____

Selection 21.5: Interpreting in Jail

I don't like to interpret in jail because you have to drive so far to get there. What's more, to get there you must drive over a high bridge that's very narrow. I don't like high narrow bridges; they scare me. If they moved the jail to another part of town, I'd be happy to go there on a regular basis, but I don't think they'll do that.

_____
_____
_____
_____

Selection 21.6: Great Boss

I have a great boss. She has twenty-eight people under her and manages to keep all of them happy. When her subordinates go to her with their problems, she helps them solve them. I've been working with her for six years, and during that time no one has quit. She's always straight with everyone, and because of that I think people enjoy working for her.

_____
_____
_____
_____

Selection 21.7: Stolen Identity

Today you have to be careful using the computer because people can steal your identity. Have you read in the newspaper where people had their IDs stolen, their money taken, and been billed for things they didn't buy? It has become a serious problem. If you decide to pay your bills on the computer, be sure you have a secure site.

_____
_____
_____
_____

Selection 21.8: I Think It's Going to Rain

I think it's going to rain soon. The sky's getting dark and there's a strong wind blowing from the north. I was going to go to the library, but if it rains I'll stay home. I don't want to get my books and papers wet trying to get from the library to my car. I'll wait an hour and see if the sky clears. If it does, I'll be on my way.

_____
_____
_____
_____

Free Expressive Practice: Create your own selection here. Try to include at least one sentence that has a rhetorical question in it.

_____
_____
_____
_____

Additional Ways to Form Negatives

Chapters 6 and 11 described ways to express negatives in ASL. The sign NONE can be combined with SEE NONE and HEAR NONE to indicate that the individual hasn't seen or heard anything. The sign NOT can be combined with GO or STUDENT to indicate the signer isn't going and he or she is not a student.

The signs NEVER and NOTHING can also be used as negatives to convey denial. In these instances the phrases ME HIT BOY NOTHING ME or ME TAKE BOOK NEVER ME are expressed in English as "I didn't hit the boy" and "I never took the book." As with other negatives in ASL, the non-manual behavior (shaking the head from side to side) accompanies the negative sign and may continue throughout the signed sentence.

Keep in mind that negative signs can be placed before the verb or at the end of the sentence. However, they are frequently placed at the end of sentences; this is particularly true in artistic or dramatic sign presentations in which negation almost always occurs at the end of the sentences. When the signer wants to emphasize the negative nature of the sentence, the negative sign can be signed before the verb and again at the end of the sentence. When produced in this manner, emphasis is often placed on the negation that occurs at the end of the sentence (Baker & Cokely, 1980, p. 149).

Several sentences below provide the opportunity to incorporate the signs NOT and NEVER. Change these English sentences into ASL and practice signing them.

 EXAMPLE 22.0

Nanci doesn't like ice cream. It doesn't matter what flavor it is or what kind it is, she just doesn't like it. She never goes to Dairy Queen or Brusters. When her friends ask her to go with them to get ice cream, she goes but she doesn't order it. Instead she orders a drink. We're all different, I guess.

    t   neg   neg

ICE-CREAM, fs-NANCI NOT-LIKE. fs-FLAVOR, KIND ANYWAY. IX-rt-she NOT CRAZY

                            t   neg

FOR ICE-CREAM. IX-rt GO-TO fs-DAIRY fs-QUEEN, fs-BRUSTERS NEVER.

 cond

HAPPEN POSS-Nanci FRIEND ASK-TO-she JOIN COME ALONG-WITH GET

                     neg

ICE-CREAM, IX-rt-she TEND NOT GET ICE-CREAM. IX-rt-she TEND BUY DRINK.

PEOPLE TEND YOUR DIFFERENT++(shrug).

Selection 22.1: The Mistake

Last night the police told me to get in the police car, and they took me to jail. They told me that I'd stolen some money and that I took another man's car. I told them I hadn't taken any money and that I had never stolen a car. After several hours another cop brought in a second man who looked like me. They saw him stealing money, so they let me go. I was so relieved to be released.

_____

_____

_____

_____

Selection 22.2: Mom's Stroke

Last year Mom had a stroke. Until then she had been in good health. She'd never had a cold, been sick with the flu, or even run a temperature. All of a sudden without warning she felt dizzy and fell to the floor. We immediately called 911. The EMTs arrived and weren't sure what was wrong with her. They took her to the hospital, kept her for three weeks, and determined she'd had a stroke.

_____

_____

_____

_____

Selection 22.3: Picture of Health

My Aunt Kate's the picture of health. She's 103 years old, stands 4'10", weighs 80 pounds, and is very sharp. She has never smoked or drunk. Until she turned 100 she walked every day and played the piano at church every Sunday. She's never too busy to talk about the "good old days." I love to listen to her.

_____

_____

_____

_____

Selection 22.4: New Experience

Last year I got sick with the flu. That was a new experience for me. I stay healthy. I exercise every day—you know I walk/run three miles, I eat healthy food, never eat junk food, and I enjoy life. One morning I woke up, my head hurt, I felt hot, and I was very tired. I went to the doctor, and he told me I had the flu. I was surprised; it was a new bad experience for me.

_____

_____

_____

_____

Selection 22.5: Ambulance Driver

Billy wants to be an ambulance driver when he grows up. He thinks it would be neat to respond to 911 calls and help people out. His grandfather had a heart attack a year ago. If it hadn't been for the ambulance, he would have died. He said sick people wouldn't bother him. He wants to be able to take people's temperature, blood pressure, and rush them to the hospital.

85

CHAPTER 22

Additional
Ways to Form
Negatives

PART I

PART II

PART III

PART IV

_____

_____

_____

_____

Selection 22.6: Weightlifting Class

I plan to take a weightlifting class next fall at the college. I've heard that the instructor is really skilled at helping students build muscle. I've never lifted weights before. I want to learn how to lift weights with my legs, do knee bends with weights on my shoulders, and improve my appearance. I also think this class will help me lose weight. What do you think?

_____

_____

_____

_____

Selection 22.7: The Baby's Sick

Margaret's baby's only 6 weeks old. Last night he started to cough and run a temperature. He'd never been sick before. He cried and cried and couldn't sleep. Margaret got worried and put the baby in the car and took him to the emergency room. The doctor checked him over and said he had an ear infection. He said that was common in babies. He gave him some medicine and sent them home.

_____

_____

_____

_____

Selection 22.8: Ole Dakota

Dakota's not a small dog. He is a Weimaraner and weighs about seventy-five pounds. He's getting old, and sometimes he's not very friendly. When the other dogs try to play with him, he snaps at them. He doesn't seem to have the patience he needs to be around puppies. He's a very handsome dog, he just isn't very smart.

_____

_____

_____

_____

Free Expressive Practice: Create your own selection here. Use at least two negatives in your sentences.

_____

_____

_____

_____

Additional Work Signing Topics

Designating a topic for discussion frequently occurs in ASL. Chapter 3 described how the grammatical feature of topic/comment is used to identify what the signer wants to discuss and then comment on the object. You recall that in these instances the eyebrows are raised and the head is tilted up and back slightly as the topic is identified, followed by the lowering of the eyebrows for the comment. Clauses can also function as topics. In these cases the same facial grammar is followed.

Several of the sentences below include clauses that are designed to be signed as topic/comment. Change the English into ASL and practice signing the sentences.

 EXAMPLE 23.0

We have so many family pictures in our house. Our house is full of them! My mom just loves pictures. Every wall is taken up with pictures of our family. All of my sisters and I danced when we were younger, and over her piano she has fifty-seven dance pictures at various ages. We really have a lot of pictures.

MY HOUSE HAVE FAMILY PICTURES MANY++. HOUSE, FULL PICTURES.

     ‾‾‾t‾‾‾   ‾‾‾t‾‾‾

PICTURE, MY MOM LOVE-IT. WALL++, FAMILY PICTURE CL:BB-there++.

          ‾‾‾‾‾‾when‾‾‾‾‾‾   ‾‾‾t‾‾‾

PAST ME, MY SISTER YOUNG, WE DANCE. OUR MOTHER PIANO HAVE,

  ‾‾‾t‾‾‾   ‾‾‾‾‾‾‾rhet-q‾‾‾‾‾‾‾

WALL IX-there HAVE. DANCE PICTURE ALL-TOGETHER HOW MANY FIFTY-SEVEN

CL:BB-there++, HAVE ME MY SISTER WE AGE VARIOUS. PICTURE++ HAVE MANY WE.

Selection 23.1: Josh's Job

I didn't know that Josh quit his job. I saw a mutual friend last week, and he told me that he quit and now he plans to work for the new company, Dillard's, that's setting up its building now. Did you see in the newspaper that it expects to open its doors in August? He should earn more money and have better benefits.

_____

_____

_____

_____

87

CHAPTER 23
....
Additional Work
Signing Topics

PART I

PART II

PART III

PART IV

Selection 23.2: Out of Africa

Several years ago my husband and I saw the movie, *Out of Africa*. We both really liked it. The countryside was beautiful, and I loved watching the animals, especially the lions, tigers, and elephants out in the wild. I especially enjoyed watching the sunsets. They were so full of color: red, orange, and gold. I would love to visit Africa someday.

_____

_____

_____

_____

Selection 23.3: Our Government

It seems as if our nation is having problems. The government can't seem to agree on anything. The House of Representatives has one idea and the Senate has another. On some issues the Vice President has been voting just so the budget won't get frozen. It's really no one's fault. The people in charge of the country all seem to have different ideas.

_____

_____

_____

_____

Selection 23.4: The Freeway

When I was driving home from work yesterday, I saw an awful accident on the freeway. It happened at about five o'clock, right during rush hour. The sun was coming in the drivers' windows, and they couldn't see. The first car thought someone was cutting in front of her and hit her brakes. Then several cars behind her ran into her. Watch the news tonight for the full story.

_____

_____

_____

_____

Selection 23.5: The Game

Do you know who won the soccer game yesterday? Two really good teams were playing. When I left, the game had been going for three hours and I couldn't stay any longer. I hope Tia's team won. She's such a bad loser. All of the players are going to the pub after the game. I'll try to catch up with all of you there later.

_____

_____

_____

_____

Selection 23.6: World Problems

Of all of the problems in the world today I think child hunger is the worst. Poverty's never good, but when it affects children it's awful. I can't imagine not being able to feed your children, can you? Here in this country many children today arrive at school hungry. They eat a free breakfast and lunch, but at night some get no dinner.

_____

_____

_____

_____

Selection 23.7: The *Did You Know* Magazine

Do you read the *Did You Know* magazine? I refuse to read it. So many of their stories are exaggerated and full of lies. I can't imagine how they get permission to print them. One of the worst stories they had on the front of their magazine was about the boy with three heads. Who reads that stuff? How do they stay in business?

_____

_____

_____

_____

Selection 23.8: Ugly Brown Toads

I hate big, ugly, brown toads. They're not cute, they can get in your house, and then they're hard to get out. Recently a toad got in my daughter's house. It was hopping all over the living room. We had to walk behind it to make it hop toward the front door so we could get it out. I don't know what I'd have done if it turned and hopped the other way.

_____

_____

_____

_____

Free Expressive Practice: Create your own selection here. When you write your selection, make sure you can set it up in a topic/comment format.

_____

_____

_____

_____

Classifiers That Show Movement and Distance

In Chapters 3 and 7 there was a limited discussion about classifiers and how they are used as descriptive adjectives (Size and Shape Specifiers, SASS), as in TABLE DIRTY fs-DUST CL:G-thick layer, and how they are used to represent nouns and pronouns, as in CAR CL:3 NEAR TREE CL:3-car-next-to-TREE. Further information was provided in Chapter 10 regarding how classifiers are used within predicate phrases as adjectives and adverbs. Classifiers can be used in conjunction with directional verbs to clarify the activity. The English sentence, "Please give me a glass of water" can be signed in ASL as follows: WATER, CL:C-glass CL:C-give-to-me PLEASE. In this sentence the classifier handshape, CL:C moves toward the signer initiating the request.

Classifiers can also be used to describe lines of people, objects that move on conveyer belts, and the flow of liquid. As with all classifiers, once the person or object is identified and the activity is described, the classifier can be signed. When indicating lines of people or the flow of liquid, the CL:44 can be utilized. The English sentence, "I went to the Tim McGraw concert and had to wait in a long line" can be signed in ASL as follows: fs-TIM fs-MCGRAW MUSIC ME GO-TO. WAIT-circular++ PEOPLE CL:44-long-line-of. In these instances, a line of people waiting to buy a ticket for a game, papers moving through a machine, or water coming from the tap can be depicted. See Figure 24.1 for an example.

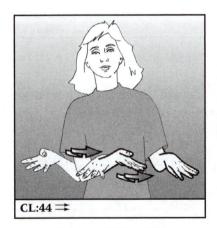

CL:44 ⇉

Indicates objects moving by, such as paper through a copying machine, newspapers through a press, or cars through an assembly line.

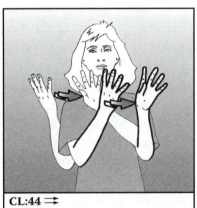

CL:44 ⇒

Indicates people filing past.

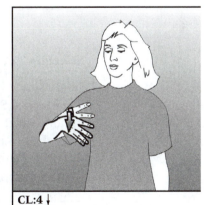

CL:4 ↓

Indicates a flow of liquid such as toner pouring from a bottle or water from a tap.

FIGURE 24.1 Example of Classifier CL:44 and CL:4. Used to Represent Moving People and Objects (CL:44) and a Flow of Liquid (CL:4)

Source: From Humphries, Tom, & Carol Padden, *Learning American Sign Language,* 2/e. Published by Allyn and Bacon, Boston, MA. Copyright © 2004 by Pearson Education. Reprinted by permission of the publisher.

Classifiers can also be used to indicate length and width. In these instances, the index finger of the nondominant hand (CL:1) is used to hold the starting point while the index finger of the dominant hand (CL:1) traces the height or width. The sentence "Draw a line six inches tall" is thus represented in ASL as YOUR PAPER DRAW LINE 1X-lf-hand-here CL:1-rt-hand-path-extend-to-here 1X-start-point TO 1X-end point MEASURE SIX fs-INCH.

Change the following selections into ASL and then practice signing them.

 ### EXAMPLE 24.0

My friend Kat has a leak in her living room ceiling. When it rains hard, the ceiling leaks like a faucet. She needs a new roof, but she can't afford one right now. She hopes by next summer she'll be able to get it fixed.

MY FRIEND fs-KAT POSS-Kat LIVING ROOM fs-CEILING CL:BB-above-head-extent-of-

                                                ___when clause___

ceiling HAVE fs-LEAK CL:4-leak++. RAIN++, fs-CEILING WATER CL:4-leak++

              ___t___   ___neg___

SAME-AS fs-FAUCET. fs-ROOF NEW IX-rt-she NEED AFFORD CAN'T. FUTURE SUMMER IX-rt-she HOPE #FIX fs-ROOF CAN.

Selection 24.1: The Wooden Box

My sister and her husband make beautiful things with wood. One Christmas they made each of my daughters a wooden box. They used both light and dark wood. Each box is about ten inches long and five inches wide. Although they're all the same size, they all look different because of the way they designed them. None of them look as if they came off an assembly line.

_____

_____

_____

_____

Selection 24.2: Cindy's Family

Cindy's married and has three children, two boys and one girl. Cindy's about five foot six. She married a man who's six foot six. All of the children have their father's height. Her daughter's six feet tall. Both of the boys are over six feet. They drive a big car so all of them have leg room. When her children were little, they used to line up to see who would get to sit in the front seat in which there was more room.

_____

_____

_____

_____

Selection 24.3: The Mechanic

Donna wants to be a mechanic, but she's so awkward when it comes to tools. She tries to use a screwdriver when she should use a wrench. She doesn't

91

CHAPTER 24
Classifiers That
Show Movement
and Distance

PART I

PART II

PART III

PART IV

know how to use a drill, and she hit her finger using a hammer. One time she poked a hole in a pipe she was trying to fix and the water came pouring out. I'm afraid she'll destroy anything she tries to fix. Maybe she should change her career goal.

_____

_____

_____

_____

Selection 24.4: Day After Thanksgiving

Have you ever gone shopping the day after Thanksgiving? I have and I'll never do it again. The lines are so long, the people act crazy, and it's hard to find what you're looking for. My friend Marie loves to shop the day after Thanksgiving. She's not a morning person but gets up early that morning to go shopping with her mom. They both love it.

_____

_____

_____

_____

Selection 24.5: The Coffee Table

Debbie recently bought a new coffee table for her family room. I think it's made with cherry wood, and it's rather large. I think it is about thirty-six inches across and almost 60 inches long. The legs curve out at the top and come down. It almost looks like a short dining room table. I think six people could eat around it.

_____

_____

_____

_____

Selection 24.6: Libby Glass

Harold works for Libby Glass. He's one of the glass inspectors. All day he and the other workers stand on both sides of a huge conveyer belt. On the belt are hundreds of glasses. As the glasses come by, he looks for glasses that have imperfections. When he finds one that isn't perfect, he takes it off the belt and puts it in a box. It's a tedious job but it pays well.

_____

_____

_____

_____

Selection 24.7: The Yellow Kitchen

Ann really wanted her kitchen painted yellow. Her grandmother had a yellow kitchen, her mother had a yellow kitchen, so when she got married she decided she wanted one too. So, she went and bought the paint, and her husband started to paint the walls. It was bright yellow—it looked like Big Bird. They had to add white paint to it several times, mix it, and finally it was the color she wanted.

_____

_____

_____

_____

_____

Selection 24.8: Favorite Holiday

What's your favorite holiday? Do you like Thanksgiving, Easter, Hanukkah, or Christmas? Of all the holidays, I think I like Thanksgiving the best. It isn't materialistic, and people focus on what they're thankful for instead of what they should buy. Every Thanksgiving we wait in the long grocery store lines to buy our food, but its worth it on Thanksgiving when we all sit around the table and enjoy each other's company.

_____

_____

_____

_____

Free Expressive Practice: Create your own selection here. In your selection either make use of the CL:44 or the CL:1 classifier.

_____

_____

_____

_____

Selections for Intermediate ASL Students

CHAPTER 1

Additional Work with Topic/Comment

Within the syntax of American Sign Language there are several sentence structures that are used to convey information. One commonly used structure is referred to as topic/comment. As you will recall from Chapter 5, within this structure the topic can be a person, an object, a place, time, an event, or a combination of these. The signer decides what the topic will be based on the context of the discussion and what immediately preceded the statement (Baker & Cokely, 1980, p. 159).

Sometimes the topic or topicalized segments are preceded by the signs KNOW-THAT, YOU KNOW, or KNOW. KNOW-THAT and YOU KNOW are signed when the signer is relatively sure the person he or she is conversing with is familiar with the topic. KNOW can be signed when the signer is not sure the person is familiar with the topic. Although these signs are not used to introduce every topic, they can and are used as introductory signs (Baker & Cokely, 1980, p. 161).

When signing sentences incorporating this sentence structure, the eyebrows are raised while simultaneously producing the sign or signs that represent the topic. The eyebrows are then lowered when the comment is made.

Keep in mind that the subject in an English sentence is not always the topic of a sentence signed in ASL. For example, in the English sentence, "The man jumped on the alligator," the subject in the English sentence would be "the man." However, when you examine this same sentence in ASL, the signer would run into difficulty setting up the man first as the topic and then trying to get the alligator under him for him to jump on. Based on context clues, the signer determines if he or she wants to introduce the subject or the object of the English sentence first. As seen in the example above, this is influenced in part by the context of the discussion and by what the individual wants to communicate (Borden, 1996, p. 37).

In the following selections, practice the appropriate facial grammar while conveying the information contained in the sentences.

Selection 1.1: Meeting at the Deaf Club

We'll go to the meeting at the Deaf Club tomorrow. The goal of the meeting is to organize the upcoming fundraiser so a needy child can go to Camp Juliana this summer. Some of the members have already sent me their ideas on how we can raise the money. Everything from car washes to bake sales. Our club really wants to help. That's the best camp. They have classes in Deaf culture, a variety of sports, as well as arts and crafts.

_____

_____

_____

Selection 1.2: Phil's New House

Phil recently built a new house. It's spacious, well built, and beautiful. The house is located on about ten acres of land. It has two stories, and altogether, including both the main floor and the upstairs, it has about 3400 square feet. Downstairs there's a living room, family room, kitchen, bathroom, laundry room, and dining room. On the second floor there are three bedrooms and two more bathrooms. In addition, the house has two fireplaces, one upstairs in the bedroom and one downstairs in the living room.

_____

_____

_____

_____

_____

Selection 1.3: The Metro

Have you seen Nikki's Geo Metro? It's a very small, short, and round car that looks like a roller skate. It has two doors and is white with a black zigzag line on the side. Her radio antenna's bent to the right and has a pink flower on the top. Inside on the mirror hang four strands of beads: Two are pink and two are red. Her car's small, but it's cheap to drive, and with all the driving she does that's important.

_____

_____

_____

_____

_____

Selection 1.4: Sue's Pennsylvania Home

Sue used to live in Pennsylvania. She had a three-story house. The house was made of wood and painted light green. It had a big front porch that went around three sides of the house. It really had three floors. The living room, dining room, kitchen, and four bedrooms were located on the main floor. The laundry room was located in the basement, and the attic had been changed into a family room.

_____

_____

_____

_____

Selection 1.5: Jeff's Living Room

You should see Jeff's living room. It's huge! The walls are all painted light gray, and he has all different-sized pictures hung all over the walls. All of the pictures have black frames. He has three couches set up in a U-shape across from the fireplace. The couches are in darker gray with black and white wavy lines.

He has different colored pillows on the couches. Some are black, others are red, and a few are light gray. On one wall, there are white bookshelves with books and candles on them. He also has two black floor lamps. It's neat!

_____

_____

_____

_____

_____

_____

Selection 1.6: The Messy Office

That office is so messy. When you go in, you see piles of newspapers and magazines everywhere on one side of the room on the floor. There are also several piles of old books, papers, and equipment. On the other side of the office, there are broken chairs, tables, and lights. It's a real junky office. Someone needs to come in and first throw away the newspapers and magazines and, second, organize the books. The third thing she should do is either fix the broken furniture or throw it out.

_____

_____

_____

_____

_____

_____

Selection 1.7: Baking Fish

A week ago on Friday my daughter decided to bake some fish. She went to the store, bought some cod, and brought it home to prepare. First she washed it and put it in a 9" × 13" pan. Then she got a bowl and mixed together mayonnaise, salt, pepper, and sweet pickles. She spread the mixture on the fish. Then she baked it for thirty minutes. It was ok to eat but a little sweet for my taste.

_____

_____

_____

_____

_____

Selection 1.8: Going to the Prom

High school proms can be very important to high school students. For girls, in particular, there's a lot involved in getting ready for the big night. First, the girl must find the perfect dress, and that often entails weeks of shopping. Second, she must find the right pair of shoes and accessories to go with it—you know, the perfect necklace and earrings to match. Third, she must decide how she'll have her hair fixed, make an appointment, and allow enough time to not only get her hair done but her nails as well. It can be a real ordeal but is something that most high school students look forward to.

_____

_____

_____

_____

_____

Selection 1.9: Summer Travel Plans

When the semester's over, I plan to do some traveling. First I want to go and visit my friend in Chicago. I haven't seen her in about ten years. We taught together in Pennsylvania, but that was a long time ago. Second, I plan to travel to Washington, DC. I love to visit historical places, and Washington's one of my favorites. I'll go to the Capitol, the White House, and the Smithsonian. The third trip I'll take is with my husband and my children to Colorado to visit their grandparents. It will be a busy summer.

_____

_____

_____

_____

Selection 1.10: Marcie's Shopping Trip

Marcie was hungry yesterday, and she had a headache. She decided she should go to the store and get something to eat. She thought that might make her headache go away. She drove to the store, went in and bought hamburger, French fries, bread, chips, candy bars, and cookies. She paid sixteen dollars. Then she went home and cooked the hamburgers. When she was finished cooking, she ate two hamburgers, some fries, and four candy bars. Then her headache was gone but her tummy hurt.

_____

_____

_____

_____

PART I

PART II

PART III

PART IV

Establishing Reference Using Pointing

In ASL the index finger is frequently used to mark a reference point for individuals, animals, objects, or geographic locations. Reference points may be arbitrarily established in the signing space to allow the signer to mark the relative real-life location of referents (persons, places, or things) as well as those previously established by the signer during the course of the conversation.

Indexing, that is, pointing to establish a reference, can also be used to establish relationships between two or more persons, places, or things. In instances where the relationship between the two objects is obvious, it is usually unnecessary to specify the relationship. However, when clarifying the distance between two towns or where one individual is located in relation to another individual, the signer can establish the first location with his or her nondominant hand, and then reference the second location with his or her dominant hand. For example, in this way one can show where Colorado is in relation to Utah and Arizona or where Calandra is standing in relation to James.

When using indexing for establishing referents, the signer will also use eye gaze to briefly glance to the location being established with the pointing gesture; however, sometimes eye gaze may be used alone to establish reference points in the sign space (Newell, 2006).

Selection 2.1: Where's the VR Office?

You know where the VR office is, right? Well, once you're on Patterson Street, you will see the university on your right. Across the street from the university is the Skinner Building. The Vocational Rehabilitation office is in that building on the second floor. When you enter the building, look for the elevator, and go up to the second floor. It's the first door on your right when you exit the elevator.

_____

_____

_____

_____

_____

 ### Selection 2.2: The Gym

Yolanda loves to go to the gym. It's close to her house, and it only takes her about thirty minutes to get there. When you go in the front doors, there's a hall on the right where the swimming pool's located. The pool has a fence all around it. If you go down the hall to your left when you enter, you will find

99

CHAPTER 2
....
Establishing
Reference Using
Pointing

PART I

PART II

PART III

PART IV

three big rooms with exercise equipment. Across the hall from the exercise rooms are two changing rooms with showers, one for men and one for women.

_____
_____
_____
_____
_____

Selection 2.3: Juan's Apartment

Juan's apartment's really cool. Even though it only has one bedroom, it's nice and spacious. When you go in, you'll see a huge window on the wall facing you. Under the window is a king-sized bed. To the left and the right of the bed are two nightstands. On the wall to your right as you enter the room is an entertainment center that has several shelves. The shelves on the right are full of pictures. The shelves on the left have some candles and pottery bowls. The closet is on the left wall. It's a walk-in closet, and there is more than enough room for his clothes and shoes.

_____
_____
_____
_____
_____

Selection 2.4: Margaret's Flower Bed

Margaret worked in the horticulture department at the school for the deaf for years. She grew beautiful plants and flowers and helped the students gain a great appreciation for gardening. Now she's retired and lives at home with her husband. She spends time with her own garden.

When you go out her back door, you see a beautiful rock garden on your left. In the center of the yard she has a pond with plants all around it, and on the right side of her yard, running the full length, are rose bushes. Of all the things in her yard, the pond is my favorite.

_____
_____
_____
_____
_____

Selection 2.5: Prekindergarten Classrooms

David is a preschool teacher at the Alabama School for the Deaf. This is his first year, and he's teaching 4-year-olds for the first time. Two weeks before school started he set up his classroom. He has his big alphabet rug in the center of the room for shared reading. Each of the children can pick a letter to sit on. His housekeeping area is close to the rug. This is where the little ones can play in the play kitchen, set the table, and have make-believe tea parties. The art center is close to the long row of windows and the sink. This is a wonderful place

100

PART II
....
Selections for
Intermediate
ASL Students

in case spills happen. Bookcases with blocks line the side wall inside the classroom door. The room has two whiteboards—one in the front and one in the back of the room. David can use one for his word wall, and one can be used for hanging up student work. It is such a bright, cheerful room.

_____

_____

_____

_____

_____

Selection 2.6: Triangular Streets

Have you ever noticed that some cities are set up with their city blocks designed in triangles rather than square blocks? Frequently, this occurs in old railroad towns where trains entered the rail station from several different points of origin. In these towns, you can get lost easily looking for various businesses. For example, the bank might be located in the bottom left-hand corner of one triangle, and the grocery store might be located in the top center area of another triangle. In order to get from one location to another, you have to travel down several side streets to arrive at your destination.

_____

_____

_____

_____

_____

Selection 2.7: Carol's Travels

Carol has to travel extensively this summer. She's leaving from Orlando and will fly to Chicago. After she stays there for a few days, she'll get back on the plane and fly to San Diego. She wants to visit her sister and take a short vacation. While she's in San Diego, they plan to drive down the coast to Los Angeles and go to Disneyland. Then they'll go up to San Francisco and do some shopping. When they're finished, she'll hop back on the plane and head for Orlando again. Once she lands, she can drive four hours north toward her home.

_____

_____

_____

_____

_____

Selection 2.8: Lines and Segments

Did you know that a mathematical line goes on and on in both directions? If we want to show just a part of a line, we draw a line segment, sometimes referred to as a segment. A segment has two endpoints. Sometimes these endpoints are labeled with letters. One end can be labeled A and the other end B. We can also label different segments along one line. Suppose you have a line that is 12 centimeters long and you want to divide it into six equal segments.

101

CHAPTER 2
....
Establishing
Reference Using
Pointing

You could measure every 2 cm and add a letter to represent each of the 2 cm. Your letters would be placed along the line like this.

_____

_____

_____

_____

_____

Selection 2.9: Vera's Plants

The plants in Vera's kitchen look so nice. She has eight of them in the window above her sink. On the far left is a bromide and next to it is ivy. Then she has five African violets. Each of them is a little bit different. The first one is fuchsia color, the second one is white, the third has ruffled edges and is pink and white, the fourth one is purple, and the fifth one is lavender. The last plant on the shelf is a flowering cactus. None of the plants is large, and they all look so pretty.

_____

_____

_____

_____

_____

Using Semantic Classifiers to Mark Location and Movement

Classifiers are an integral part of American Sign Language (ASL). Some are used to represent nouns and their location and movement within predicates in sentences. Others are used as predicate adjectives. When functioning as predicate adjectives, they are referred to as Size and Shape Specifiers (SASS) (Cokely & Baker-Shenk, 1991). In this instance, they are used to describe specific physical characteristics of nouns within the predicate phrase.

Semantic classifiers (SCL) are used to mark locations and indicate movement (Mikos, Smith, & Lentz, 2001). Every classifier predicate has a location in three-dimensional space that represents the actual point in real three-dimensional space where the noun is located. For example, when a signer wants to indicate the exact point where a car is located, the sign CAR would be followed by the CL:3-there (Valli & Lucas, 2000, p. 83). Continuing with this example, once the location of the car is established, a semantic classifier is used to describe how and where the car moved from one location to another: CL:3-rt-move-toward-lf.

Semantic classifiers are also used to show how an individual moves. Individuals can walk across a room, fall down, pick themselves up, and keep going. By changing the palm orientation the signer can describe if a person is facing toward or away from him or her or standing sideways (Mikos, Smith, & Lentz, 2001, p. xiv).

 Selection 3.1: Alan's Family Room

Alan's family room is so cool! When you walk in, the first thing that catches your eye is the sliding glass wall that looks out on the ocean. It's thirty-six feet long, and the glass goes floor to ceiling. The glass wall is adjacent to a huge rock fireplace. It takes up another full wall. Facing the fireplace is a massive sectional with an end table at each end. In the far right-hand corner of the room is a TV with four comfy chairs. If you walk out through the sliding glass doors, you can walk back and forth on the forty-foot deck and have a magnificent view.

_____

_____

_____

_____

_____

Selection 3.2: Walls

What do you have hanging on your bedroom walls? Some people have walls full of family pictures. Other people use their walls to put up shelves and put candles on them. Shamika uses a combination of both. The wall to the left of

103

CHAPTER 3
....
Using Semantic
Classifiers to Mark
Location and
Movement

PART I

PART II

PART III

PART IV

her door has a big window that lets in a lot of sun. Across from that wall she has put up four shelves that are filled with plants. She has a real variety of large and small plants, and they all seem to do well in the sun. The wall in between is full of family pictures. It's really cozy for a dorm room. When her door is open, people walking by like to stop and look in.

_____

_____

_____

_____

_____

Selection 3.3: Silent Dinner at the Mall

On the second Saturday of the month, our local Deaf community has a silent dinner at the mall. I usually drive up to the entrance to the food court and walk in so my car will be close to the exit when I'm ready to pull out and drive home. Last week I was heading toward the food court when a man came walking toward me waving excitedly. Oh, my gosh! It was an old friend of mine from twenty years ago. We hugged and went and sat around the circle with so many of our friends. About thirty minutes after we got there, I started to notice new folks walking slowly to the group—some came up alone, some in twos and threes. They were new students from the sign language class. We welcomed them into the group for their first silent dinner.

_____

_____

_____

_____

_____

Selection 3.4: Earthquakes

Earthquakes can be so damaging. My friend Cara lives in California, and she tells the story about the one that hit her area when she was growing up. It was awful. She describes glasses falling out of the kitchen cupboards and breaking, pictures falling off the walls, and huge cracks appearing in the walls, floors, and ceiling. She also talks about light fixtures falling from the ceiling and shattering. One of the worst parts of the story is her describing the chest of drawers that fell on her brother; thank goodness he wasn't seriously hurt.

_____

_____

_____

_____

_____

Selection 3.5: The Turtle Tree

Paul lives around a small lake in a town not too far from here. There are several trees around the lake that have been recently planted. However, there's one tree that's growing in the shallow part of the lake, and that's where the turtles like to live. Some days you can walk by the lake and see about twenty-five turtles on various parts of the tree. Some stay on the lower branches while a few climb higher. When Paul walks his dog close to the tree, the turtles on the lower branches all fall off their branches and end up in the water.

_____

_____

_____

_____

_____

_____

Selection 3.6: Newborn Nursery

Have you ever looked in the window of the newborn nursery at your hospital? It's a fun place to visit if you like babies. Usually the nursery has three or four rows of bassinets where the babies sleep. They're all wrapped neatly in blankets, and many of them have little caps on their heads. Nurses come in and out regularly and turn the babies from their tummies to their backs. They change their diapers and make sure they're all comfortable.

_____

_____

_____

_____

_____

Selection 3.7: The Stage

Have you ever been to a performance by the National Theatre of the Deaf? If not, you should try to go when the touring company comes to your area. They're awesome! Like all stage productions, scenery decorates the stage and can be moved easily to change rooms or moods. Actors enter and exit the stage and perform their lines—sometimes facing each other and sometimes facing the crowd. A voice interpreter's usually placed in the wings for hearing folks who aren't fluent in ASL.

_____

_____

_____

_____

_____

Selection 3.8: Messy Roommate

I have a messy roommate. She leaves dishes all over the coffee table in the living room. I can't stand it! So many days I come back from class, find her mess, carry it back into the kitchen, and put it in the dishwasher. She leaves plates with food on them from the night before and glasses with half-finished drinks. I've talked with her about it but she just turns and walks away. I can't wait until my lease is up so I can move.

105

CHAPTER 3
....
Using Semantic
Classifiers to Mark
Location and
Movement

PART I

PART II

PART III

PART IV

_____

_____

_____

_____

_____

Selection 3.9: Airports and Weather Delays

Have you ever gotten stuck in an airport when they're having bad weather? Sometimes when that happens, they have to ground all of the planes and not let any more land. It creates a big mess for all of the travelers. You can walk up and down the terminal and see plane after plane in a row. Then, when they can fly again, the runways are backed up with as many as thirty planes waiting to take off.

_____

_____

_____

_____

_____

Selection 3.10: Rearranging the Library

The library where Tom works has recently added a new addition. Now the librarians have been asked to relocate a lot of the books. In some sections, Tom only has to move a couple of books, so he just pulls them off the shelf and walks them into the new room. For other sections, he has to pull down stacks and carries them in to the new area. When he has to move several stacks of books, he pulls them off the shelf, stacks them on a cart, and rolls them into the new addition.

_____

_____

_____

_____

_____

Time

In Part I, information was presented in Chapter 17 about time and how it is expressed in ASL. A general description of how the body serves as a reference point for a time line was discussed, demonstrating how time signs are produced in forward or backward directions depending on the time frame indicating past or future. In addition, morning, noon, afternoon, and night are signed with respect to the horizon, thus presenting a visual representation of where the sun is located throughout the various times of the day.

When describing multiple weeks, months, and years that will occur in the future or did occur in the past, the numbers 2 through 9 can be incorporated while making the sign. For example, when signing 3-MONTH FROM NOW, 9-WEEK-PAST the number becomes part of the sign and the time line is used to show whether it is past or future. In the event that an activity has not taken place or is not yet completed, the sign NOT-YET can be signed to convey this concept.

You will recall from Part One, Chapter 8, that the sign FINISH can also be used in sentences to indicate that an action has been completed. In these instances the sign FINISH can indicate that one has finished taking a shower, walking the dog, or attending a meeting. FINISH can be signed either before the verb or at the end of the predicate phrase. For example, if the signer wants to convey that she went to the movie, she could sign it as either, ME FINISH GO-TO MOVIE or ME GO-TO MOVIE FINISH. In this example the sign FINISH functions in a manner similar to the English word "already" (Borden, 1996, p. 27).

Selection 4.1: Picking Up the Speaker

The NAD convention starts tomorrow and I can't wait. So many of my old friends from FSDB will be there. I've been on the planning committee this year, and it's my job to pick up the speaker. So, I'd better leave in about two hours to drive to the airport so I can pick him up. He's an old friend of mine, and I haven't seen him since we both graduated seven years ago. It'll be fun to catch up on old times. I'm just glad I'm the one who gets to pick him up. I hope his plane arrives on time, and we can get out of town before the traffic becomes too bad.

_____

_____

_____

_____

_____

_____

Selection 4.2: Exciting Times

In seven months, my roommate's getting married, and she has asked me to be her maid of honor. I've got so many things to do to help her out. In three

107

CHAPTER 4
Time

PART I

PART II

PART III

PART IV

months, I need to start planning a bridal shower for her. I think she wants a kitchen shower because she doesn't have many cooking utensils or pots and pans. Last month we shopped for our bridesmaids' dresses and that was fun. A month before the wedding I've got to write my speech for the toast, because it will be my responsibility to give one. This is so neat! I really like the guy she's going to marry.

_____

_____

_____

_____

_____

_____

Selection 4.3: The Puppy

Dontal got a new puppy from the pound a few weeks ago. When he took him to the vet, he was told that he'd probably be a big dog and weigh about 120 pounds. This scared Dontal because he wasn't expecting such a big dog. He decided after hearing this that he should take the dog to obedience school. He called around and found that one of the pet stores has an obedience class that lasts for eight weeks. It meets weekly every Wednesday for one hour. When the dog's three months old, he can start classes, so he signed him up. In two months, they'll begin.

_____

_____

_____

_____

_____

_____

Selection 4.4: Old Friends

Yesterday I ran into Pat and Mike. I hadn't seen them for ten years. The two of them became business partners three years ago. Their company is designed to help party goers. If someone needs help organizing a party, they're the ones to call. They only need a week's notice. They also provide entertainment for parties, designated drivers, and help with the cleanup when the parties are over. They anticipate in three years that they'll have to hire two more employees. Business is booming, and before long they'll have more than they can handle.

_____

_____

_____

_____

_____

_____

Selection 4.5: Getting Ready to Graduate

Have you gone through the graduation process? One year in advance you have to complete your graduation check. Then six months later you have to meet

108

PART II
....
Selections for
Intermediate
ASL Students

with your advisor and make sure you've completed all of your classes. Three months before the big day, you go to the registrar and have someone do one final check. Then, one month in advance, you send out your invitations. Once all of this is completed, you're ready for the big day. It always seems like a lot of paper work when you're doing it, but once you walk across the stage, it's well worth it.

_____

_____

_____

_____

_____

Selection 4.6: Cleaning the Apartment

I've got to clean my apartment this Saturday. It will take all morning to gather up the trash, scrub the floors, and clean the bathroom and kitchen. I'll need an hour or two in the afternoon to vacuum, dust, and do the laundry. The dust is an inch thick, and I have a huge pile of laundry. I've been out of town for the past two weekends, and as a result I'm really behind. I think by the time I spend all day cleaning up, I'll need a day just to recuperate. Next time, I won't get so far behind with my cleaning. I don't like to give up a full day when I could be hanging out having fun with my friends.

_____

_____

_____

_____

_____

Selection 4.7: Chairperson for GAD

Tom's the chairperson this year for the Georgia Association for the Deaf Convention. It's his job to plan the activities for the conference. One year in advance, he must secure the site, book a block of hotel rooms, contact the caterers, and begin the publicity campaign. Nine months before it's held, he must send out the call for presenters. Six months in advance, he must let speakers know that their proposals are accepted. During the weeks right before the Convention, he must make an onsite visit and ensure that everything's ready to go.

_____

_____

_____

_____

_____

Selection 4.8: RID *Views*

Are you a member of RID? If you are, then you receive the *Views* monthly. That's the best publication. Monthly, they have interesting articles. Once a year they feature different topics that pertain to educational interpreters, judicial interpreters, as well as other areas of specialization. Every two years, RID holds its national convention, and for months before the conference there are numerous advertisements about it. If you're not a member, you should join. It only takes five minutes to fill out the application online. If you haven't done it already, I suggest that you do it now.

Selection 4.9: The Plastic Lizard

My friends Becca and Terri are terrified of little lizards. The other day I dropped a plastic lizard someone had given me on the kitchen floor by mistake as I was hurrying out the door. Later, while I was gone, Becca came into the kitchen and spotted the lizard. She was so scared, she ran and asked the neighbor girl if she would get it out of the kitchen. When the girl bent down to get it she realized right away that it was a toy. Boy, did Becca feel like an idiot. When I came back that afternoon, she wanted to know why I would play a trick on her.

Selection 4.10: Sleepless Night

Mitch said he didn't sleep well at all last night. He said he went to bed around midnight and tossed and turned for hours. It seemed that every thirty minutes he was awake. At three in the morning, he still hadn't fallen asleep. This morning, when the alarm went off at 5:30, it was all he could do to get out of bed. He got up, drank four cups of coffee, and headed for class. He said it was all he could do to keep his eyes open. He'll be so glad when his classes are finished and he can go home this afternoon and take a nap. Don't you hate it when you have nights like that?

Listing, Grouping, Prioritizing

When listing, grouping, and prioritizing items in ASL, the topic is usually established first and is then followed by listing, grouping, or prioritizing details that relate to the topic. Establishing categories or describing details can be done by ranking the items on the signer's nondominant hand or setting up groups in space. Rank order on the hand can be used to describe the most popular names of children, movies one wants to see, or the order of the tasks that need to be completed. This can involve the steps required to write a paper, errands that need to be run, or ingredients needed for a recipe.

Signers establish referents on the nondominant hand in one of two ways. They either point to a particular finger on the nondominant hand, usually starting with the thumb and then signing or fingerspelling the referent, or by raising the first nondominant finger and then signing or fingerspelling the referent. In this respect, additional fingers are raised as subsequent referents are identified (Baker & Cokely, 1980, p. 235).

When listing five referents, signers start with the thumb and proceed consecutively until the referents have been identified. When there are only two, three, or four referents in a list, signers sometimes begin with the index finger on the nondominant hand, pointing to as many fingers as are necessary. Up to ten referents can be established on the nondominant hand by signing the numbers 6 through 9 before pointing to the referent and shaking the number ten before pointing to the thumb, thus distinguishing it from the first referent (Baker & Cokely, 1980, p. 235).

Sometimes categories are listed on the nondominant hand and are then set up in space. Depending on the types of categories being discussed, the signer will set them up in space either horizontally or vertically. While layers of the earth might lend themselves to a vertical use of space, stages in human development along a continuum might be more appropriately placed horizontally. When setting up items or details horizontally, the first category is set up beginning on the signer's left side with subsequent groups being set up on a horizontal plane in front of the signer's body and ending on the right side of the signer's body. Descriptions of categories of books, classes, or farm animals can be presented in this manner.

Items can be prioritized using rank order beginning with the first topic of importance and continuing on down the list. The majority of time, when these items are signed in ASL, the signer begins with the first item signed at eye level with subsequent topics on the list being placed in descending order vertically. However, in those instances when the items being prioritized and the topic being discussed involve levels of advancement, the signer can establish the first item slightly above waist level and then set up the following levels or items in ascending order vertically, thus reflecting their order of importance or location. This use of space is appropriate when describing promotional levels, stories of a house, or floors in an office building, thus allowing for clarification of information.

Selection 5.1: ASL Textbooks

There're many outstanding ASL textbooks: *Learning American Sign Language*, *Signing Naturally*, and *ASL at Work*, to name just a few. *Learning American Sign Language* and *Signing Naturally* have been in print for a long time. *ASL at Work* is a new text that has some nice features. The first two books have two or more authors. The third book has multiple authors. They're all great resources. When students are serious about learning sign language, it's critical that they have an instructor work with them who can demonstrate how the language is used. Otherwise, if left on their own, students make many sign errors while trying to master the language.

_____
_____
_____
_____
_____
_____

Selection 5.2: Cooking Terms

Are you familiar with cooking terms? There are five terms that you should be familiar with so you can be a good cook: baste, braise, julienne, marinate, and roux. When you baste something, you moisten it with liquid during cooking, using a spoon or a baster. To braise means to brown your meat in fat and then cook it slowly with just a little bit of liquid. Julienne refers to foods that are cut into very thin, long strips; marinate means to soak food in a liquid to add flavor, and a roux is a mixture of fat and flour sautéed together and then added to liquid to thicken it. Oh, and there's another useful cooking term, sauté. That means to fry in a manner similar to stir frying. Sauté is a French word that means "to jump." I guess foods that are sautéed sort of "jump around" in the pan.

_____
_____
_____
_____
_____
_____

Selection 5.3: Proficiency Levels

Regardless of what skill you want to master, whether it's in sports, a musical instrument, or just learning a new skill, there are usually categories in which all of us can be placed. If you're a "newbie" and have never attempted the skill, you're usually placed in the novice category. Those with some experience are usually grouped in the beginning category, and people with slightly more experience are placed in the intermediate group. Depending on groupings and skill levels, those who have mastered the skill are usually placed in the category for advanced or proficient practitioners.

_____
_____
_____

112

PART II
....
Selections for
Intermediate
ASL Students

Selection 5.4: ASL and Sign Systems

ASL is the language of choice within the Deaf community. However, in educational settings, when teaching English grammar and syntax, the teacher may find certain features of English sign systems useful in combination with ASL. The ability to code switch between ASL and English-like signing is essential for teachers of deaf students. Often when Deaf and hearing people interact a form of ASL called Contact Signing, a mixture of ASL signs and English word order, will be used.

_____

_____

_____

_____

_____

_____

_____

Selection 5.5: Officers at the Club for the Deaf

Our community has a very active Deaf Club. Annually, they elect a president, president elect, or vice president, a secretary, treasurer, a historian, and a director of public relations. The president presides over all of the meetings, and the president elect serves as the president's right-hand person, learning the ropes for when he or she assumes the presidency. The secretary, treasurer, and historian do traditional duties delegated to individuals serving in these roles, and the director of public relations keeps the website current and works with the secretary promoting current events.

_____

_____

_____

_____

_____

_____

_____

Selection 5.6: Socioeconomic Status in the United States

Socioeconomic status, otherwise known as SES, in the United States is determined by level of income and number of family members. You can be classified as living in poverty, placed in the low income group, the middle class, the upper middle class, or the upper class. People move between these levels as they generate more income, have more children, or their children leave home and become independent. Sometimes one's true SES isn't accurately reflected in the government's statistics.

113

CHAPTER 5
....
Listing, Grouping,
Prioritizing

PART I

PART II

PART III

PART IV

_____

_____

_____

_____

_____

_____

Selection 5.7: Types of Hearing Aids

Modern technology has revolutionized the types of hearing aids we have today. Although, in the past, some people preferred the powerful body aids, for the most part they haven't been used for decades. Today, more and more folks are turning toward digital technology and aids that are programmable to meet their needs. Behind the ear, in the ear, and cochlear implants have all come of age. Each type of aid has its own strengths and weaknesses. However, as the TV ad used to say, "We've come a long way, baby."

_____

_____

_____

_____

_____

_____

Selection 5.8: Categories of Dogs

Let's talk about some of the categories of dogs. For ease, we can separate them out into the small, medium, medium large, and large categories. Dogs in the small category usually weigh between two and ten pounds. In the medium category are dogs that range from eleven to the mid-twenty-pound figure. While some only weigh eleven pounds, others top the scale at twenty-five. The medium large group is reserved for dogs twenty-six to fifty pounds, and dogs in the large group can weigh anywhere between fifty-one and one hundred pounds. Do you have a dog? How much does he weigh? Would you put him in a category on the light end or the heavy end?

_____

_____

_____

_____

_____

_____

_____

Selection 5.9: Shapes

Do you know how many different kinds of shapes there are? Five basic kinds stand out in my mind. There are squares, circles, triangles, rectangles, and diamonds. Think of all the things that are square—boxes, tables, napkins, just to name a few. Lollipops, pancakes, and doughnuts are all round, while cookies and street signs can be made in all the basic shapes. Beds, books, and copy paper are rectangular, while Chinese lanterns and marquis diamonds can take on the diamond shape. What's your favorite shape?

_____

_____

_____

_____

_____

_____

Selection 5:10: Stages of Development

All of us go through various stages of development on our way to adulthood. If you've studied Erik Erikson, you know that he believes there are eight stages in development that we all experience. Starting with birth through infancy, he describes conflicts that arise during each of the developmental stages that must be resolved for a healthy personality to emerge. Beginning with infancy and concluding with the "golden years," he describes along the way why some of us feel fulfilled in our twilight years while others experience a sense of discontent.

_____

_____

_____

_____

_____

Role Shifting

In English the interaction between two or more individuals is often communicated through indirect discourse. For example, "Molly said she was going to the store after lunch." This sentence reports what Molly said. The narrator stays in the voice of narrator and reports in an indirect discourse style what Molly said (Newell, 2006).

When signers produce narratives that include two or more persons, they use direct address and assume the role of each character in the interaction. By shifting the torso of the body slightly to the left or right and using eye gaze to focus the eyes in the same direction, the signer is able to indicate who or what is in a specific location. While in that position, everything the signer does or says reflects what that person does or says (Baker & Cokely, 1980, p. 272). In essence, the signer assumes the role and becomes the person.

Eye gaze plays an important function in role shifting. It provides signers with a mechanism to indicate who the signer and who the recipient of the information are while also showing height relationships between individuals engaged in the conversation. As two or more individuals converse, eye gaze can shift to indicate who is the taller of the two by looking upward and downward. Therefore, when a teacher is standing and talking to a student who is sitting down, the eye gaze would be downward for the teacher and upward for the student.

Selection 6.1: What's Up?

Joe saw Jason at the Club House last Saturday and asked him how he was doing. Jason said that he was just trying to figure out where they had put all of the trophies when they remodeled the Club House. Joe asked him if he had looked in the closet in the back room. He told him he thought that's where he had seen them last. Jason said that he hadn't looked there yet but he'd give it a try. He also told Joe that if he didn't have anything he needed to do right then that perhaps he could stay and give him a hand. Joe said he'd be happy to stay and help for a while.

_____

_____

_____

_____

_____

_____

Selection 6.2: Mowing the Yard

Connie saw Oscar when she was out walking her dog. It was the perfect opportunity to see if he'd help her. She asked Oscar if he'd help her mow the yard on Monday. She explained that Rich was remodeling the bathroom and didn't have time to do it. Oscar said he'd be happy to come over and help and asked her what time she'd like him to stop by. She said it would be great if they could start around eight. She didn't think it would take more than an hour with both of them mowing. Oscar said that was a good idea, because they'd be finished before it got too hot. Connie agreed with him. She told him when they were finished, she'd shower, go to the store, and pick up the things she needed for the cookout that night and invited him to come. He said that was a great idea and he'd see her then.

_____

_____

_____

_____

_____

_____

Selection 6.3: The Gorgeous Woman

The other day I asked my friend who that gorgeous woman was. I described her at great length. I asked him if he knew who the tall shapely lady with the long brown hair and the blue eyes was. I told him I thought she was really hot! He asked me if I was talking about the one who was wearing the brown V-neck sleeveless sweater with the small copper coins accenting the V, the turquoise skirt, and heels. I let him know that that was who I was talking about. Boy, was I embarrassed when he told me that he knew her, and that she was his mother! Talk about open mouth and insert foot.

_____

_____

_____

_____

_____

_____

Selection 6.4: Ritual for Deciding What to Eat

My friends go through the same ritual every day trying to decide what to eat. One of them starts by asking the others what they want to eat for dinner. The others will reply that they don't care, and ask her what she wants to eat. This usually generates a response like, "I don't care as long as it doesn't have eyes, a tail, or feathers," which means, no meat, fish, or poultry. This is followed by, "OK, then I guess we'll just have salad and hummus again." Seems to me it would be easier if one of them just asked the others if they'd like to have salad and hummus for dinner.

_____

_____

_____

_____

_____

_____

117

CHAPTER 6
....
Role Shifting

PART I

PART II

PART III

PART IV

Selection 6.5: Buying a New Car

As we entered the used car lot, the salesman approached us and asked my dad what we were looking for. Before my dad could speak up, I replied that I'd like a little red sports car that was cute and would make me look sexy. Then my dad spoke up and said we were interested in the little white Geo Metro with the black racing stripe because it would get good mileage. Can you guess which car the man showed us?

_____

_____

_____

_____

_____

Selection 6.6: Where's George?

I ran into Marilyn this afternoon, and she asked me if I'd seen George. She said she'd been looking for him for the past hour. I told her to go and ask Jennifer if she knew where he was because I'd seen her talking to him earlier in the day. So Marilyn drove over to Jennifer's house to ask her. When she asked Jennifer if she knew where George was, she said she did. She told Marilyn that he had gotten a call from his uncle, who told him that his aunt had taken a fall in the house and he couldn't get her up. He asked George if he'd come up and help him. Jennifer said he'd left about an hour ago so he should be back pretty soon. Marilyn thanked her and asked her to tell him to come and see her when he got back. Jennifer said she'd be happy to relay the message.

_____

_____

_____

_____

_____

_____

Selection 6.7: Fireworks

Mom asked Monique if she was going to stay home and watch the Fourth of July fireworks on TV. Monique told her that she wasn't planning on staying home. She thought she'd go out to Mike and Angela's. She told her mom that they usually invite a bunch of people over for a cookout and then do fireworks after it gets dark. Monique asked her mom if she wanted to go with her. Her mom declined; she told her she needed to stay home and get some work done. Besides, she said they'd be doing fireworks at the lake as well as on TV so she'd probably go outside, catch the ones at the lake, and keep the TV on for those in Washington. She told Monique to have fun.

_____

_____

_____

_____

_____

_____

Selection 6.8: Going to the Store

Bob came in from outside and saw Loedge sitting at the table. Bob asked him if he was going to the store later. Loedge told him he was because he needed to grab some steak for dinner. He told him he was cooking out later. Bob asked him if when he went if he'd pick up some chips for him. Bob told him that he ran out yesterday and Leah was coming over tonight and that the dill pickle chips were her favorite. Loedge said he'd be happy grab some and asked him if he wanted a small or a large bag. Bob told him he better get a large one because he liked them too. Loedge said it wasn't a problem, that he'd get them when he got the steak.

Selection 6.9: Speedy Strength Workout

Blair asked Landon if he had seen the speedy strength workout that was in the paper. Blair said she had looked at it the other day but wasn't sure if it was a good one and asked Landon what he thought. Landon said he hadn't seen it yet and asked what part of the paper it was in. Blair said she thought it was in the sports section. According to the paper, it's supposed to take ten minutes, and they say if you do it three days a week it can help prevent bone loss and also heart disease and diabetes. Landon said he'd look at it when he got back from class. He said he had to take off. Blair said she'd be interested to see what he thought and that she'd find it and leave it on the table for him.

Selection 6.10: What Did You Think of the Movie?

Denise saw Joetta a little while ago and asked her if she went to the Dollar Movie Theater yesterday. Joetta said she had. Denise wanted to know what she'd seen. Joetta told her she saw the movie *Stick It!* Denise wanted to know if it was any good. Joetta said it was ok, but she was glad she didn't go when it was in the regular theater. She said she wouldn't watch it again, and she wouldn't recommend it to anyone. Denise asked her what it was about. She said it was about a girl with an attitude problem and gymnastics; they used NCAA champions to film it, so the gymnastics was good but the storyline was weak. She told her to save her money.

Contrasting and Comparing

Information sharing frequently involves making comparisons and contrasting one event, activity, or situation with another. When describing comparisons in ASL, space is used to establish relationships, thus allowing the signer to effectively contrast the information. When two individuals are described, the signer usually begins by setting the first person up on the nondominant side of the body and identifying who the individual is. A second individual can be placed on the dominant side, thus allowing for ease in referencing who or what the signer is referring to. When pointing or referring to each of the individuals, the signer shifts the torso slightly from one side to the other and focuses his or her eye gaze in the direction of the individual while employing a slight body shift. Usually right-handed signers will begin their comparison on the left side of their bodies, while left-handed signers will begin on their right side (Smith, Lentz, & Mikos, 1988a,b, p. 59).

The same holds true when establishing two events, locations, or activities that the signer wants to compare. By identifying both topics, the signer can proceed by using indexing to refer to the events that are being contrasted or compared.

Selection 7.1: Pros and Cons of Small Town Living

There are pros and cons to living in a small town. On the positive side, there isn't much traffic, houses are usually less expensive, and it takes less time to get from one place to another. You usually know most of your neighbors and the people who run the local businesses. Whenever you need something, you can count on your neighbors and the local business owners for help. And if someone can't help you, he or she usually knows someone who can and will call that person for you. However, there are negatives to living in a small town. Some of the things that come to mind are that you have to drive to go shopping, to go to a movie, or to go to a nice restaurant. If you're working on a project and you run out of materials, frequently you have to drive between thirty and fifty miles to get more supplies. Even though there are cons to living in a small town, I still think I prefer living in one.

_____

_____

_____

_____

_____

_____

Selection 7.2: Living in the Desert

Living in a desert climate is so different from living in the southeast. The desert's dry with very little humidity. Although the days can get very hot, when the sun goes down, it is usually cool, if not cold, at night. The vegetation is different, too. This part of the country receives very little rain, so many yards have rock gardens instead of grass, and cacti dominate the area. In the Southeast, it is very humid. Usually it rains frequently during the year and everything stays green. Grass, plants, flowers, and trees seem to grow in abundance. It is both hot and humid in the summer. At night, the temperatures may drop in the seventies but the humidity can stay between 90 and 100 percent. Of the two climates, where would you prefer to live?

_____
_____
_____
_____
_____
_____

Selection 7.3: Sunrise Suzie/Night Owl Nick

Are you a day person or a night person? Some of my friends prefer to go to bed early and get up with the sun, or at least pretty early in the morning. They feel they're their most productive early in the day. Suzie is one of them. She's in bed by 10:00 and up by 4:30. By 8:00 she's worked out, had her shower, and has started her job. Then I have other friends like Nick who can't begin to start working until at least 10:00 at night. They stay up working until the wee hours of the morning, sometimes not going to bed until 3:00 or 4:00 A.M. The early birds love the sunshine, while the night owls are nocturnal creatures who seem to work best in the dark.

_____
_____
_____
_____
_____
_____

Selection 7.4: Two-Year Versus Four-Year Colleges

When students graduate from high school, do you think they should go to a two-year or a four-year college? Two-year programs usually are on smaller campuses, have smaller class sizes, and can serve as a good transition between high school and college. Four-year programs typically offer more of a collegiate environment. Although the class sizes are usually larger, they offer a variety of clubs and organizations that appeal to almost everyone. Oftentimes two-year programs are cheaper, although they don't offer dorms or campus housing. Which setting do you think is best?

121

CHAPTER 7
....
Contrasting and
Comparing

PART I

PART II

PART III

PART IV

_____

_____

_____

_____

_____

_____

Selection 7.5: Residential Schools and Inclusion

Throughout the United States you will find a variety of school settings in which students who are deaf or hard of hearing receive their education. For years many deaf students went to the residential school for the deaf in their state. These schools provided them with a learning environment specifically designed to meet their needs. Today about 83 percent of deaf and hard of hearing students receive their education in public school classrooms designed for hearing students. In the residential schools, there are some Deaf instructors. In the public schools, students receive a lot of their instruction through an interpreter.

_____

_____

_____

_____

_____

_____

Selection 7.6: Summer or Winter Vacations

Do you prefer summer or winter vacations? Summer vacations provide opportunities to be outdoors. If you like to swim, boat, fish, hike, walk on the beach, or rollerblade, this might be for you. Winter vacations offer chances to snow ski, ice skate, play in the snow, or go snow boarding. People who live in the north often prefer summer vacations where they can get outside and into the warm climates. Folks who live in the south often prefer mountains in the winter where they can ski, snow board, ice skate, and sit around a fireplace and watch it snow.

_____

_____

_____

_____

_____

_____

Selection 7.7: Downsizing

Randy recently moved from a large apartment into a small apartment so he could save money. Now he's trying to find a place to put everything. His large apartment had many closets and cupboards and a ceiling fan in every room. The small apartment only has two closets and only a few cupboards. What's more, in his former apartment, he had a nice-size kitchen with room for a kitchen table. The new one has a tiny kitchen and a little eating area next to

122

PART II
....
Selections for
Intermediate
ASL Students

the living room. His large apartment had three bedrooms, but the small one only has one. In the large one, he had two showers; now he has one. He's trying to figure out where to put all his stuff.

_____

_____

_____

_____

_____

Selection 7.8: Healthy Eating

Myra loves to eat healthy food. She refuses to eat anything fried, and never keeps junk food in her house. Her healthy list includes foods like vegetables, dairy products, nuts, legumes, peanut butter, and so forth. Her junk food list includes potato chips, candy, red meat, cookies, and bacon. She steams or boils all of her vegetables and bakes or grills her chicken and fish. She snacks on rice or soy cakes, and she only drinks water—anything like Coke or Pepsi is delegated to the junk food list. You'd think with her healthy eating that she'd be thin, but she's not. Go figure.

_____

_____

_____

_____

_____

_____

Selection 7.9: Thanksgiving and Christmas

I like all holidays but I think Thanksgiving and Christmas are two of my favorites. While I like them both, I have very different thoughts when I think about them. When I think of Thanksgiving, I immediately think first of spending a day with family and friends and then I think about all of the things that I'm thankful for. Then my thoughts turn to food, and I think of turkey, stuffing, sweet potatoes, and pumpkin pie. Christmas makes me think of church first, followed by thoughts of family and coming together to spend as much time as possible with loved ones. Then my thoughts turn to Christmas trees, decorations, snow, presents, and Santa Claus. Which of the two holidays do you like best? If I had to pick one, it would be a hard choice to make. What about you?

_____

_____

_____

_____

_____

_____

Selection 7.10: Pete's Heritage

Pete has a very interesting heritage that he has inherited from two different parts of the family—his mom's side and his dad's side. On his mom's side of the family he has ancestors that came from Ireland and Germany. His grandmother on his mom's side is Irish. She has beautiful blue eyes and a beautiful personality to match. His mom's dad is German. He has very strong Nordic features and is a very sensitive guy. His dad's mom came from Egypt. She has beautiful dark features and is very quiet. His grandfather on his dad's side is from Greece. His coloring looks a lot like his wife. They are a striking couple. Which side of the family do you think Pete favors?

_____

_____

_____

_____

_____

Instrument Classifiers

In previous chapters classifiers were introduced. As you will recall, they can be used to describe people and objects and to indicate pronoun placement and movement (see Part I, Chapters 7, 10, and 24). Classifiers can also show how something is handled, held, or used (Newell et al., in press). These classifiers are referred to as instrument classifiers (ICLs). Once objects are identified, signers can use instrument classifiers to pull a cord on a ceiling fan, grab the handle on the refrigerator and open and close it, and adjust a dimmer switch to get more or less light. With these classifiers, the predicate phrase shows agreement with the noun, represented through the handshape showing how the object is handled, held, or used.

When using instrument classifiers, it is essential that the signer set up the object and then "look at" it when describing how it would look if you could actually see the item being discussed. As with other descriptive classifiers, the non-dominant hand serves as the reference point when describing how something is attached or used (Lentz, Mikos, & Smith, 1992).

Once an object is identified, instrument classifiers, found in predicate phrases, allow the signer to express how the object is handled or how it works. These classifiers change handshapes demonstrating how the object is picked up, put, and placed. For example, by using appropriate ICL handshapes the signer can appropriately pick up and pour liquid from a pitcher by its handle, move a trash can, or open and close an oven. Signers can also use ICL to pick up a box, a piece of paper, a paper clip, or a glass. In these uses, the handshapes for each object handled would be different. But, they would all mean "pick up."

Selection 8.1: Baking the Cake

Bonnie, please turn on the oven to 350 degrees so we can bake the cake. When the oven's hot, please put it in so it can start baking. Once you do that, will you please get the pitcher out of the cupboard and make some sweet tea and put it in the refrigerator? Then it'll have a chance to chill before dinner. While you do that, I'll start unloading the dishwasher. I can't believe how much stuff's in it! But, I'll put all of the glasses, plates, and pots and pans away while you make the tea. Between the two of us we should get everything done before it's time to start dinner.

_____

_____

_____

_____

_____

_____

Selection 8.2: The Bottom Fell Out of the Box

The other day I decided that I just had to clean up around my computer. So I got a big box, took the lid off, and started to dump stuff in it. I put in a couple of books, a handful of pens and pencils, some old magazines, a couple of spray cans used to clean dust off the computer, and some paper clips. Dumb me! I forgot to check the bottom of the box to make sure it was strong enough to hold everything. Well, you guessed it—I picked it up to move it, and the bottom fell out. The pens and pencils went everywhere; so did the paper clips. The cans rolled across the room, and the magazines went in five different directions. After I taped up the bottom of the box, I spent the next fifteen minutes picking up paper clips, pens and pencils, and magazines. Next time I'll look before I throw stuff in a box.

_____

_____

_____

_____

_____

_____

Selection 8.3: Ross and Mike's Fishing Trip

Saturday Ross and Mike went out on the fishing boat. They had to get up at 3:00 in the morning to drive to the beach. Then the man took them out on the boat all day from 7:00 in the morning until 3:00 in the afternoon. They used poles and nets to bring in the fish. Some of the fish were so large it took two hands to pull them onto the boat. Others were small enough they could easily use one hand to take them off the hook. They stacked all of the fish up in a cooler filled with ice to bring them home. When they got home, it took both of them using both hands holding onto the handles on each end of the cooler to get it in the house. Sounds like good eating to me.

_____

_____

_____

_____

_____

_____

Selection 8.4: Assembling the Bookshelves

Shelby recently asked me to help him put his bookshelves together. The shelves were in a big box and weighed a ton. They had to be assembled using a screwdriver and a hammer. First, we pulled each of the shelves out of the box. Then, we took out the dowels. We had to slide the dowels in the holes on each of the shelves. Next, we screwed on the two black iron decorations they included for the sides. The iron decorations were kind of neat. They were shaped like backward Ss. They had made six holes in each of the pieces of iron and gave us some screws so we could attach one of the pieces of iron to each side of the bookcase. Once we used the screwdriver to get them on, we took the hammer and put the cardboard back on. It was definitely a two-person job.

126

PART II
....
Selections for
Intermediate
ASL Students

_____
_____
_____
_____
_____

Selection 8.5: Tanya's Cooking Show

Tanya has a cooking show on TV, kind of like some of the ones you see on those channels that feature food. She makes a variety of things for the home viewer to see. All of her ingredients have to be put in those clear glass containers so the people at home can see what and how she is adding things. She has small glass cups for salt and other spices. She has medium ones for rice and chopped vegetables and large ones for pasta and meat. Once she starts cooking, she starts by pouring all of the ingredients from the large containers into her pans on the stove. Then she adds the ingredients from the medium and small containers. It's fun to watch.

_____
_____
_____
_____
_____

Selection 8.6: Gail's Halloween Decorations

Gail loves to decorate at Halloween. She has a gigantic orange metal pumpkin that she puts on her front porch. It doesn't weigh much, but it takes both hands to move it. Then she puts cling stickers with ghosts, spider webs, and skeletons on her windows. She finishes her decorations by draping two-inch strips of crepe paper from one side of the roof to the other. Then she sets out big ceramic bowls filled with candy inside the front door.

_____
_____
_____
_____
_____

Selection 8.7: Uncle Charlie's Beer Steins

Uncle Charlie has a really neat collection of beer steins. Some have rounded handles, others have rectangular handles, and some have very intricately designed handles. While some have tops that can be removed, others have an extension on the lid that when pressed on makes the top come up. Some of the steins are short and round and others are tall and narrow. My favorite ones are the ones with the massive handles. They're a "real man's" stein.

_____
_____
_____
_____
_____

Selection 8.8: Mrs. Wishey Washey's Tub

Have you ever read the stories about Mrs. Wishey Washey? She is a delightful woman who always has a story to tell. One of her trademarks is her tub that she uses to wash her clothes in. It is a large metal tub with two handles, one on each side. You know, the old-fashioned kind. She carries the tub to her table outside, uses a pitcher to fill it with water, and then adds her soap. She then puts in her scrub board with all of the louvers so she can rub her clothes up and down on them to get them clean. I think my washing machine works better. What do you think?

_____

_____

_____

_____

_____

_____

Selection 8.9: Reid Has a New Squirt Gun

Have you seen Reid's new squirt gun? It's awesome! It's bright red and has a long barrel. The handle is shaped like a quarter moon, and it makes it easy for him to get his fingers around it. It has a trigger designed for little hands. It's white, plastic, and about a half-inch thick. The rubber plug that you take out to put the water in is also designed for little hands. He can use his thumb and index finger to pull it out, then he can put in the water and stick it back in. He really likes it.

_____

_____

_____

_____

_____

_____

Selection 8.10: Jar of Kitchen Tools

All good cooks have a jar of kitchen tools on the counter next to the stove. Kelly's jar is plum colored and about twelve inches tall. In her jar she has a spatula with a plastic handle and a metal plate with holes in it to let liquid out when she turns her food. She also has a plastic spoon with prongs to lift spaghetti out of a pot. In her jar are several wooden spoons with long handles with varying shapes—some are completely round while others are flat across the spoon portion. She has three different-sized whisks—you know, with wire handles and then thin wires that are all joined together—to mix eggs for omelets and egg whites for meringues.

_____

_____

_____

_____

_____

_____

Characterization

Role shifting was previously described in Part II, Chapter 6. You will recall that role shifting is used to assume the role of the persons interacting in a dialogue, thus permitting signers to indicate who is speaking to whom by first referencing the individuals and then subsequently shifting their shoulders in the direction in which the person is located. By using role shifting and eye gaze, it becomes apparent who is speaking throughout the duration of the conversation.

Characterization is often a vital part of role shifting. When conveying the spirit of the message, signers frequently take on characteristics of the individual who originally conveyed the information by expressing what he or she said as well as how it was said. In these instances, the attitudes, emotions, and sentiments are displayed. Through characterization, signers capture the mannerisms and the feelings of the person they are describing, providing the listener with the full flavor of the message.

Role shifting with characterization is a very effective tool in ASL. It can be used to show a child's frustration in dealing with a parent or peer, a subordinate's asking the boss for a raise, or a dialogue that takes place between two close friends or family members. As explained in Part II, Chapter 6, by using direct address and assuming the role of each character in the interaction, everything the signer says or does reflects what that person says or does. Through this use of direct discourse, the person can state directly what the person said using first person.

Several dialogues below provide the opportunity to incorporate characterization and role shifting. Change these English sentences into ASL and practice signing them.

Selection 9.1: Shonda's Nephew

I saw Shonda yesterday in the grocery store. She had her nephew with her—you know, he's only 3 and not well behaved. He was sitting in the cart, and as we were talking he kept looking up at her and saying he wanted some candy. His aunt told him "No" because it was too close to lunch time. He yelled that he wanted candy. Back and forth it went. Finally he screamed, "I'm going to tell my mommy you're mean!" With that she said she had to go and left.

_____

_____

_____

_____

_____

_____

Selection 9.2: Miss Prim and Proper

Who is the new chick who moved in next door to you? I saw her outside yesterday. She stands so straight she looks like she could break, and when she walks she takes such short little steps. Her hair is always perfect; it comes straight down and just flips out a little on the ends. Her glasses pinch the edge of her nose and she looks over them. It almost looks like she's always looking down on you. When I talked to her yesterday, she stood up and seemed even taller, looked over her glasses at me, and in a clipped voice said, "I don't talk to strangers." "What's that all about?" I said.

_____

_____

_____

_____

_____

_____

Selection 9.3: Great Aunt Mildred

My great aunt Mildred is 90 years old. She is short, a little slumped over, and has lived in the South all her life. When she talks to you, she tilts her head to the side and purses her lips between words. She talks very slowly. You know, she has a southern drawl and it takes her thirty seconds to say "How are you?" because she stretches it out and it sounds like, "Hooooooow arrrrrrrre yoooooooo?" Whenever you go to visit with her, you plan to stay at least an hour if you want to really talk with her.

_____

_____

_____

_____

_____

_____

Selection 9.4: Asking for a Date

Did you see Joe Cool over there hitting on that girl? He sauntered over to her like he was the coolest dude around. As he towered over her, you could just see Mr. Macho feeding her his well-practiced lines. She looked up at him, like are you for real, batted her eyelashes, and said something I couldn't hear. Then he turned to leave, and the look on his face when he walked away said it all—looks like he didn't make it to first base.

_____

_____

_____

_____

_____

_____

PART I

PART II

PART III

PART IV

Selection 9.5: Brian

Brian is the new hire at work. He's a real country fan and thinks he looks like a real cowboy. He wears tight-fitting jeans, western shirts, and cowboy boots. What's more, he loves to turn the radio to the local country station and sing along. It wouldn't be so bad but he can't carry a tune. He sings everything on one note. One of the guys at work asked him how many years of singing lessons he'd had, trying to be funny. Brian took it as a compliment and told him none, that he was just a natural. He honestly didn't get it. My desk is directly across from his, so I get the full benefit of his voice or lack thereof. I may be asking for ear plugs for my birthday.

_____

_____

_____

_____

_____

_____

Selection 9.6: Stories Children Like

I think all children like the story about the three little pigs and the big bad wolf. They especially seem to like it when their dads read it to them with a lot of expression. I used to love it when my dad would puff up his chest and say, "Little pig, let me come in or I'll huff and I'll puff and I'll blow your house in!" Then in a frightened little voice he would cower and say, "Not by the hair on your chinny chin chin! You can't come in." It was great! Kids today still seem to enjoy that story.

_____

_____

_____

_____

_____

_____

Selection 9.7: Imitating the Teacher

Jackie was imitating her favorite teacher from the California School for the Deaf the other day. I laughed so hard my sides hurt. You should have seen her describe him. Mr. X was a paunchy man with thinning hair that stood straight up on top of his head when the wind would blow. He would walk in the room like a house on fire, sign as fast as he could go, but the best part was that she said he had the habit of burping, and when he did all you could smell was onions, and all the kids would back up. He was an awesome teacher.

_____

_____

_____

_____

_____

_____

Selection 9.8: Deaf Olympics

Who was the guy who won the freestyle swimming event at the 1976 Deaf Olympics? Do you know who I'm talking about? You know, he was about 6'2" with brown curly hair, and a perfect V-shape body. He would take his place by the side of the pool, look his opponents up and down, slap the sides of his face, and then stick out his tongue. Someone asked him why he went through that ritual every time he was ready to compete, and he said it was for good luck. It must have worked. He was a real champion.

_____

_____

_____

_____

_____

_____

Selection 9.9: Driving Home

I was driving home last week from Atlanta when some guy pulled in front of me and cut me off and then slowed way down. I was furious! I couldn't get around him, so I honked my horn, shook my fist out the window, and hollered, "Didn't you see me? What's wrong with you?" It really made me mad. I could have lost my front bumper. I could have slammed on my brakes and the person behind me could have rear ended me. Man, what was he thinking?

_____

_____

_____

_____

_____

Selection 9.10: I Have to Go Home

Some of my friends and I were having a great time and thought it would be fun to go to the paint ball park and play some dodge ball. That's when my phone rang. It was my mom. "I need your help. Your brother was just in a car accident, and they're taking him to the hospital," she said. I asked her which one. You could hear the fear in her voice when she answered, "I'm not sure, but I think it's serious." I told her I would start heading toward the house. "Let me know when you find out where he is," I said, choking back tears as I spoke.

_____

_____

_____

_____

_____

More Work with Conjunctions

As you will recall from previous chapters, the sign FINISH can be used in multiple ways to express information. In Part I, Chapter 14, the discussion examined how FINISH can be used as a conjunction to indicate one action following upon another. When used in this manner, several activities can be joined together, making it easy for the listener to follow the sequence. This chapter will focus on the signs FRUSTRATE, HIT, WRONG, and HAPPEN and how they can also be used as conjunctions.

The sign FRUSTRATE indicates unexpected obstacles that may occur, thus influencing an event; HIT can be signed to indicate something occurred that was not expected, but when it occurred, it contributed to a positive outcome. The sign WRONG is used as a conjunction to indicate that something happened suddenly, unexpectedly, and without warning, while HAPPEN and FIND are signed to express events or discoveries that occurred that were either not expected to happen or that one did not expect to find out about (Humphries & Padden, 2004, p. 191).

While signing the selections that follow, change the English text into ASL and practice signing the sentences. Several of these selections contain opportunities to use conjunctions.

Selection 10.1: Getting to the UPS Store

Saturday I hurried to disassemble a piece of equipment I wanted to get in a box to ship via UPS. I started to dissemble it about 10:45 and thought that the UPS store was only open until noon, so I hurried to get it in the box, tape it up, and take it to the store. I arrived only to find that the store wasn't open on Saturday so I couldn't mail it. Then I remembered I had been there on a Friday before, not on a Saturday.

_____

_____

_____

_____

_____

Selection 10.2: Walk Around the Lake

Maureen decided to take a walk around the lake. When she got about halfway around, the sky opened up, and it started to pour. It just came down in buckets. She decided she'd better jog back to the house before it got any worse. When she got back to the house, she realized she had locked the door and left the key inside. It just wasn't her day. Fortunately, she could stay in the carport

133

CHAPTER 10
....
More Work with
Conjunctions

PART I

PART II

PART III

PART IV

and wait a few minutes for her roommate to get back from class. Then she could get in.

_____

_____

_____

_____

_____

_____

Selection 10.3: Nikki's News

Yesterday was Nikki's birthday. She invited several of her friends to meet her and her husband at a restaurant for dinner. She told all of them that she had some exciting news to share. While they were all there eating, they discovered that she is pregnant and expecting her first child in May. She and her husband are both so happy. They had been trying for months to start a family, and now it seems as if they're going to be parents. She promised to keep all of her friends posted on her progress.

_____

_____

_____

_____

_____

_____

Selection 10.4: The Soccer Game

Do you like to play soccer or watch it on TV? Did you see any of the World Cup games when they were played this past year? Some of the players are absolutely awesome! I couldn't keep up with them, I know that. The sport moves so fast, and even when players are alert, they can find themselves getting hit in the face with the ball or colliding with other players. It's interesting to keep track of the brackets and try to predict who will win and who will be eliminated because of player injuries and careless mistakes.

_____

_____

_____

_____

_____

Selection 10.5: Visit to the Doctor's Office

Last week I was waiting for my grandfather in the waiting room at the doctor's office. A good friend of ours came in with his grandfather and sat down and chatted with me while his grandfather went in for his appointment. I was shocked to find out that his grandpa had cancer. He looks like a picture of health; you would never know he was sick. My friend told me that he had started to have bad headaches, and when they went to check it out, they found he had a brain tumor that was malignant. He had planned a trip to Europe but now he won't be able to go.

134

PART II
....
Selections for
Intermediate
ASL Students

_____
_____
_____
_____
_____
_____

Selection 10.6: The Concert

Saturday I went to the theater and waited in a very long line to buy tickets for the concert next month. When I got to the front of the line, they were out of tickets. At first, I was really depressed, but then it hit me that I knew someone who had connections. I drove home and called my friend to see if she could help get me a couple of tickets. It was then that I learned that my friend didn't work for that company any more. She had switched jobs last year. It just wasn't my day—so much for the concert.

_____
_____
_____
_____
_____
_____

Selection 10.7: The Rollerblading Accident

Two years ago, while I was rollerblading, one of my wheels fell off and I had a terrible accident. I was going pretty fast when I lost the wheel. Then I lost control, flipped over a curb, went through a fence, and was stopped by a tree. It was a horrible experience. I broke my left leg, my right arm, and fractured three of my ribs. I couldn't go to work for a month. Since that time, I've given up rollerblading. I just can't afford another accident. My friends tell me I should get back on them but I doubt that I will.

_____
_____
_____
_____
_____
_____

Selection 10.8: We're Related

About a month ago my girlfriend and I went to a party for someone she used to work with. I decided to go sit on the patio for awhile with some of the older men who happened to be there. As we were shooting the bull, I realized that two of those old codgers were related to my grandmother. Who would have known? These guys were my grandmother's cousins. I had no idea there would be anyone there I would know, let alone be related to. After we chewed the fat for a while, I went looking for my girlfriend.

_____

_____

_____

_____

_____

_____

Selection 10.9: I Studied for the Wrong Test

Have you ever gotten your wires crossed and read all the wrong material before you showed up to take a test? That's exactly what happened to me last week. I don't know what I thought the teacher said, but obviously I misunderstood. I spent the weekend reading, making notes, and memorizing information. When I showed up on the test day, I was totally dumbfounded to see the questions in front of me. I had prepared chapters sixteen through eighteen, and the test was on eighteen through twenty-one. How did I get so far off track? Who knows?

_____

_____

_____

_____

Active/Passive Voice

Sentences constructed in both active and passive voice appear in the English language. According to Mulderig and Elsbree (1990), "a verb is said to be in the active voice when the grammatical subject of a sentence does the action presented in its predicate. . . ." Examples of verbs or sentences written in active voice include: "She painted the picture. He evaluated her ability to paint. The art critics praised her work." In these sentences, the subjects perform the actions that the verbs describe. Generally, sentences written or spoken using active voice are very clear and concise, making it easy for the reader/listener to determine who or what was involved in the activity described by the active verb.

Although most sentences are structured in active voice, there are occasions when the persons or things acted upon in a sentence are more important than the one who acts. In these sentences the object or the recipient of the action is placed in the subject position. The verbs in these sentences are referred to as passive voice (Mulderig & Elsbree, 1990, p. 132). Sometimes passive voice is used when a speaker wants to be diplomatic; it can also be used when the person who did something in the sentence can be left unstated. Examples of sentences written in passive voice include: "Her performance was nominated for a Golden Globe Award. Only exceptional Deaf athletes are selected for the Hall of Fame." In these sentences the people who nominated these individuals for their awards are less important than the individuals' performances.

Passive verbs are also used when the doer of the action of a sentence is unknown as in "Joel's car was apparently stolen during the night" or "The dog was abandoned on the country road."

There are two types of passive voice sentences: overt and covert. For example, "William was hit" is a passive voice sentence. One can determine that it is written in passive voice because the words "by his friend" could be added to the sentence. Overt passive voice sentences include the person who did the action in a "by" prepositional phrase. For example, "William was hit by Paul." A covert passive voice sentence will not include the "by" phrase, but you can determine if a sentence is written in passive voice if you can add a "by" phrase (Newell, 2006).

Even though there are times when it is necessary to write or speak using passive voice, these sentences are generally less concise than active verbs, thus obscuring the true action in the sentence, creating ambiguity and wordy sentences.

In ASL, most sentences are structured in active voice. Therefore, when interpreters/transliterators are faced with sentences structured in passive voice, they may be faced with the challenge of signing the sentences in a way that accurately conveys the meaning. Although some passive sentences can be signed adhering to the structure of the English language, others require restructuring in order to facilitate meaning and clarity. When faced with sentences presented in passive voice, it is critical that the interpreter/transliterator allows sufficient time to process the information and determine if the sentence needs to be restructured in active voice.

In the following paragraphs, pay particular attention to those sentences written in passive voice. Determine whether the sentences can be signed following

English word order or if they need to be restructured in order to achieve message equivalence.

137

CHAPTER 11
....
Active/Passive
Voice

PART I

PART II

PART III

PART IV

Selection 11.1: Miss Deaf Montana

Jane was selected to be Miss Deaf Montana. During the year, she'll attend several functions and talk with deaf students throughout the state. She's so excited about her new role. She was picked because of her dynamic personality and will be an excellent role model for young Deaf girls. I'm really happy for her. I've known her since we were both at the school for the deaf. She really has a great personality!

_____

_____

_____

_____

_____

Selection 11.2: Burglary on Elm Street

Our apartment was burglarized yesterday. They took our TV, microwave, and some change that was on the kitchen counter. I think they must have heard the neighbors next door coming home, so they left in a hurry. The police came and we filed a report. Fortunately, nothing of real value was taken. The police assured us they'd do everything possible to catch the thief.

_____

_____

_____

_____

_____

Selection 11.3: Grooming the Dog

We've got to give the dog a bath. I don't know what he got into, but he's pretty smelly. I guess I shouldn't have let him off his leash in the park, but he was having such a good time. He must have rolled in something. Mom usually has him groomed by Pampered Pets, but they're not open today. If we use some of the shampoo that was made for eliminating strong odors, we should be okay. I guess we should get started. If this doesn't work, we'll have to go to Plan B.

_____

_____

_____

_____

_____

Selection 11.4: Cakes for Christmas

My friend Lynn has a cake business, and she's been extremely busy. She had to hire some extra help for the holidays. Four high school girls have been hired to help her out because she wants to be able to fill all of the cake orders. The cakes are between ten and thirteen layers high. Some of the cakes are frosted

138

PART II
....
Selections for
Intermediate
ASL Students

by Lynn and some are done by the girls. I picked up my cake yesterday. While I was there, fifteen other cakes were picked up. She really has a busy but lucrative business.

_____

_____

_____

_____

_____

Selection 11.5: Painting Grandma's House

For weeks we've been talking about how grandma's house needs to be painted. Finally, the color of the paint was picked. Now Gerard can start painting. The house isn't too big, so it shouldn't take too long to finish the job once he gets started. The house was last painted thirty years ago, so it really needs it. The painting was supposed to get underway last week, but the weather didn't cooperate. It rained for four days in a row. It'll be nice when he can start the job and get it finished.

_____

_____

_____

_____

_____

_____

Selection 11.6: Picking Blueberries

Picking blueberries is hard work. Some of the best blueberries are grown in Maine. These berries have been picked by people who live in the area as well as visitors who like to come to Maine in July and August. Many a blueberry has been picked by my friend Cara. She likes to wear a long-sleeved shirt, long pants, and gloves before she attacks the bushes. She loves to take the berries and put them in pancakes. Yum!

_____

_____

_____

_____

_____

_____

 ### Selection 11.7: Tommy's Soccer Game

Tommy loves to play soccer. He loves to run and kick the ball and play with his friends. Every Monday and Wednesday he has practice, and usually there's a game every Saturday morning. Last week he was playing when a ball kicked by a boy hit him in the face. The next day the right side of his face was very swollen. But it didn't slow him down. Not for a minute. He was ready to play again the following Monday when they had practice. Maybe when he's older he'll be picked by a college team to play with them.

139

CHAPTER 11
....
Active/Passive
Voice

PART I

PART II

PART III

PART IV

_____

_____

_____

_____

_____

_____

Selection 11.8: Voyages of Sea Captains

In the 1700s, whaling captains went out to sea for several months or years. Sometimes, they were accompanied by their wives on the voyage. Charlotte Smith spent four years aboard her husband's whaling ship. During the months at sea, Charlotte became pregnant and was temporarily left in Chile by her husband to have their son. Months later, her husband picked up Charlotte and their son, and they headed to the African coast. It was there that the sounds of whales were heard by Charlotte.

_____

_____

_____

_____

_____

_____

Selection 11.9: Potato Farmers

Did you know that only half of the potatoes grown in the United States are grown by farmers living in Idaho? The rest of the potatoes are grown by farmers living throughout the country. Many of the farms today have been handed down from great-grandfathers and great, great-grandfathers who were given the land by government officials during the days when the Homestead Act was authorized. While some of the existing farms will be handed down to the boys in the family, others will be sold and bought by the highest bidder.

_____

_____

_____

_____

_____

_____

Selection 11.10: The Picnic

On a sunny spring afternoon, it was decided by mom that we should go for a picnic. She packed chicken, potato salad, fruit, chips, cookies, and enough drinks for six people, and we headed for the park. Once we arrived, the quilt was spread on the grass, and the food was set up. When we finished eating, we kicked off our shoes and socks and ran to the stream to wade in the water. Then we played hide and go seek until it was late in the afternoon. Finally mom called to all of us and told us it was time to pack everything up and head for the house. It was the best picnic, and a good time was had by all.

140

PART II
....
Selections for
Intermediate
ASL Students

_____
_____
_____
_____
_____
_____

Selection 11.11: The Birthday Surprise

On the morning of Dawn's eighth birthday she was woken up by her mom, who told her she had a surprise for her. For as long as she could remember she had been telling her parents that she wanted a kitty. Sure enough, her parents had gotten her one. It was beautiful, with long white fur and big green eyes. Dawn was so excited; the cat was what she had always wanted. She picked her new kitty up and ran down the street to show it to her friend Shelby. She would be excited too!

_____
_____
_____
_____
_____

CHAPTER 12

Sequencing

Teachers of the deaf, interpreters, and tutors working in educational settings may be faced daily with classes in mathematics, science, social studies, and English. While some of these classes lend themselves to a lecture format, others are interactive in nature, requiring students to work together to solve word problems and conduct science experiments. Those facilitating communication must be able to convey word problems and the steps involved in experiments in a manner that makes sense visually for students who are deaf.

The following selections have been included to provide practice material similar to the content found in these academic subjects. When signing them in ASL, signers are encouraged to use their sign space appropriately and to use ordinal numbers and classifiers when necessary. Pay particular attention to the narratives as you determine how they can be signed for optimum clarity.

Selection 12.1: The Experiment

Today we're going to do an experiment. First, wad up a dry paper towel and tape it to the inside of the plastic cup. Next, fill the sink with water. Now turn the cup upside down and slowly push it straight down into the water. Now bring the cup straight up and out of the water. Take out the paper towel and examine it. How does it look? What do you think happened? Why does it look the way that it does? What did you learn from this experiment?

_____

_____

_____

_____

_____

Selection 12.2: Design Your Own Boat

We're going to figure out what size boat we need to carry a load of something across the water. Think about the type of boat you'll design. Decide what materials you'll use. What do you want your boat to look like? What type of load will your boat carry? Now figure out how you will measure the mass of your boat and your cargo. Make sure you can explain how you will design your boat so it can float on water. You will need to describe your materials and what cargo your boat will carry.

_____

_____

_____

_____

_____

142

PART II
....
Selections for
Intermediate
ASL Students

Selection 12.3: Understanding Collisions

Let's explore what happens when things collide. Pick a partner, then stand about two meters away from your partner facing each other. Slowly roll a baseball on the floor toward your partner. At the same time, have your partner quickly roll a tennis ball into your baseball. Watch what happens when the balls collide. Write a paragraph in your science journal about what you observed. Explain why you think what you observed happened.

_____

_____

_____

_____

_____

Selection 12.4: Can You Solve These Problems?

Today we're going to solve three problems. The first problem is about a bee. A bee flies 30 meters north of the hive, then 15 meters east, 10 meters west, and 5 meters south. How far north and east of the hive is it now? Explain how you calculated your answer. The second problem is about a squirrel. A squirrel has 27 acorns. It eats 3 acorns a day. How many days will the acorns last? And the third problem is about Ron: Ron eats 3 candy bars a day. How many candy bars does he eat in a week?

_____

_____

_____

_____

_____

Selection 12.5: Let's Solve Some More Math Problems

There were some birds sitting on the telephone wire when the sun came up. About an hour later 64 more birds came. Then there were 123 birds sitting on the wire. How many birds were sitting on the wire when the sun came up? Here's another problem for you. Jeanne has a beautiful necklace. Every third bead on her necklace is blue. There are 161 beads in her necklace. How many beads are blue? This is a hint: Think in groups of three.

_____

_____

_____

_____

_____

Selection 12.6: Writing About You

When we write a story about us, it becomes part of our autobiography. Before you write today, think about a personal experience that you want to share. Why do you want to share this experience? What makes it memorable? Jot down a few notes then write your first draft. When you're done, ask a friend to read what you've written. Then revise your story, proofread it, and turn it in so it can be graded.

_____
_____
_____
_____
_____

Selection 12.7: Fractions

The word *fraction* means part. So, if we want to divide something into two equal parts, we could represent one of those parts by the fraction $\frac{1}{2}$. The 2 on the bottom represents the total number of parts, and the 1 on the top is a part of the total.

_____
_____
_____
_____
_____

Selection 12.8: Solving Word Problems

Listen to the following information and see if you can solve the problem. Jot down important information as you hear it so you can use it to help you figure out the answer. This is the problem: The school elections took place last Wednesday. Shelley, Juan, and Katrina all ran for president. Shelley got 156 votes and Juan received 115 votes. Katrina received 46 more votes than Juan. How many votes did Katrina get? Who won the election? How did you arrive at your answer?

_____
_____
_____
_____
_____

Selection 12.9: Independent and Dependent Clauses

Remember yesterday we talked about the difference between independent and dependent clauses? Let's review those differences. An independent clause is a group of words that has a subject and a predicate. It can stand alone as a sentence because it expresses a complete thought. A dependent clause starts with words like *before, after, when, because, who*, or *which*. This clause cannot stand alone. It depends on the independent clause for meaning. Listen to the next two groups of words. Tell me which ones are the independent clauses and which ones are the dependent clauses.

_____
_____
_____
_____
_____
_____

Selection 12.10: Steps in Division

There are four steps we follow when we divide. First, we divide; second, we multiply; third, we subtract; and fourth, we bring down. Now suppose we want to divide 187 into 5 equal groups. Follow the steps and try to solve the problem. Now, let's try another one. Suppose we have 320 pieces of gum, and we want to give each of our 10 friends equal amounts of gum. Use the steps again and try to solve the problem. You can use the same steps with word problems. Try this one. Twenty players in the school band divide into groups of 5. How many groups do they make?

_____

_____

_____

_____

_____

Practice Selections: Grouping, Comparing, Directional Verbs

The following selections in this chapter and those included in Chapters 14 through 20 contain selections of varying length and provide additional source material to practice translation, interpreting, or transliterating. The content found in these selections has been designed to provide opportunities to practice referencing, role shifting, listing, using classifiers, as well as several of the other features found in ASL.

Selection 13.1: High School Subcultures

In any high school three subcultures exist in the larger school environment. The three groups are quite different, and almost every student can be identified with one of them. The first group is the delinquent subculture. This one is the least popular of the three groups. The delinquent group despises school. They hate the faculty, staff, and symbols of authority. The second group is the academic subculture comprised of hard-working students who value their education. The third major student group is the social status or the fun subculture. These students care most about looks, clothes, and cars. For this group, social status is the most important thing in the world. Needless to say, frequently the third group is the most popular of the three.

_____
_____
_____
_____
_____
_____

Selection 13.2: Gun Control

Few issues generate more heated debate than gun control. Most of the controversy has centered around the sale of handguns that can be concealed easily because they are usually the types of weapons used in armed robberies and murders. For that reason, while it is often easy to buy a rifle, many localities ban private ownership of handguns or require owners to get licenses from the police. Advocates of gun control argue that these restrictions do not go far enough. For example, they feel that selling handguns through the mail should be abolished. Their opponents maintain that further restrictions would prevent law-abiding citizens from buying guns for protection or recreation. Such debates have continued for years with both sides appealing through emotion rather than reason. Because neither side attempts to understand the other, it has been difficult to reach a rational public consensus.

_____

_____

_____

_____

_____

Selection 13.3: Maggie O'Brien

Although Maggie O'Brien has hiked and skied in frigid weather, her greatest risk from cold was when her car broke down in a rural area during a winter storm. The temperature fell well below zero. At first she stayed in her car and waited for help, but she was so cold that she couldn't stop shaking. She hoped that moving around would warm her up, so she began to walk briskly toward the nearest town. Walking did warm her up at first, but it also drained what little energy she had. She knew that her body was quickly losing heat. As she struggled against the wind, she started to feel disoriented. She was afraid her low body temperature had begun to affect her brain, and if she didn't get help soon she would become too tired and confused to save herself. Luckily, it wasn't long before a car came plodding through the snow, and the driver insisted that Maggie get in. The driver took her to a nearby diner, and once she drank some hot tea, warmed up, and rested, she felt better. However, she knew that she'd been lucky; she could have frozen to death. Her experience taught her a valuable lesson. Now, during the winter months she always carries a blanket, a cell phone, and candy bars with her in the car.

_____

_____

_____

_____

_____

Selection 13.4: Library Assistant

When I was a part-time library assistant at our local high school, I worked the Friday afternoon shift. In the middle of an unusually hectic and complicated morning of running errands, I realized that I would never make it to work by 12:30. I tried several times to call the high school but kept getting busy signals. So I decided to just keep going and explain later since I had never been late before. When I finally arrived at the library at 1:10, the librarian shot a glance at me and then looked up at the wall clock. "I was in the neighborhood so I thought I'd drop in," I quipped. We both laughed and I went right to work. The librarian never asked me to explain but I made a point of getting to work the following Monday forty-five minutes early.

_____

_____

_____

_____

_____

147

CHAPTER 13

Practice Selections:
Grouping,
Comparing,
Directional Verbs

PART I

PART II

PART III

PART IV

Selection 13.5: Mark

When Mark began his first full-time job, he immediately got a credit card, and new furniture was his first purchase. Then he began to buy expensive clothes that he couldn't afford. While still in school, he bought impressive gifts for his parents and his girlfriend. Several months passed before Mark realized that he owed an enormous amount of money. To make matters worse, his car broke down. A stack of bills soon seemed to be due at once. Mark tried to cut back on his purchases. Then he realized he had to cut up his credit card to prevent his use of it. He also began keeping a careful record of his spending. He had no idea where his money had gone until then. He hated to admit to his family and friends that he had to get his budget under control. However, his girlfriend said she didn't mind inexpensive dates, and his parents were proud of his growing maturity.

_____

_____

_____

_____

_____

_____

_____

Selection 13.6: Media Influence Teens

A young girl looks at a fashion magazine and sees clothes modeled by women who weigh 115 pounds although they are nearly six feet tall. She receives a teen doll as a present and studies its proportions. The doll has legs nearly two-thirds the length of its body. It also has a tiny waist and nonexistent hips or thighs. She goes to the movies, and the heroines on the screen resemble adolescent boys rather than mature women. Her favorite TV shows are filled with commercials showing attractive men and women. The commercials are for weight loss programs. These programs insist that the person must be slender to be attractive. By the time the girl reaches her teens, she has been thoroughly brainwashed. The media have given her the same messages over and over. They all say to be thin is the only acceptable option.

_____

_____

_____

_____

_____

Selection 13.7: Flea Market

If you have ever been to a flea market, you know that Americans love to collect things. In fact, shopping at flea markets has become a social event, just like activities at county fairs once were. When you go the market, you'll usually see long tables where the sellers have displayed glassware, old magazines, records, and anything else that can be collected. While people do their shopping, they can buy and munch on hot dogs, sodas, ice cream, and local food favorites. Business begins early in the morning and lasts until late in the afternoon. In the morning, prices are high. However, they usually get lower later in the day. As closing time approaches, the prices get even lower. The really smart shopper does a lot of browsing but doesn't buy anything until the end of the day and then arrives home with real bargains.

_____
_____
_____
_____
_____
_____

Selection 13.8: Playing in the Leaves

Michael's job is to rake all of the leaves in the yard so his dad can bag them up and get rid of them. One day Michael had just finished raking the leaves into a big pile when Scott showed up. Scott asked if he could run and jump in the leaves. Michael thought it would be ok so he told him to go ahead. It looked like so much fun that soon both Michael and Scott were jumping in the leaves, throwing them up in the air, and having a great time. Before they knew it, there were leaves everywhere. Michael's pile was quickly reduced to a small mound. Scott felt bad when he realized what he had done, so he grabbed a rake and helped Michael rake them back up.

_____
_____
_____
_____
_____
_____

Selection 13.9: Snowball Fight

Have you ever had a snowball fight? We used to have them all the time when we were kids. When it first started to snow, we'd run out and test it to see if it was dry or wet snow. Dry snow was great for skiers but not for making snowballs. If it was a good wet snow, we knew we were all set. Sometimes we would build a snow fort or a wall of snow to hide behind before we started. Other times we would make snowballs just as fast as we could and pelt each other with them. We could entertain ourselves for hours throwing snowballs at each other. Once in a while, we would build a snowman and then see who could knock him down with their snowballs. It was always fun to play in the snow.

_____
_____
_____
_____
_____
_____

149

CHAPTER 13
....
Practice Selections:
Grouping,
Comparing,
Directional Verbs

PART I

PART II

PART III

PART IV

Selection 13.10: Feed the Ducks

Sarah's mom loves to take Sarah and her brother to the park and let them feed the ducks. Before they go, their mom takes all of their old bread, tears it into small pieces, and puts it into two bags, one for Sarah and one for her brother. Once they get to the park, they feed the ducks. Sarah grabs handfuls of the bread and throws it out for the ducks. The ducks come quacking toward the bread. Sarah doesn't like them to get too close because they scare her, so she usually throws her bread down and runs back and stands by the car so she can just watch them. Her brother has a different approach to feeding them. He likes to stand in the middle of the ducks and just throw a little bit of bread out at a time. He's not afraid of them at all. The ducks all gather around him quacking as if to say hurry up, feed me!

_____

_____

_____

_____

_____

_____

Selection 13.11: Rascal and Coco

I have two wonderful cats—Rascal and Coco. Rascal's nine and Coco's seven. Several years ago I rescued them from the animal shelter. Rascal's a sleek black kitty with orange eyes, and he lives up to his name. Sometimes he hides in the cabinets, and when Coco walks by, he bats at her when she's not looking. When she turns around, he ducks back in the cupboard. He also loves to chase his stuffed toy mice. The mice are various colors—green, blue, orange, and pink. Sometimes I toss a toy mouse across the room and Rascal will bring it back, but this game is only interesting to Rascal for a short time. Coco doesn't play the same games. She doesn't even like toy mice. Coco's a fluffy cat; her tummy and paws are white, her body is light gray with apricot patches. One of her front legs is apricot and the other is gray, but her back legs are white. She's a lap cat and will sit and let you scratch her ears while she naps, but if she decides she's comfortable, don't try to shift her while she's snoozing or she'll hop off of your lap in a hurry. The two cats are good friends. Sometimes I'll wake up and they're both curled up next to me. It's great to have such wonderful and entertaining pets.

_____

_____

_____

_____

_____

_____

CHAPTER 14

Practice Selections: Pronouns, Locations, Classifiers

Selection 14.1: Skydiving

My friend Mary Susan went skydiving on her twenty-second birthday. She had wanted to do this for a long time, so as a birthday present to herself, she set it up. She did a tandem jump with one of the instructors, and she had a blast! They went up in the plane, and then they jumped out at the same time. After pulling the cord, their parachutes opened, and they just drifted down through the air. The instructor had a camera and took pictures of them on the way down. Someone else in the plane took a picture as they jumped out and another one as their chutes opened. Mary Susan said it was exhilarating—she said it was just like floating on air. She said she'd do it again in a heartbeat! Would you ever like to do that? I had a friend who did it in college. She liked it so much she went back several times and eventually ended up marrying the instructor. She loved it!

_____

_____

_____

_____

_____

_____

Selection 14.2: Blackie

When we were growing up, we had a dog named Blackie. He probably weighed between fifty and sixty pounds and was tied outside because my mom didn't want a dog in the house. We were all little kids at the time so he seemed like a very big dog. None of us kids liked him because he always jumped on us when we went in or out of the house. We never played with him much because he was too rough and he'd always knock you over. Anyway, one year on Mother's Day he broke his rope and ran off. None of us were sad, and none of us went looking for him. He was one dog that we were glad to see run off. You know it's funny, he never came back—I'm sure he found a good home—maybe on a farm.

_____

_____

_____

_____

_____

Selection 14.3: The Bumper

My friend Ruth came in the other day and was talking about her new car. She's only had it for a few months, and she's still trying to get used to its length. It's about a foot or two longer than her last car. You see, she went from a little sports car to a big Cadillac. She just can't quite figure out how to park it. The other day she pulled into a parking spot and wanted to be sure she got in far enough so no one would bump the end of her car. She didn't realize she had pulled in so far that she had hooked her bumper over a concrete pylon. Later, when got ready to leave and she backed up, she pulled the bumper loose from the front of her car. All the way home it wobbled back and forth and made a horrible rattling sound. Now she's got to take it into the shop and get it fixed. I hope she learns how to gauge the length of her car soon before she loses something.

_____

_____

_____

_____

_____

_____

_____

_____

Selection 14.4: Toto and the Frog

I never realized that Toto was such a common name for a dog until I had one named Toto. Anyway, this story isn't about my dog, Toto, it's about some friends of ours. Several years ago some of our friends got a puppy for their son. Their little guy had wanted a dog for a long time, so when they got Toto, their son quickly became attached to him. One Saturday morning their son and the dog Toto were playing outside in the backyard. It had rained the night before, and baby frogs were hopping all over the ground. Toto spotted the frogs, started to chase them, and in a single gulp swallowed one of the baby frogs. You could see Toto's tummy moving in and out as frog hopped around. Our friends, knowing that frogs can be poisonous, quickly got the dog to throw up before he got sick. Once Toto threw up, the frog hopped away. Can you believe it? It was still alive!

_____

_____

_____

_____

_____

_____

_____

Selection 14.5: The Bat

When we lived in Pennsylvania, we had an upstairs window that didn't have a screen on it. One summer evening, my husband opened the window because the house was hot and he thought it would help cool the house down. Soon after he opened the window, a bat flew into the house. It circled the living room and the kitchen. My husband thought he could knock it down with a broom and then get it back outside. So he chased it around the house trying

152

PART II
....
Selections for
Intermediate
ASL Students

to stun it. Because bats have radar this wasn't a successful technique. Finally, it hit him that he had some starter fluid out in the garage. He went out got the can of starter fluid and sprayed the bat. The ether in it anesthetized the bat. Sure enough, it worked. The bat fell to the floor, and he was able to toss him back outside with the broom. After that we never opened that upstairs window again.

_____

_____

_____

_____

_____

_____

_____

Selection 14.6: Clowns at the Circus

Do you like to go to the circus? I like to go to the old-fashioned ones that are still held under the big tent. We used to call those the Big Top. I love to watch the clowns because they're so funny. It seems that every circus has at least three kinds of clowns. One is tall and thin—you know, I think they walk around on stilts. One is short and round—the costume must have a wire around the middle the way it comes out, and one always has a big plastic flower on his jacket that when he pushes the center of it, it will shoot water at you. All of them seem to have big red noses and brightly colored hair. Usually the one that is tall has an orange wig, the short one wears a rainbow-colored wig, and the one with the flower is usually bald. I do love the clowns at the circus. Do you?

_____

_____

_____

_____

_____

_____

_____

Selection 14.7: Mr. Wimber's Grocery Store

Did you grow up in a small town or a big town? I grew up in a small town, and one of my fondest memories is when we used to walk about four blocks down the street to Mr. Wimber's grocery store. We lived on Twelfth Street and Sixteenth Avenue, and the grocery store was located on Twelfth and Twelfth, so it was only a few short blocks from our house. The best part about his store was that he had penny candy. Down in the big glass case you could see licorice, gum drops, circus peanuts, rock candy, and taffy. We would go stand at the counter and point to the different kinds of candy and tell him how many pieces of each kind we wanted. Then when our mom was finished getting the few things that she needed, we would take our little bags of candy and eat our treats on the walk back home.

_____
_____
_____
_____
_____
_____

Selection 14.8: Making the Perfect Pizza

Chris can make a pretty awesome pizza. He makes his dough from scratch and then flips it from hand to hand just like you see the chefs do in restaurants or on TV. Once he stretches out his dough on a round stone—he doesn't use a pizza pan—he's ready to add the toppings. He starts with a mixture of tomato sauce seasoned with herbs and spices, and then the fun begins. He puts everything on his pizza. First he cooks sausage. Once it's browned, he crumbles it up and sprinkles it all over the top. Next, he puts on the pepperoni, the mushrooms, and the onions. Then he adds some sliced black olives, and last comes the cheese. He uses two different kinds, mozzarella and provolone. He piles his on about an inch thick. He sets his oven to about 400 degrees. Once it bakes for about thirty minutes, he pulls it out and cuts it. It's the most delicious pizza you'll ever eat.

_____
_____
_____
_____
_____
_____
_____

Selection 14.9: Unloading the Dishwasher

Mona has a real knack for unloading the dishwasher. First, she takes out all of the dinner plates and puts them in a stack. Next, she takes the salad plates and stacks them on top of the dinner plates. These are followed by the bread plates. Once she's stacked up the three different sizes of plates, she starts with the bowls. She puts the serving bowls on top of the stack of plates, and then puts the soup bowls and the small fruit bowls inside of them. This makes for a pretty big stack. You'd think she'd just carry that across the kitchen and put the plates and bowls away, but no, she starts stacking the glasses. Once she has a stack of about five or six twelve-ounce glasses stacked inside the fruit bowls, she carries her first stack across the kitchen and starts putting them in the cupboard. She continues to make additional stacks of glasses, putting five or six in a stack and then carrying about three stacks at a time. It's a wonder she doesn't break anything. When she's done with the plates, bowls, and glasses, she starts on the silverware and the pots and pans. I've tried to tell her she can make more than one trip, but she doesn't listen.

_____
_____
_____
_____
_____
_____
_____

Selection 14.10: Spiders

There are all different kinds of spiders, but all of them have eight legs, a head, and a body. There are both small and large spiders and those in between. Most people like spiders best when they stay outside. Garden spiders are big, yellow and black, and eat lots of insects. They're a good kind of spider to have. Daddy long leg spiders have very thin legs and also eat lots of insects. When my friend finds them in her house, she catches them in a jar and takes them outside so they can continue to eat bugs. Brown recluse spiders and black widows are poisonous, so you want to avoid them. Have you ever noticed how intricate a spider's web is? After it rains, or when the sun hits a web just right, you can see the design spun by the spider. Webs can reach across several feet or they can be very small. Some have been known to be five or six feet across and equally as large in height. Those are the ones you want to avoid walking into, or you can find yourself covered with sticky pieces of the web.

_____
_____
_____
_____
_____
_____
_____
_____
_____

Practice Selections: Descriptive Adjectives, Classifiers, Conjunctions

 Selection 15.1: Storm Stick

Umbrellas are great! Especially if it's pouring rain and you have to go outside and don't want to get soaked. Have you ever been on Times Square in New York City on a rainy day? There are so many different kinds of umbrellas, big, small, plain black, different colors, and those covered with prints, stripes, flowers, and even slogans. Some of them even have ruffles around the edges. Did you know that they even go by different names? A popular name for the umbrella in England is a bumbershoot. One day I heard two ladies talking, and they used a term to refer to an umbrella that I had never heard of. They were standing in line waiting to buy a drink, and I was behind them. One of them turned to the other and said, "Myrtle, look it's raining, and I forgot my storm stick!" I must admit I'd never heard it called that before.

_____

_____

_____

_____

_____

_____

_____

Selection 15.2: The Car Accident

Did you hear what happened to Lynn's car? It's almost funny, but I guess not really. She was driving home from class the other day, thinking about what she had to do and not paying a lot of attention to the cars around her. She started into the intersection when a car going the opposite direction failed to stop at the stop sign and broadsided her. That's not the funny part. Both Lynn and the woman driving the other car were going pretty slow, and the when the woman hit Lynn's car she caved in the passenger door. The woman's car had a broken headlight and glass was all over the street. After the woman hit her, she put her car in reverse, rolled down her window and yelled, "Did I hit you or did I stop in time?" Lynn got out of her car and told the woman that she had hit her.

With that the woman stuck out her head and said something to the effect that it didn't look very bad and drove off. Can you believe it? Poor Lynn, that's the second time her car was hit in a week.

_____

_____

_____

_____

_____

_____

_____

Selection 15.3: Eating at the Old Train Station

Do you live in Pittsburgh, or have you ever had a chance to visit there? Like most cities, it has a charm all its own. In the downtown area is the old train station. It was built in the 1800s, and it really is a sight to see. The train station has been restored and converted into a beautiful restaurant. When you enter, there's a piano bar on your left. As you continue into the main area of what used to be the train station, you enter the main dining room. Up on the ceiling as well as around the room are the original stained-glass windows. There are over a thousand of these windows. Each window is made with yellow glass and is probably two feet by two feet. The original beams have been refurbished and are still standing. If you like historic places and delicious food, this is a place you might want to visit.

_____

_____

_____

_____

_____

_____

_____

Selection 15.4: The Electricity Goes Off

Have you ever had to get up real early in the morning to get somewhere on time? Some of us have early jobs that force us to get up before the sun comes up, get ready, and head out the door. Businessmen as well as other folks sometimes have to catch early morning flights, so they have to get up early to make it to the airport. The other day one of my friends had an early morning flight. She knew she'd have to get up by 3:30 in the morning just to get ready and make it to the airport on time. She got up, showered, and was getting ready to dry her hair when the electricity went off all over her part of town. She called the power company, but they said it wouldn't be back on for over an hour. What was she going to do? Being the resourceful person that she is, she loaded her suitcase in the car, drove to the airport, and when she arrived, she went in the ladies room, dried her hair, and then checked in. Has that ever happened to you?

157

CHAPTER 15

Practice Selections:
Descriptive
Adjectives,
Classifiers,
Conjunctions

PART I

PART II

PART III

PART IV

_____

_____

_____

_____

_____

_____

_____

Selection 15.5: Foton's Table

Foton is a man who is in the habit of following routines. Now all of us have routines, but if his daily pattern gets thrown off, it ruins his whole day. He has a habit of going to the same restaurant every morning. He goes in, orders a cup of coffee and a bagel, and gives the cashier his money. He always gives her three dollars, and she always gives him forty-six cents back in change. Then he takes his bagel, walks over to the toaster, and when it pops up, he sits down at the same table to eat his breakfast. He likes a particular small round table close to the fireplace. One morning I went into the same restaurant, got there before him, and sat at his table. When he arrived, you could tell by he look on his face it wasn't going to be a good day. Next time I won't take his table. I wouldn't want to be responsible for ruining anyone's day.

_____

_____

_____

_____

_____

_____

_____

_____

Selection 15.6: The Iron Pattern on the Rug

Have you ever done something that when you look back on it you say to yourself "oh my gosh, that was really stupid!"? A few years ago I had one of those experiences. I was in a hurry to go somewhere, and I realized the sweater I wanted to wear needed to be ironed—it had a wrinkle just in the middle of the front of it. Because I was in a hurry, I decided I wouldn't take time to set up the ironing board. Instead I decided I'd just iron the sweater on the floor. I thought it would only take a minute, and I could be out the door. So I found an outlet in the hallway, put my sweater on the floor, and turned on the iron. I quickly put the iron on my sweater and the wrinkle disappeared. However, when I lifted the sweater up, there was a perfectly shaped imprint of the iron on the carpet. I about died. I had to wake up my husband and tell him what I did. He was great! He cut a piece of carpet out of the closet and replaced it with the iron imprint in the hall. What a dumb thing to do—I'll never do that again.

_____

_____

_____

_____

_____

_____

_____

Selection 15.7: Coffee, Tea, or Hot Chocolate?

On cold rainy or snowy days, do you have a preference for what you like to drink? If someone offers you coffee, tea, or hot chocolate, what do you usually pick? Some people love coffee—they can drink two or three pots of coffee a day. That's a lot. Some people like sugar and cream in it, but others prefer it black with nothing it in. John makes very strong coffee, and you have to be tough to drink it. Other people are real tea drinkers and prefer it plain, while others have to add sugar or cream to their cup before they drink it. I worked with a Deaf man from England one time, and he made such strong tea. He would boil multiple tea bags on the stove for about thirty minutes, and he was probably the only one who could drink it that way. Once in a while, nothing tastes better than a cup of hot chocolate. It's great with either some marshmallows or a little bit of whipped cream on the top.

_____

_____

_____

_____

_____

_____

_____

_____

Selection 15.8: Watching the Train

Are you a train watcher? All of us get stuck sometimes waiting at the crossing gates for the train to go by, but if you're not in a hurry and can just sit back and count the cars or look and see what's in them, it can be fun. There was a train that went by the school recently, and it had a variety of cars. Some of the cars were filled to the top with coal, others had long narrow pipes stacked to the top, and others had flat beds with equipment tied on them. There were some that were closed in so you couldn't see what was in them. It was a very long train; the engine must have pulled fifty or sixty cars. James and Bobby were talking about the train. James said when he grew up he'd like to be the engineer and have an important job. Bobby said he'd rather ride in the caboose and get to see the people smile because he was the last car. He said that his mom was always happier to see the end of the train instead of the beginning.

159

CHAPTER 15
....
Practice Selections:
Descriptive
Adjectives,
Classifiers,
Conjunctions

Selection 15.9: The Rowing Team

Have you ever watched rowing teams on TV, or maybe you've had a chance to see them in person? Some colleges have rowing teams. There are teams for both men and women. The boats are long, and there are several people on a team. All of them must row together at the same time, and the object obviously is to get your boat from point A to point B before your opponents. This sport takes a lot of upper body strength, hours of training, and a lot of hard work. Everyone on the team has to pull his or her weight; you can't have any slackers. It's a sport that people sign up for if they have a real love of water and they love to work out. The shoulders on the competitors are well developed. They alternate between working out in the gym and working out in the boat as a team. I could never be part of a team, but I sure enjoy watching them compete.

Selection 15.10: Devices for the Deaf and Hard of Hearing

Are you familiar with the devices designed for deaf and hard of hearing people? There are both visual and audible telephone signalers that alert the person when the phone is ringing. While some are used in conjunction with a light, sending out a flashing light, others sound a horn when the phone rings. Personal FM systems are available for use in classrooms, churches, or for special occasions when the individual needs enhanced listening capabilities. Pocket TTYs with VCO (Voice Carry Over) and HCO (Hearing Carry Over) are also combined into one portable device, making it convenient for users to take it with them and use with cell phones. There are also a variety of alarm clocks and other warning devices available that are designed for individuals with varying degrees of hearing loss.

Selection 15.11: My Favorite Clock

My wall clock is one of the favorite things in my house. It was a Christmas present from my sister. The clock is a rectangular shape and has a cat painted on it. But that's just the beginning. The cat's a cheerful yellow with bright orange stripes; he has long whiskers and is wearing lavender sunglasses. He's sitting outside on a bright, sunny day. His tail is separate from the clock's face, and it twitches back and forth all day long. The hour and minute hands are black with purple polka dots. The second hand's red and has zigzags. I keep this treasure on the wall so I can look at it often, because it makes me smile when I do. I'll always keep my clock somewhere special in my house.

_____

_____

_____

_____

_____

_____

_____

CHAPTER 16

Practice Selections: Topic/Comment

Selection 16.1: Professional Wrestling Matches Versus High School Wrestling Matches

Are you a fan of the professional wrestling matches that you can go and see in person—you know, that ones that air on TV? Fans of this type of wrestling love to watch all the hype as the brightly dressed wrestlers enter the ring and the match starts. These professionally trained athletes usually draw fairly large crowds wherever they go. But this sport is very different from the matches you will see at the high school level. At the high school level, these athletes wear the school uniform, come to the mat with very little fanfare, and focus on beating their opponent. Many of them enjoy the challenge of the sport and have little if any desire to draw attention to themselves like the professional wrestlers. Do you like wrestling? Did you ever wrestle in high school?

_____

_____

_____

_____

_____

_____

_____

_____

Selection 16.2: Ice Floating Down the River

Do you live where it gets so cold in the winter that the lakes and rivers freeze over? If it stays very cold for several weeks, many of these lakes and rivers form thick ice, providing a nice surface for ice skating and ice fishing. Then as the weather starts to warm up, the ice either melts or begins to break apart. All different sizes and shapes of ice can be seen floating down large rivers in late winter or early spring. If you've never seen it before, it's quite spectacular. Large and small chunks of ice irregular in shape float quickly to the mouth of the river. One time I had a chance to see the Ohio River with chunks of ice moving downstream. I'd never seen that before. It was pretty cool to just watch the ice for hours as it moved downstream.

162

PART II
....
Selections for
Intermediate
ASL Students

_____

Selection 16.3: Soup or Juice?

When I was growing up, it used to be a special treat to go with my parents to the American Legion Hall for dinner. They had a restaurant there, and as I recall the food was delicious. Well, one time when we went, I think my brother was about 10 or 11 at the time, the waitress came over and was taking our orders. When she got to my brother—I guess he hadn't been listening to what she asked the rest of us—anyway, she asked him if he wanted soup or juice. He thought hard for a few seconds, and then he said, "Sure, I'll have some of that super juice." It was pretty funny. The waitress only smiled and then asked him again. I can't remember now what he ordered, but for a while at our house we had fun asking him if he wanted some super juice.

_____

Selection 16.4: Fruit Anyone?

Apples, bananas, grapes, oranges, plums, and watermelon—those are only a few of the kinds of fruit my mom keeps in her refrigerator. While some people are chocoholics, my mom is a true fruitaholic. It's nothing for her to eat both an orange and a banana in the morning, have an apple in the afternoon, and in the evening after dinner eat a huge bowl of watermelon. I've never seen anyone who likes fruit that much. One time a friend of ours—her dad grew watermelons—brought six of them over to the house and lined them all up in a row next to the refrigerator. One by one they disappeared; not one of them went to waste. I've seen my mom eat a whole half of a melon in a day all by herself. I don't think I could do that, could you?

_____

Selection 16.5: Files in the Doctor's Office

Have you ever noticed all of the files in the doctor's office? There are just rows and rows of files, and all of them have different-colored tabs. Some of them are red for patients who see one doctor, others are blue for patients who see another doctor, and so forth. Although they keep all the files in alphabetical order, they are color-coded, so if the nurse wants to pull her patients for the day she can make sure that the files she is pulling are the right ones. One of my friends is a nurse. She was telling me that there is one woman who comes in who has the same name as three other patients, but they all see different doctors. Before they went to color coding, it was easy to get in a hurry and pull the wrong file. Imagine the doctor thinking he's going in to see a 23-year-old when the woman sitting in front of him is in her fifties.

_____

_____

_____

_____

_____

_____

_____

Selection 16.6: Contacts and Glasses

Do you need glasses? If you did, would you wear glasses or contacts? You know they make hard, soft, and disposable contacts. People who even need bifocals can now wear contacts. I've heard they take a little getting used to, but once you do, they're great. Some people really prefer glasses. They like some of the newer frames and have several pair to go with their different outfits. Some people have deep-set eyes, and glasses just look better on them. Gail only needs glasses for reading. I can't tell you how many different pairs she has. She keeps one pair by her reading chair, another pair in the family room for reading the mail, and of course a pair in her purse for when she's out. Whenever she sees a new pair that she likes, she just picks them up. She's the only person I know who coordinates her glasses to go with her outfits.

_____

_____

_____

_____

_____

_____

Selection 16.7: Tiling the Bathroom Floor

If you decide you want to tile your bathroom floor, there are some things you should pay attention to so that you'll be happy with your floor when the project is completed. First, make sure that the floor is level and smooth before you start. Second, as you lay your tile, make sure you use spacers so you have equal space between each of the tiles. Third, go back once the tile is set and put the grout in between the tiles. Within several days you want to seal the grout so it

164

PART II
....
Selections for
Intermediate
ASL Students

won't become dirty or discolored. Tile comes in a variety of colors and so does grout. It can take several days to complete a project like this, depending on the size of the room, but once the project is completed it can provide you with a beautiful floor for years to come.

_____

_____

_____

_____

_____

_____

_____

_____

Selection 16.8: The Picture in the Art Museum

Art museums provide the public with a variety of paintings, sculptures, and other works of art that the curator deems have merit. Some art museums collect classic paintings, while others look to new artists and modern art to fill their walls. Recently, some friends told me about an art museum they went into. One of the pictures really caught their eyes. It was painted on a rather large canvas, and was a representation of cubes. The painting was done on a gray background. In the upper right-hand corner, there was a large rectangle outlined in red that kind of resembled a keyboard from a piano. On the left side, running down almost the entire left side of the painting, was a rose rectangular shape, and in the center was a green square that filled the remaining canvas. That was it. They wondered what the picture was doing there.

_____

_____

_____

_____

_____

_____

_____

_____

Selection 16.9: Autism

Have you ever known someone with autism or read much about it? Doctors have studied this disability, and as with other medical challenges, they are constantly coming up with new information and new findings. While these individuals may exhibit classic behaviors of repetitive movements and periodically hitting themselves, they are discovering that some of these individuals are very bright people. Distracted by the amount of stimulation in the environment, they struggle with conforming to the social behaviors expected by society. However, when permitted to function in their own space and using a variety of communication techniques, they are able to express their thoughts and feelings. As the medical profession continues to conduct research in the area, it is hoped that they will shed new light on this disability.

_____

_____

_____

_____

_____

_____

_____

Selection 16.10: Concentration

Have you ever played the card game Concentration? You take a deck of cards—
you can use decks with pictures or the typical deck of cards with numbers, diamonds, clubs, spades, and hearts. It's important that you have two of each kind
of card to start with. The object of the game is to shuffle the cards and then lay
them out on the floor face down in usually about four rows with eight to ten
cards in a row. The first person starts by turning over two cards. If they match,
the person has a pair and can turn over two additional cards. He or she gets to
continue until the cards turned over don't match. Then it's the next person's
turn to try. That's where the name Concentration comes from—by remember-
ing where they saw the cards, people can go back to the right row and make
the match. Whoever has the most pairs at the end of the game wins. It's a great
game, and it really helps you work on your memory.

_____

_____

_____

_____

_____

_____

_____

Practice Selections:
Sequencing, Comparing, Time

Selection 17.1: How to Write a Good Business Letter

There are several steps that are important in writing a good business letter. First, make sure you have the person's contact information correct that you are sending your letter to, including the spelling of the individual's name, his or her title, and the address. This is called the heading. After the greeting—you know, "Dear Mr., Mrs., Ms., or Miss"—put a colon. Begin your letter by stating the reason that you're writing it; be succinct. After you state your purpose, provide the person with additional background information or with questions you might have. If this is a cover letter for a job, you will want to include exactly what position you're applying for and why you think you're qualified. In your concluding paragraph, be sure to thank the person for his or her time and consideration. As a final step, make sure to proofread your letter for any typos or grammatical errors before you send it. When you're finished, sign it and put it in the mail.

_____

_____

_____

_____

_____

_____

_____

Selection 17.2: Beach Plums

Are you from the Cape Cod area? If you are, you probably know about beach plums. My grandparents live on Cape Cod, and every summer my parents would take me to visit them. Many times when we were there, the beach plums would be ready to be picked, and we would gather them for my grandmother. Now, if you've never seen them, beach plums are small compared to a big purple plum. They're somewhere between the size of a kumquat and a large strawberry; they're a little tart to the taste but delicious in jelly. Beach plums grow on more of a bush than a tree. As kids, when we'd pick them, grandma would tell us not to eat them, because there never were many of the plums and she needed as many as possible to make her jelly. This summer I'm going back up to visit my grandmother. I do hope the beach plums will be ready and she will make us some jelly.

_____
_____
_____
_____
_____
_____
_____

Selection 17.3: Using the Internet to Cook

Jeff is a great cook; I think he's going to go to culinary arts school when he finishes high school, at least that's what he talking about. His parents support his
dream to become a chef, so they're always buying him books with new and
different recipes in them. Last week he was looking for a recipe to cook salmon.
He wanted to make a special kind of sauce, and he couldn't seem to find the
recipe he wanted in any of his books. So he decided to surf the Web and see
what he could find. He found one site that had lists and lists of different kinds
of sauces. It was awesome! Some of these recipes asked for ingredients that
he'd never heard of, let alone used before. He found what he wanted and went
off to get the salmon, while thinking the whole time he had a lot to learn if he
was going to be a chef.

_____
_____
_____
_____
_____
_____
_____
_____

Selection 17.4: The Packrat

Do you know what a packrat is? It's a person who packs up or keeps everything he or she has ever received and never throws anything away. Sabrina's
mom really fits that description. Sabrina warned me about her before she took
me home with her the first time. Listening to her description I thought she was
exaggerating, but from the minute we walked in the front door, I realized she
hadn't made any of it up. As we went in the front door, I noticed immediately
the stacks of newspapers and magazines that were everywhere. There was a
path leading through the living room to the couch and the chairs and then on
to the kitchen. But, other than the path, all of the floor space was taken up by
stacks of newspapers, magazines, and books. The stacks varied in height, with
some of them being anywhere from three to five feet tall. I have to admit I had
never seen anything like it. When we made our way to the bedroom where
we were going to sleep, we found piles of clothes everywhere. Just like someone had folded the laundry but never put it away. Sabrina said her mom has
always been this way. She's a delightful woman; she just likes to save everything and doesn't put anything away.

168

PART II
....
Selections for
Intermediate
ASL Students

_____
_____
_____
_____
_____
_____
_____

Selection 17.5: Setting Up the Classroom

Have you ever noticed the difference between classrooms set up specifically for deaf students as compared to those who can hear? When you go into a typical general education classroom, you usually see the teacher's desk at the front or the back of the room and the students' desks all lined up neatly in rows. When you go into a classroom set up for deaf students, you will frequently find the desks set up in a semi-circle or a U-shape so all of the students can see not only the teacher, but each other. That way, when the answers to questions are signed, everyone can see the response. In pre-K and kindergarten classrooms, teachers of both hearing and deaf students frequently have children sit on one side around a kidney- or a semi-circular-shaped table. The teacher sits on the opposite side of the table and can easily view the students' work. That makes it easy for instruction and for responding to student questions.

_____
_____
_____
_____
_____
_____
_____

Selection 17.6: Photosynthesis

Today we're going to talk about photosynthesis. Do any of you know what the word means? Who can tell me what this is? Photosynthesis is a process that involves the sun and plants. This is the process that is responsible for helping leaves on plants turn green. Let's talk about what happens. When sunlight shines down on the earth, all of the plants change the CO_2 (carbon dioxide) into carbohydrates. The energy for this process to occur comes from the sun. During the process, the plants absorb red light and blue light; however, plants do not absorb yellow and green light; therefore the yellow and the green light either pass through the plants or are reflected off them, and that's why plants are green. Do you have any questions? Do you understand now how this happens?

_____
_____
_____
_____
_____
_____

169

CHAPTER 17
....
Practice Selections:
Sequencing,
Comparing, Time

PART I

PART II

PART III

PART IV

Selection 17.7: Plug-in Heaters for Cars

About a month ago I was sitting behind two ladies who were talking about Alaska. The one woman said her son lives in Fairbanks, and she went on to say that in the winter there are many days when the temperature is thirty-six degrees below zero. It was interesting listening to her talk about the plug-in heaters for cars. She said in her son's garage he had a heater that he plugged his car into every day when he got home. Then when he was ready to leave in the morning, his engine would be ready. But that wasn't the most fascinating part. She went on to say that when you would drive downtown, it looked like parking meters lining the street, but in reality what you were looking at were more of the plug-in heaters. When people would go downtown, they would pull up, turn off their cars, and plug them in before going inside to take care of their business. I had never heard of that. Interesting!

_____
_____
_____
_____
_____
_____
_____

Selection 17.8: Fallingwater

Are you familiar with Fallingwater? It's one of the famous houses designed by Frank Lloyd Wright. Located about an hour from Pittsburgh, it's a sight to see. In order to get there, you have to travel on a two-lane highway because it's located out in the country. Built on a rock overhanging a waterfall, the view from the house is spectacular! In the spring and summer, you can see the waterfall cascading down. In the winter, the temperature frequently drops low enough that icicles form on everything, and that's beautiful too. The house was built in the late 1930s and was designed so well that it remains in relatively good condition today. If you ever are in the area, take time to visit this architectural wonder.

_____
_____
_____
_____
_____
_____

Selection 17.9: Forming Concepts in Math

Several months ago, a woman from Sweden presented a paper on how deaf children develop concept formations in math. She summarized a study she had done with fourth-grade deaf students who were learning to multiply. As part of the study, the students were presented with the following problem: There are seven children, and each one was told that he or she can have three apples. How many apples altogether would you need so the seven children can each have three? She presented the problem in different modalities, through sign language, through using manipulatives, through using paper and pencil, and through writing. She explained how, by watching the students sign and how they used the language, she could determine their mastery of the content. When they used paper and pencil, many of them drew pictures of the children and the apples and then drew lines to them. It was really interesting.

_____

_____

_____

_____

_____

_____

_____

Selection 17.10: Hybrid Cars

Do you own a hybrid car? Do you know anyone who does? Hybrid cars use both gasoline and electricity to get you where you're going. They are designed to help save on fuel and are supposed to be better for the environment. Some people driving these cars say they're getting between forty-six to forty-eight miles to the gallon. That's better than what most cars get that just run on gas alone. When the cars first came out, people thought they would get better gas mileage, but because people are driving them at faster speeds and using both air conditioning and heating, the number of miles per gallon drops. When the cars first came out, some were advertised at getting sixty miles per gallon, or mpg, but in reality that was too high. Now the sticker prices on the cars reflect a lower mpg and people have a better idea of what to expect if they decide to buy one of the hybrids.

_____

_____

_____

_____

_____

_____

_____

_____

_____

Practice Selections: Categorization, Classifiers, Questions

Selection 18.1: Spelunking

Friends of mine love to go spelunking. They put on their hats with lights, pack water and snacks, and head into the caves. For years, they've been exploring a variety of caves all over the United States. They think it's great fun to crawl on their hands and knees looking at stalactites and stalagmites. Recently, they were in France, and they went to visit a famous cave in the heart of France. They said it's well known throughout the world and that visitors come year-round to travel down inside the cave and travel by boat to see its hidden lakes. The name of the cave is Padirac. To get into the cave, visitors go down in an elevator. Once they reach a certain level, they walk down to where the boats are located. Then, traveling by boat, they go about a quarter of a mile. Then they get off the boat and explore the river and lakes and the bottom. They said it was awesome!

_____
_____
_____
_____
_____
_____
_____

Selection 18.2: Writing a Persuasive Paragraph

When you're writing a persuasive paragraph, you want to persuade your audience to accept your idea. When writing this type of a paragraph, you need to start with a topic sentence and then support it with reasons why someone should support what you're saying. You can either present the most important reason first or build up to it and save it for last. When writing a persuasive paragraph, you need to separate out facts from opinions. Facts are information that can be documented. Opinions are how you and others feel about them. For example, when talking about clothes, a fact can be documented by stating how many pairs of jeans a company sells every year. An opinion would be that teenagers think they're cool. Think of who your audience is before you begin to write.

172

PART II
....
Selections for
Intermediate
ASL Students

_____
_____
_____
_____
_____
_____

Selection 18.3: Poetry

There are all different kinds of poetry and many famous poets. Anytime you see lines grouped together in a poem you have a stanza. A haiku is a Japanese poem that has seventeen syllables, arranged in three lines. This is very traditional poetry in Japan. Many times a haiku will describe a scene in nature; sometimes it can express strong feelings. e.e. cummings is a famous U.S. poet. When you read his poetry, you will find that he never used capital letters; everything was written in lower case. His poetry is very easy to spot for that reason. Robert Frost is another famous U.S. poet. Many of you are familiar with his poem "The Road Not Taken." While some poetry contains a lot of alliteration and similes, other poetry rhymes and is appealing to children. Do you like poetry? Do you have a favorite poet? I have several.

_____
_____
_____
_____
_____
_____
_____

Selection 18.4: Geography

When you hear the word *geography*, what does it make you think of? The word *geography* actually comes from a Greek word that means to write about the earth. Some people think of maps when they think of the word geography, but it actually involves much more than that. This subject not only looks at the earth's features but also the people and how they live in different parts of the world. Geographers use a lot of different ways to describe the earth and its inhabitants. They draw maps, take pictures, and interview the people. The information they gather is put into books. When you go to the encyclopedia and you look up a country and read the description of the land and the people, what you read has been gathered by geographers. These people scrutinize the earth to see what changes are taking place to provide the rest of us with up-to-date information.

_____
_____
_____
_____
_____
_____

173

CHAPTER 18
....
Practice Selections:
Categorization,
Classifiers, Questions

Selection 18.5: Hot Air Balloon Ride

Have you ever been up in a hot air balloon? If so, did you like it? Several years ago Kim was telling me that she wanted to do something special for her husband for his birthday, so she called a man who takes people up in hot air balloons. She said he was great! He told her that she could pack a picnic lunch, and he'd take them up. He said it was up to them how much they wanted to swoop up and down in the sky or if they just wanted to stay at one level. The day of the ride, Kim packed the lunch and told her husband to get in the car for his birthday surprise. They went out to the field where they met the man who would take them up, and off they went on their adventure. Kim said it was wonderful—they stayed in the air for about two hours, and then he brought them back down. I asked her if she'd do it again and she said definitely!

_____

_____

_____

_____

_____

_____

Selection 18.6: Chicken Houses

Tiffany's dad and her brother have raised chickens for years. They start with the biddies and then raise them until they're full grown. They raise thousands of chickens at a time. If you've never been to a chicken house, it's quite an experience. Chicken houses vary in size and length but are set up in very much the same way. In between, where the chickens move around, there are long rows where food and water are dispensed. When the biddies first arrive, there is plenty of room in the chicken house, but as they grow it gets very crowded. Maybe you've driven by chicken houses and noticed the smell. I must admit they don't smell very good, especially in the summertime. I don't think I could ever be a chicken farmer, but I have great respect for farmers in general. It's very hard work and the hours are long. It takes a special person to farm today.

_____

_____

_____

_____

_____

_____

Selection 18.7: View from the Launch Pad

People living in Florida close to the Cape have easy access to rocket launchings. Many of these people get up early on the day of the launch and drive within three miles of the site to have a good view. Cars and buses line the side of the road, and people get out eager for the count down to begin. In the early morning light, the spectators pull out their binoculars and peer nervously at the launch site. Once they hear the radio announcer counting down they really

174

PART II
....
Selections for
Intermediate
ASL Students

get excited. As the steam shoots downward and the flames ignite the sky, all eyes look upward to watch the rocket ascend into the sky. People stand in awe as the huge rocket goes up in space. As the rocket goes up, the earth shakes and vibrations are felt for miles. As it goes miles into the sky, it becomes smaller and smaller. People watch quietly until it leaves their view. Then they get in their cars and head for home.

_____

_____

_____

_____

_____

_____

_____

Selection 18.8: Mime

Marcel Marceau has a reputation for being one of the greatest mimes of all time. He mastered the art of conveying so much information through facial expressions, gestures, and body movements. Never uttering a word, he captivated his audience with his performance. Mimes frequently dress all in black or black and white stripes and have their faces painted white. Their lips are frequently red, and makeup around the eyes provides added expression. They delight crowds by telling stories—some of which are humorous and others that tug at our sympathies. When we watch mimes, we are able to supply our own dialogue. It gives us a chance to basically write the script and come up with what we think the actor is thinking or doing. It's a great way for us to use our imaginations. There are a number of games on the market today that require pantomime. Those playing have the chance to act situations out and try to guess what the other players are trying to describe.

_____

_____

_____

_____

_____

_____

_____

Selection 18.9: Comparing and Contrasting

Sometimes, middle school teachers ask their students to write paragraphs that compare and contrast something. Students are encouraged to think of two different routes from their homes to the mall and compare the pros and cons of using each of the routes. Other times they're asked to group books according to fiction and nonfiction and list the titles of books they know under each category. Assignments that students usually enjoy writing about might include why the sport they like is superior to a sport someone else likes, why one kind of food tastes better than another, or why you should go to one restaurant or fast food place over another. It's always interesting to read these papers—you gain lots of insights into students in middle school.

175

CHAPTER 18
....
Practice Selections:
Categorization,
Classifiers, Questions

PART I

PART II

PART III

PART IV

_____

_____

_____

_____

_____

_____

_____

Selection 18.10: What Animal Would You Be?

Ms. Megghan recently asked her students to name some of their favorite animals. The students came up with dogs, cats, lions, turtles, tigers, bears, and penguins. Then she asked them to imagine that for a day they could be any animal in the world. She told them to make a list of all of the character traits their animal would have. Would they be big or small? Would they be fast or slow? Would they be friendly or scary? After they had their list compiled of all of the characteristics, she told them to write a short paragraph describing the animal, without telling what the animal was. Then, once they were finished, she had each student read his or her paragraph to the class and had their classmates guess which animal they described that they'd like to be. It was a lot of fun to listen to their papers.

_____

_____

_____

_____

_____

_____

_____

_____

Practice Selections: Directional Verbs, Classifiers, Sequencing

Selection 19.1: Amelia Earhart

Amelia Earhart was the first woman to fly across the Atlantic. She made this historic flight in 1932. What an accomplishment this was for her! She traveled from Canada in a tiny plane, often flying in the dark when she couldn't see anything. When she landed successfully in Europe, she immediately became an American heroine. She was a very brave pilot; she was the first one try a solo flight across the United States. She also flew from Hawaii to California. She set an outstanding example for other pilots as well as for women. When she tried a solo flight around the world, her plane disappeared. Search parties looked for her but never found her or her plane. She will always be remembered for her achievements and for her bravery.

_____

_____

_____

_____

_____

_____

_____

 Selection 19.2: Solid Geometry

There is a special kind of math called solid geometry. In solid geometry, we study shapes, and each shape has a special name. All of you probably have balls at home—soccer balls, basketballs, or even tennis balls. In solid geometry the shape of these balls is referred to as a sphere. It doesn't matter if it is the size of a Ping-Pong ball, or a giant medicine ball, it is still a sphere. Cans from the grocery store that are filled with vegetables, soda, or fruit are referred to as cylinders in solid geometry. What else can you think of that is shaped like a cylinder? Another shape commonly referred to in solid geometry is the cube. Who can tell me what a cube would look like? That's right, a box. Sometimes you can find boxes of sugar cubes in the store. There is another shape, and that is a cone. You've all seen ice cream cones—you know, the ones with the pointed bottoms, the sugar cones. All of these are shapes you will learn about in solid geometry class.

177

CHAPTER 19

Practice Selections:
Directional Verbs,
Classifiers,
Sequencing

PART I

PART II

PART III

PART IV

_____
_____
_____
_____
_____
_____
_____

Selection 19.3: Trees

Did you know that you can tell the age of a tree? Do you know how to find out how old a tree is? Trees can't talk like people. They can't tell you how old they are, but scientists have found a way to determine the age of trees. If you look at a tree that has been cut down, you can tell how old it is. As trees grow, new wood is formed on the inside of the bark. That makes the tree grow taller and bigger. Each year one new band of wood or a new ring of wood grows, making the trunk larger. Sometimes the color of the new wood is a little different than the older wood, and different things that happen to the tree during that year, such as floods or fires, also affect the color of the ring for that year. When a tree is cut down, you can usually find out how old it is and what happened to the tree by counting and studying the rings.

_____
_____
_____
_____
_____
_____
_____

Selection 19.4: Animal Tails

If you read stories about animals, you will soon discover that one of their most useful tools is their tails. Some animals use their tails to hang on branches while they gather food. Others, like the alligator, use their powerful tails to fight off enemies. A kangaroo uses its tail for balance as it hops, and a beaver uses its tail to sound a warning and as a paddle when it's swimming. It also uses its tail to pack mud down when it is building a dam or its house. Dogs wag their tails when they're excited and put them down when they know they're in trouble. Cows and horses use their tails to keep flies away. While some animals like bears have very short tails, other animals like monkeys can have very long tails. What other animals can you think of that have tails?

_____
_____
_____
_____
_____
_____
_____

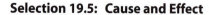

Selection 19.5: Cause and Effect

Sometimes one event alters another event. For example, maybe your plans for the weekend include a picnic at the park. For days you've been planning what you're going to pack to eat, what you plan to do once you get there, and how long you can stay. You've called your friends, and they've all made plans to come too. You've all decided to grill hamburgers and hot dogs, and there are enough of you going that you can play a game or two of frisbee. Then, once Saturday arrives and you're getting ready to load everything up in the car, the bottom falls out and it starts to rain buckets. So much for the picnic. This is a perfect example of cause and effect—the rainstorm caused you to cancel your plans. We use cause and effect connecting in solving problems everyday. By looking back on the causes of past situations and what happened, we can learn what to do and what to avoid.

_____

_____

_____

_____

_____

_____

_____

Selection 19.6: The First Horses in America

Have you ever wondered where the first horses came from, or did you imagine that they have always lived in this country? Actually, the first horses were brought to America in the 1600s by Spanish explorers. Before horses arrived in this country, the native people used dogs to help them haul heavy things. However, most of the dogs, even the larger ones, could only carry between forty or fifty pounds. The dogs were easily distracted and didn't make very good pack animals. When the Spanish explorers first arrived on this continent, some of their horses escaped and eventually made their way to the Great Plains where different tribes of Native Americans lived. At first the horses ran wild. Then the Native Americans figured out ways to tame them. They realized that the horses could carry four times as much weight as a dog, and they also learned to ride them. We have the Spanish explorers to thank for horses coming to America.

_____

_____

_____

_____

_____

_____

_____

Selection 19.7: Solar Energy

Solar energy comes from the sun's rays. Today we are finding more and more ways to use energy from the sun to heat our homes and keep us warm. In some parts of the country you will find a number of houses that have large solar pan-

179

CHAPTER 19

Practice Selections:
Directional Verbs,
Classifiers,
Sequencing

PART I

PART II

PART III

PART IV

els on their roofs. This energy is converted into electricity—it not only keeps us warm, but it also heats our water. While some homes only have one or two solar panels, others have several. Today, solar energy is more expensive to use than fossil fuel. However, as fossil fuels become less and less abundant, we will look for additional ways to harness solar energy to generate electricity that might not be as expensive.

_____

_____

_____

_____

_____

_____

_____

Selection 19.8: Mixing Colors

Mr. Gould wanted to teach his students about colors. One day, after they had finished drawing their pictures, he told them they could paint them. When the students came to his desk, they only found three different colors: red, blue, and yellow. One of the children had a lot of grass drawn on his paper and didn't see any green paint. Another child said that her favorite color was purple, but there wasn't any purple there either. Mr. Gould asked the students if any of them knew how to make the colors that they wanted from the paint cans. One of the children said he knew what to do—he said we need to mix them. Mr. Gould asked him to show him how. He mixed a little blue with some yellow and kept adding a little of each until he got the right color. Then Mr. Gould asked who knew how to make purple. Several of the children experimented with mixing two colors together until they found out the right combination to make that shade.

_____

_____

_____

_____

_____

_____

_____

Selection 19.9: How to Make a Paper Fan

When I was a little girl, my mother taught us how to make paper fans for hot summer days when there wasn't a breeze blowing. She gave each of us a heavy sheet of paper twice as long as it was wide. First, she told us to fold the short side of the paper an inch from the edge. Next, she told us to turn the paper over and fold it an inch from the edge. Then she told us to keep repeating the process from side to side until we came to the far side of the paper. She told us the folds would look like stair steps. When we got our paper all folded, she told us to hold the bottom edge of the folded paper in one hand and to smooth out the edges with our other hand. Then she told us to scotch tape the bottom edge or base of the fan so it would stay in place. That was the first kind of fan I ever had.

180

PART II
....

Selections for
Intermediate
ASL Students

_____

_____

_____

_____

_____

_____

_____

Selection 19.10: Making Beanbags

You can buy beanbags in the stores today in a variety of sizes, shapes, colors, and animals. Did you also know that you can make your own? If you want to experiment with making some, get some dried white beans, about a half a pound for each beanbag. Get some food coloring that you can use to color them. Next divide the beans into four equal parts. In each bowl put a different color—a few drops should be enough. Next drop some of the beans into each bowl and stir them so they're colored on all sides. After the beans have soaked up the colors let them dry. Once dried, you can put them in snack-size plastic bags. You may want to double bag them for extra strength. Once bagged up, they're great fun to toss in the air, or toss them into a bowl at the end of a room. Making homemade beanbags can be a fun project to do on a rainy day.

_____

_____

_____

_____

_____

_____

_____

Practice Selections: Descriptive Adjectives

Selection 20.1: Doing Laundry

For people who have never done their own laundry, doing it for the first time can be a real experience. Sometimes, when students go away to college and live on their own for the first time, it is also the first time that they're faced with doing their own laundry. Sometimes a helpful mom or dad will give their son or daughter directives before he or she leaves home; sometimes a roommate provides helpful suggestions. College students quickly learn how to sort clothes by color, what can and can't go in the dryer, when to use bleach and when to avoid it, and other helpful hints that will help keep their clothes looking nice. It usually only takes one load of pink underwear and most folks catch on, realize what they did wrong, and they don't make the same mistake again. Once the basics are mastered, doing the laundry becomes a piece of cake.

_____

_____

_____

_____

_____

_____

_____

Selection 20.2: Pelicans

Pelicans are one of the larger members of the bird family. They are very tall, and their beaks can be as long as a child's arm or longer. Under a pelican's big beak is a pouch made of skin, and this is what the pelican uses to store the fish that it catches. Pelicans can fly and swim and look very graceful in the air or when they're swimming. However, to see them walking on the shore you would laugh at how awkward they look. They usually live and fish together in groups. Flying in a straight line, they swoop down on schools of fish and gather them up in their powerful beaks, storing the fish in their pouches. When the mother pelican comes back from a flight, she opens her beak, and the baby will then stick its head in the mother's pouch and eat the fish. Pelicans live on the beach in homes that they've built with sand and dirt, using sticks for a roof.

182

PART II
....
Selections for
Intermediate
ASL Students

_____
_____
_____
_____
_____
_____
_____

Selection 20.3: Making Snowmen

If you don't live in a climate that has snow, there are several different things children can use to make snowmen. You can pop popcorn and use that, or you can use cotton balls. There are several things you need to get before you make your snowman. First, get a piece of paper to glue it onto. Get some glue and something you can use for eyes, a nose, buttons, and a mouth. If you are using popcorn, once it is popped you can begin by drawing three circles on your paper. The bottom one should be large, the middle one medium sized, and the top one should be small. Take your popcorn or your cotton balls and begin gluing them in the circles. Once all of the circles are filled, you can either add food or use construction paper for the eyes, nose, mouth, and buttons. Raisins, cloves, small gumdrops, and thin licorice all work well for these details.

_____
_____
_____
_____
_____
_____
_____

Selection 20.4: Owls

How many of you have seen a real owl? Owls live almost everywhere, in the north, south, east, and west. While some are very large, others are quite small. Owls can see better at night than during the day, so they do their hunting when it's dark. They quietly swoop down on their prey and catch it with their long, strong claws. Owls can't turn their eyes. The only way they can see things around them is by turning their heads and looking. Sometimes they turn their heads so fast that you don't even realize that they moved. Different kinds of owls make different kinds of sounds. Some make sounds that are pleasant to our ears. Others seem to sound very sad. Most of the time owls sleep high up in trees on branches during the day. They wait until dark to search for food and explore their surroundings.

_____
_____
_____
_____
_____
_____

183

CHAPTER 20
....
Practice Selections:
Descriptive
Adjectives

Selection 20.5: Fun Ways to Measure Things

Have you ever tried to measure something without a ruler or a yardstick? Hundreds of years ago people used parts of the body to measure things. The width of a man's thumb was an inch, and the length of his foot was a foot. Today elementary school teachers sometimes have children measure distance from one location to another by having them walk heel-to-toe from their chairs to a designated spot across the room. This gives the children a chance to count while they walk. Teachers can have them walk from their chairs to several different locations and then compare the distance between their chairs and the different locations in the room. These can then be displayed on a graph for the children to see what the closest location to their chairs is and what is the farthest away.

_____

_____

_____

_____

_____

_____

Selection 20.6: Seeing Things Through a Microscope

Microscopes are a special kind of magnifying glass, and when you look through them you can see things that you'd never be able to see without the magnification. Under a microscope you can see tiny plants and animals that you can't see with your eyes alone. Scientists and students use microscopes to learn what things are made of and to see germs. When you look through a microscope, you have to adjust the lens so you get a clear view of what's on the slide. It's amazing what you can see—even if you're just looking at a grain of salt or a drop of water. Scientists use very, very powerful microscopes to look at cells. Although students' microscopes aren't as powerful, they can still see tiny creatures and plants in pond water by viewing them under the lens.

_____

_____

_____

_____

_____

_____

Selection 20.7: Mirrors

What would we do without mirrors? Mirrors help us see who's behind us when we're backing up a car. Mirrors also let us see the cars behind us so when we want to change lanes we can. Mirrors let us know if our hair is parted straight or if it's standing on end. We also use them to see if our faces are clean and if our clothes fit right. If you go to a carnival or a fair, you can find mirrors to make you look tall and thin or short and fat. You can also find mirrors to make you look curvy. Mirrors can be used to reflect the sun and start a fire if you don't have a match. There are so many uses for mirrors that I honestly think we'd be lost without them.

_____

_____

_____

_____

_____

_____

_____

Selection 20.8: Piggy Banks

Piggy banks come in all shapes and sizes. Originally, many of them were made in the shape of a pig, and that's where they got their name. Today there are as many different kinds of piggy banks as there are animals. Some are shaped like giraffes with very long necks. Others are made in the shape of dogs and cats. I've even seen piggy banks that look like a turtle. While some are brightly painted, others are made with an iridescent glaze—you know, that white substance that seems to reflect a variety of pastel colors? Regardless of the shape of the bank, all of them share one thing in common—they all have a slot in the top where you can drop the money in. Usually they also have a rubber stopper at the bottom that you can remove when you want to get your money out.

_____

_____

_____

_____

_____

_____

_____

Selection 20.9: Wheels

Have you ever noticed how many different kinds of wheels there are? There are wheels for steering the car and wheels to put on your car. Most car steering wheels are about twelve inches in diameter and are about an inch around in circumference. Without them, we couldn't steer our cars. There is a huge ferris wheel at the fair that reaches up in the air several hundred feet and has chair seats all around it. The wheel on a bicycle has spokes that are thin and made of metal, and a roller skate wheel is also made of metal, but it's much thicker. A tractor wheel is about three feet tall and about a foot across. It's made of thick rubber and designed to move through mud and tall grass. It's amazing all the different kinds of wheels that we use.

_____

_____

_____

_____

_____

185

CHAPTER 20
....
Practice Selections:
Descriptive
Adjectives

PART I

PART II

PART III

PART IV

Selection 20.10: Getting the Pig to Madison

Years ago Monique wanted to show a hog in the 4-H livestock show in Madison. A friend of hers said her father's neighbor raised pigs, and if she wanted one, he would be happy to give it to her if she'd just come and get it. The man lived in Reidsville, so one Friday we drove up and spent the night there. The next morning she picked out the pig she wanted, she put it in a cat carrier, and we drove it back to Madison. The pig stayed out at another friend's farm, and once a day we'd drive out to feed it. Rudy grew into a pretty good-sized hog, and by the time of the show she weighed about 160 pounds. She didn't win any prizes, but Monique won herdsman of the year for her ability to show it. I don't think she'll want to be a hog farmer when she grows up, but it was a good experience for her.

_____

_____

_____

_____

_____

_____

_____

_____

_____

_____

Multiple-Meaning Words, Idioms, and Vocabulary Building

Run, Down, Call, Make, Look

Language learners as well as interpreters know the value of a broad and extensive vocabulary. According to Nist and Simpson (2001), possessing an extensive vocabulary is of paramount importance for several reasons. In particular, it is directly related to reading rate and fluency, it impacts one's academic career, and it gives individuals the power and precision to express themselves both in spoken and written communication (p. 8-9).

Sign language interpreters are cognizant of the value of an extensive vocabulary in both ASL and English, recognizing that if they do not understand a word or sign, they cannot express it either through ASL or spoken English. They also acknowledge that, although dictionaries provide definitions for what words and signs mean, the context that surrounds them determines the actual meaning. Nist and Simpson (2001) describe what is involved in "conceptually knowing a word." By using an iceberg as an analogy, they compare conceptual word knowledge to the layers of an iceberg. Figure 1.1 provides an illustration of this analogy.

As illustrated in Figure 1.1, the correct definition of the word or sign appears on the surface. Below the surface, one must acquire appropriate "synonyms, antonyms, examples, and nonexamples for a word" (Nist & Simpson, 2001, p. 12). Once this level of understanding is reached, a foundation is established whereby the individual can think of additional examples of when and how the word or sign can be used.

The second layer involves obtaining an understanding of the characteristics and connotations of words and signs. This type of knowledge typically comes from reading, listening, talking with other people, and attempting to use newly acquired vocabulary. As a result, learning of this nature takes place over an extended period of time with repeated exposure to words (or signs) (p.13).

The third layer of conceptual word/sign knowledge is referred to as "personalizing words." When individuals have mastered this level of word/sign knowledge, they are able to use the word or sign in situations and forms that are different from their initial exposure to the word/sign. They understand that many words/signs can serve different functions and appear in different forms (p. 14).

Approximately 40 percent of the words found in the English language have multiple meanings. English also contains over 8,000 idioms and idiomatic phrases, thus presenting sign language interpreters with additional challenges when equalizing communication for learners trying to master the English language (Makkai, Boatner, & Gates, 2004).

Sign language interpreters encounter multiple-meaning words and idiomatic phrases on a daily basis. They are required to process the meaning of the source material quickly and accurately so that, when it is delivered in the target language, message equivalence is achieved. Therefore, selections have been included in this chapter that focus on multiple-meaning words, idiomatic phrases, and vocabulary development.

189

CHAPTER 1
Run, Down, Call,
Make, Look

PART I

PART II

PART III

PART IV

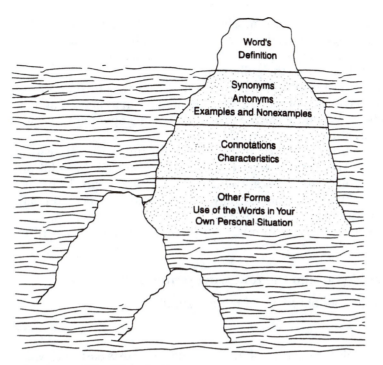

FIGURE 1.1 Conceptual Word Knowledge

Source: From Seal, Brenda Chafin, *Best Practices in Educational Interpreting.* Published by Allyn and Bacon, Boston, MA. Copyright © 1998 by Pearson Education. Reprinted by permission of the publisher.

The first ten chapters include selections that focus on multiple-meaning words. Each chapter contains five selections with one multiple-meaning word being featured in each selection. Each of the multiple-meaning words is included in boldface numerous times to provide maximum exposure to how the word can be used and how this usage affects the concept being expressed. By presenting these words multiple times within a few short paragraphs, students are challenged to practice changing concepts quickly in order to express meaning accurately. Individual sentences are also included, thus providing students with additional opportunities to focus on one meaning at a time.

Although it is unlikely that these words would ever appear so redundantly in conversations, for the purpose of developing automaticity in accurate sign production, they have been grouped intentionally in this manner throughout these passages.

The second set of chapters includes selections that contain a number of idioms and idiomatic phrases, also shown in boldface. Five idioms or phrases are included in each selection. The purpose of these chapters is to provide maximum exposure to a variety of idiomatic phrases. The goal is not to model spoken language but rather provide source material illustrating how these phrases are used and therefore how they could be signed.

The third part of the chapter focuses on both enhancing and expanding vocabulary. Selections include words that are taken from magazines, newspapers, fiction, and nonfiction providing examples of a wide variety source material. The featured words are also shown in boldface.

Selection 1.1: My Old Friend

I **ran** into an old friend of mine yesterday. He **runs** a family business in town, and as we talked, he told me he was thinking of **running** for office. I told him that I was aware of that after reading a **run down** of the candidates in the paper. My friend quickly **ran** through a list of issues he felt were critical upon which he planned to base his platform. The more he talked, the more his ideas started **running** through my head. He was concerned about the **run down** condition of several housing projects in town. He was also concerned about the river that **runs** east of town because of the pollution.

Another top priority for him was finding a way to support new businesses that seem to **run out** of money. He compared them to plays that have a short **run** on Broadway. When he started to **run down** his opponents, I told him I had to **run** as I was already late for work.

A block from the office, it started to rain, and as the rain **ran off** the gutter, I **ran** into the building. It was only then that I noticed the color on the blouse I was wearing had **run** onto my skirt and that I had a **run** in my hose. The only thing that would have made the day worse would have been if I had experienced a **run in** with my boss.

Ok, I guess I have **run** my mouth long enough about **running** into my old friend.

How would you sign the following sentences?

1. I **ran** into an old friend of mine yesterday.

   _____

2. He was also concerned about the river that **runs** east of town.

   _____

3. I **ran** into the building.

   _____

4. The new business seemed to **run out** of money.

   _____

5. Ok, I guess I have **run** my mouth long enough.

   _____

Selection 1.2: Small Town Gossip

Do you live in a small or a large town? I live in a small town, and it is pretty easy to get the low **down** on anyone or just about anything by going **down** to the corner drugstore. Yes, our town still has an old-fashioned drugstore with a soda fountain and everything. It's **downtown** on Base Street on the corner across from the florist.

The last time I was **down** there I ran into my old friend from school, Jane. She looked so **down**. I asked her what was wrong, and she said the meat packing plant where her husband works is closing **down**, and he'll be out of a job. What's more, her boss just told her they were **downsizing** where she works so they're cutting **down** on hours. Both of their incomes are going to be reduced.

I asked her how her family was doing, and she said her children were all fine but her mother had been in the hospital for about a week. She fell **down** in her kitchen and broke her hip. The doctors moved her to a hospital about fifty miles from our town, so Jane has been burning a path up and **down** the highway visiting with her and making sure that she's doing all right.

I asked Jane to put **down** the name of the hospital and her room number so I could send her some flowers. With that, I gave her a hug and turned to leave. That's when I realized that I had put my keys **down** on the counter when I went to order my drink. I went up to the counter to retrieve them when I saw two of my former students starting to chow **down**. One was giving the other the low **down** on the football game that had been played the night before.

191

CHAPTER 1
Run, Down, Call,
Make, Look

PART I

PART II

PART III

PART IV

Once I had my keys, I headed to the door and across the street to the florist. With any luck, they'd be able to get the flowers **down** to her before the sun went **down**.

How would you sign the following sentences?

1. She looked so **down**.

_____

2. Her boss told her they were **downsizing**.

_____

3. Jane has been burning a path up and **down** the highway.

_____

4. One was giving the other the low **down** on the football game.

_____

5. The company is closing **down**.

_____

Selection 1.3: Checking on Grandma

I **called** the other day to check on my grandma. She's 82 years old now and just as spunky as ever. Her real name is Eunice but we've always **called** her Mom B. When I asked Mom B what she was doing, she said she was baking cookies.

She is so funny! She said the recipe **called** for two cups of sugar but that she knew that no one needed two cups of sugar so she had reduced the recipe by a cup. I asked her what the cookies were for and she said they had **called** a meeting for the seniors at her church, and she decided she should bake something to take to the meeting.

I asked her how she was feeling, and she said she was a little tired as she hadn't slept well the night before. It seems that there was a domestic disturbance and the police had been **called** to the house next door. Grandma said the man was **calling** the woman all kinds of names, and in her opinion he had no **call** to do that. She said they carried on for a long time. Mom B thought the neighbor across the street had **called** the police.

I asked her what she thought grandpa would think if he were still alive. Grandpa had been **called** to become a preacher, and he felt everyone should try to get along. When he was living, he and Mom B used to love to **call** on people after church on Sunday. They thought that was part of the church mission.

After we talked a little while longer, I told grandma I had to go and let my dog in. It was starting to rain, and I didn't want him to get all wet. Sometimes I have to **call** his name a long time, as he's deaf in one ear and my yard is big. I told her I'd **call** her again soon. I told her I loved her and hung up the phone.

How would you sign the following sentences?

1. The police were **called** to the house next door.

_____

2. I have to **call** my dog for a long time before he'll come.

_____

3. Her name is Eunice but we **call** her Mom B.

_____

4. Mom B said he had no **call** to say that.

_____

5. The recipe **called** for two cups of sugar.

_____

 Selection 1.4: Buying a New Car

What **make** of car do you have? Mine is very old, and my friend Chris keeps telling me it doesn't **make** any sense to keep it. He said for someone who **makes** as much money as I do that I should be able to buy a new car. I keep telling him that I don't like to deal with car salesmen.

He told me he was going to come by the house on Saturday and **make** me go with him to look at some new vehicles. I told him I could never **make** any sense out of what the salespeople tell me about the benefits of new cars. They throw out so many numbers, and when I try to **make** them add up, the numbers I get are different than what they **make** them out to be.

Then when you finally **make** up your mind and decide what you want to buy, the finance guys add charges that **make** the cost of the car that much more. That really **makes** me mad, and when that happens it **makes** me want to leave. Maybe I can **make** up an excuse why I can't go. That will never work. I'll just get up early on Saturday put on some clothes and **makeup** and be ready to go. If it doesn't go well, I'll just **make** a beeline for the door and leave.

How would you sign the following sentences?

1. You need to **make** up your mind and decide what you want to buy.

_____

2. Maybe I can **make** up an excuse why I can't go.

_____

3. I guess I'll put on my **makeup** and be ready to go.

_____

4. What **make** of car do you have?

_____

5. Chris says I **make** enough money to be able to buy a new car.

_____

Selection 1.5: Rain in Florida

I live in Florida, and we get a lot of rain. Sometimes it rains so much that it causes limbs to break and fall all over the place. Then it is critical that you **look** where you're going when you walk or drive. The other night the weatherman came on TV, and he **looked** worried. He kept **looking** down at his paper, then he would **look** directly into the camera. From what he said, it **looked** like Florida was going to get hit by a hurricane, and he was concerned.

Looking back at some of the devastation hurricanes can cause, I can see why he **looked** worried. Folks who have property with windows or patio doors that **look** right out on the ocean are particularly vulnerable. I was going to **look** up on the Internet and try to find out how strong the winds must be before they can do damage.

When you **look** at the statistics, it seems that we have had more damaging storms lately than ever before in history. Today everyone has to be on the **lookout** for changing weather. Storms can come up so rapidly that many times you don't have time to **look** where you are going as you run for cover.

I'm **looking** forward to the end of hurricane season. At that time we can breathe a sigh of relief, go to the beach, **look** for shells, and enjoy the nicer side of Mother Nature.

How would you sign the following sentences?

1. He said it **looked** like Florida would get hit by a hurricane.

   _____

2. I was going to **look** up on the Internet how many hurricanes we've had.

   _____

3. Let's go to the beach and **look** for shells.

   _____

4. The weather man **looked** at his paper and then at the camera.

   _____

5. I really **look** up to rescue workers. They have their hands full after major storms.

   _____

Place, Up, Break, Fix, By

Selection 2.1: The Camping Trip

Do you like to go camping? Many of my friends really enjoy it. They look forward to the warm spring weather when they can pack their tents, sleeping bags, and hiking boots and head to the mountains. They tell me that picking the perfect **place** to go is half the fun.

Long before the first trip, they go to my friend Rob's **place** and sit around for hours planning their trip. They're all serious campers and feel that horseplay has no **place** on camping trips. They believe there is a time and **place** for everything, and camping is not the **place** for it to happen.

Julie's probably the most organized of the campers. She's great at packing and can usually find a **place** for everything. She really enjoys the outdoors. Her friend Gayle came with them one time, but she didn't know what to do, how to dress, and really in the end felt very out of **place**.

One time Kevin was organizing his gear and forgot that he had **placed** his sunglasses on the top of the truck. By the time he realized it, they had left one **place** and moved on to the next. He had no choice but to invest in a new pair when they returned.

I have learned from my friends that sometimes you must **place** your food in plastic bags so the bears won't get it. I've also learned that in some campsites you must reserve a **place** well in advance if you want to stay there. When that happens, the group meets, they decide on a date, confirm it, and they all **place** it on their calendars.

How would you sign the following sentences?

1. Gayle really felt out of **place** on the camping trip.

   _____

2. They left one **place** and moved on to the next one.

   _____

3. They will all **place** the date on their calendars.

   _____

4. According to my friends horseplay has no **place** on camping trips.

   _____

5. The camping trip will take **place** in the spring.

   _____

195

CHAPTER 2
....
Place, Up,
Break, Fix, By

PART I

PART II

PART III

PART IV

Selection 2.2: The Word "Up"

Maybe some of you have seen stories or things written about the word "**up**." It has so many different meanings in the English language, and when combined with other words, we sometimes have to ask ourselves why we really need it. I know all of you who know ASL get tickled sometimes when you realize how much more efficient ASL is in conveying the same concepts.

Think for example how you sign fed **up** and clean **up**. These concepts are communicated with single signs not two sign phrases. Think too, how you would sign sentences like the decision is **up** to you, you ran **up** a very big bill, and your time is **up**. How do you get **up** out of bed in the morning? And, why do people tear **up** papers they don't want, give **up** on great ideas, and show **up** late for class?

We can look **up** in the sky, but that is different than looking **up** something in the dictionary. We hook **up** the computer and sign **up** for classes at the gym. Sometimes we get tied **up** in traffic or tied **up** in a meeting. We fill our cars **up** with gas and line **up** to buy tickets for concerts and movies.

The list could go on and on, but I think you have a pretty good idea by now of the many ways the word **up** shows **up** in the English language.

How would you sign the following sentences?

1. I woke **up** late so then I showed **up** late for class.

   _____

2. I need to fill **up** the car with gas so if I get tied **up** in traffic I won't run out.

   _____

3. We need to hook **up** the computer so I can finish **up** some work.

   _____

4. She ran **up** a huge bill on her mom's credit card.

   _____

5. Are you going to sign **up** for the aerobics class? I am.

   _____

Selection 2.3: The Dancer

The field of professional dance is so competitive that sometimes it's hard to get a **break** and really **break** into the business. Many dancers have a secret desire to dance professionally but don't know how to **break** the news to their families. This can be especially true for male dancers. Unfortunately, in this country we still maintain certain stereotypes about males who want to dance.

One night when there was a **break** in the conversation Lyle told his folks what he wanted to do. They took the news better than he thought they would. He let them know that he would be leaving at day **break** the following day. The next morning there was a horrible storm. Lyle had to wait for three hours before there was a **break** in the weather and he could leave.

He was in a hurry to get to his first audition, but he knew if he drove fast and got a ticket, it would not bode well for him. He didn't have enough money to pay a ticket, and he heard that people who **break** the law in New York usually end up in jail. He wanted no part of that.

He arrived for his first audition and had some bad luck. He didn't see that there was some water on the stage. He slipped and would have fallen on the floor if another dancer hadn't stepped in and **broken** his fall. Had he fallen on the floor, there was a risk that he could **break** an arm or a leg. He was really lucky.

196

PART III
....
Multiple-Meaning
Words, Idioms, and
Vocabulary Building

He thanked the other dancer for **breaking** his fall. Then he decided he should take a **break,** regroup, and come back the next day and try again. Maybe tomorrow he would get his big **break.**

How would you sign the following sentences?

1. He waited for a **break** in the conversation to approach his parents.

_____

2. He had to wait until there was a **break** in the storm before he could leave.

_____

3. The other dancer saw him start to slip, stepped in, and **broke** his fall.

_____

4. It's hard to get your first big **break** in New York.

_____

5. Do you want to take your coffee **break** when I take mine?

_____

Selection 2.4: Jack of All Trades

My dad is a "Jack of all trades." He can **fix** anything. For as long as I've had the privilege of knowing him, he's possessed all of these wonderful talents. I don't know how many men are like him, but I'm sure glad my dad can do so many things.

When the car breaks down, he is the first one out there seeing what he needs to do to **fix** it. Comfortable with wrenches and motors, he usually can have the car running again in no time. His skills are not limited to cars. He is also great at **fixing** dinner. He can **fix** a "killer" omelet in no time and is a natural when it comes to **fixing** formal meals. If I didn't know better, I'd think he worked as a chef to earn a living.

He can also help **fix** a broken heart. I remember when my sister broke up with her boyfriend and moped around the house for weeks. My dad was the first one to come up with the right words and the right things to do to make her feel better.

Dad can **fix** a clogged up sink so the water will drain, he can **fix** a flat tire, and he can **fix** a great drink when we're hot and thirsty. He is also great at **fixing** my glass animals when they fall and get broken. It's amazing how he can put them back together where you can't even see where they broke.

All in all, my dad is a pretty amazing man! I guess that's why we've nick-named him "Super Mr. **Fix**-It Man."

How would you sign the following sentences?

1. He is also great at **fixing** dinner.

_____

2. Dad can **fix** a flat tire.

_____

3. He can also **fix** a broken heart.

_____

4. My dad can **fix** the car; just give him a wrench.

_____

5. Dad can **fix** the sink when it gets clogged up.

_____

Selection 2.5: Angela and Her House

Angela lives in the country in a very large house. Her house is **by** the river, and it is surrounded **by** trees. You can tell **by** looking at it that it was built **by** a French architect in the 1600s. It has tall gables and heavy French provincial doors.

We passed **by** her house earlier today on our way into town, but she wasn't home. We wanted to stop **by** and show her some pictures we had taken on our trip when we went to Europe. We flew over there but then traveled **by** train all over the countryside. We were met **by** so many wonderful people and had a fabulous time. I would go back again in a heartbeat. We just have to save our money so we can do it again.

I guess I'll have to contact her **by** phone and see when we can stop **by.** We need to see her soon because she is chairing the fundraising committee with me for the cancer drive, and we need to have our proposal finished **by** the 13th so we can meet with the committee. I just thought it would be great to kill two birds with one stone—show her the pictures and finish our proposal at the same time.

By the way, did I tell you that the last time I talked to Angela, she said she had bought some new bedroom furniture? She said she had gotten a new king-sized bed, two nightstands, and a double dresser. She placed the dresser **by** the window and the bed on the wall **by** the large plant. That's another reason why we need to go **by** and see her—to see her new furniture.

How would you sign the following sentences?

1. **By** the way, did I tell you I saw Angela yesterday?

_____

2. We live **by** the lake next to the yellow brick house.

_____

3. The book was written **by** J. K. Rowling.

_____

4. Her house is surrounded **by** oak trees.

_____

5. We have to have our proposal finished **by** the 13th.

_____

CHAPTER 3

Charge, Advance, Around, Back, Right

Selection 3.1: Charged with Murder

In today's world we all have to be careful and watch for identity theft. Identity theft can show up on your credit card or bank statements in the form of **charges** that you didn't make. You read stories all the time in the newspaper about people who have been **charged** with fraud using someone else's identity.

Last month I read a story about a man who was in **charge** of the family's medical supply business. His job was to keep track of all the things purchased by the business, all the income that came in, and all the credit card **charges** that were made by employees. It was a huge job that entailed a lot of responsibility.

The business fell on hard times, so the man began to **charge** the customers double what he had in the past. This made one customer angry, and he **charged** into the office on a cold rainy day and asked to see the man in **charge**. He was furious! He needed the supplies to take care of his terminally ill wife. He was so angry with the man behind the desk that he pulled out a revolver and shot him. The shot was fatal.

The following day the customer was arraigned in court and **charged** with first-degree murder. When the case finally went to trial, the judge **charged** the jury to consider all of the evidence. At the end of the article it stated that the jury had still not reached a consensus and was hoping to wrap everything up by the weekend.

How would you sign the following sentences?

1. The man was in **charge** of the family's medical supply business.

   _____

2. Do you check the **charges** on your bank statements monthly for fraud?

   _____

3. The man **charged** into the office and demanded to see the manager.

   _____

4. The man was **charged** with first-degree murder.

   _____

5. I think your **charge** is to be sure your team gets everything accomplished.

   _____

 Selection 3.2: The Military

Just think how much the military has changed since its inception back in the early days of this country. From foot soldiers and cannons, the military has **advanced**

into a whole new realm of technology as they use computers and satellites to **advance** their knowledge of the enemy and what strategies it needs to use to overtake them. **Advancements** in science, medicine, and technology have helped improve the way maneuvers are carried out today both on the homeland as well as abroad.

Remember in the days of Sherman and Lee, the troops would **advance** by foot or by horse. When the commander would shout "**Advance!**," the troops knew to move forward. Those who performed well and showed leadership potential quickly **advanced** up the ranks from private to lieutenant with the most outstanding candidates continuing on and becoming captains and generals.

Not all individuals support the notion that the military should engage in war. For some, the notion of violence is appalling, and they would rather focus on **advancing** the cause of peace. Sometimes these individuals hold protests in **advance** of political speeches, hoping to sway individuals to their views and their cause.

Some individuals are committed to serving our country and like the benefits of being in the armed forces. When they re-enlist, they like the fact that they get an **advance** that serves as a real bonus for them. Many of them also have their moving expenses paid for when they are required to relocate. Considering how much moving costs have **advanced** through the years, that helps make it worth it.

How would you sign the following sentences?

1. He **advanced** from private to sergeant.

   _____

2. Can I have an **advance** on my loan?

   _____

3. We have **advanced** our knowledge through science and technology.

   _____

4. Can we **advance** the time of the meeting until ten o'clock tomorrow?

   _____

5. We had **advance** warning that they were coming.

   _____

Selection 3.3: The Bride

Several years ago, my son's friend Brad got married. Brad and Kelly had grown up together and had double-dated through high school, so we considered him like one of our own. He married a girl he had dated all through high school, and we couldn't have been happier about his choice. She is a beautiful girl both inside and out.

Both Brad and his bride were about 25 when they got married. They picked a beautiful location, **around** thirty miles from Savannah. The church was small and quaint and had palm trees all **around** it. Not only was the outside picturesque, the bride had spent a great deal of time decorating on the inside. All of the pews had hurricane lamps with beautiful bows on them. Flower arrangements of calla lilies and roses had been set up every three feet **around** the semi-circular altar, and she had dropped white rose petals **around** on the aisle.

But the church was nothing compared with how beautiful the bride looked. Her blonde hair hung loosely **around** her shoulders, creating a natural but stunning look. Her strapless dress was covered with **around** 2,000 pearls and rhinestones. It must have cost a fortune. I know one of the relatives asked her mom how much the dress had cost, but her mother talked **around** the subject.

200

PART III
....
Multiple-Meaning
Words, Idioms, and
Vocabulary Building

At the reception, there were more flowers, an open bar, and a delicious dinner. When they rolled out the cake so the bride and groom could cut it, we were all amazed to see that it had to be at least seventy-two inches **around** at the base. It had six layers with fresh flowers on each one. It was lovely. They left the reception right after they cut the cake, because they had plans to travel **around** the world on their honeymoon. We left the reception **around** 10:30 and headed to a cottage close by for the night.

How would you sign the following sentences?

1. She talked **around** the subject when asked how much she paid for the dress.

   _____

2. The cake was seventy-two inches **around** at the base.

   _____

3. Her hair hung loosely **around** her shoulders.

   _____

4. There were **around** two hundred palm trees on the beach.

   _____

5. They will travel **around** the world on their honeymoon.

   _____

Selection 3.4: Politics

Getting into politics can be very difficult. Most people need financial **backing** from influential people before they can even begin their campaign. In order to get support, oftentimes candidates must make promises that they can't **back** out of later. This can prove challenging at best.

During campaign years candidates decide on issues they want to endorse. When they have the opportunity to debate these issues, they often are forced to go in through the **back** door in order to get their point across. Throughout the course of a campaign, you can usually look **back** through **back** issues of newspapers to see if the candidates changed their minds on how they feel. Sometimes these articles can be very revealing.

Oftentimes during speeches one candidate will **back** stab one of the other candidates. I hate it when that happens. I think they forget that they can't take **back** their words and that words can be very damaging. Once out of one's mouth, they can't turn their **back** on what they said.

Sometimes I think it would be fun to sneak in the **back** door of some of the candidate's headquarters, hide, and just listen to the candid remarks. It would be fun to see the person laid **back**, with his or her guard down, just airing true feelings. I know that will never happen, but it's fun to imagine.

One time I remember hearing of a politician who got mad at one of his aides when the aide talked **back** to him. The politician told him to go to the **back** of the room, sit in the chair, and just wait for him. It wasn't pleasant. All in all, politics can be an interesting game to watch and is not one the fainthearted want to play.

How would you sign the following sentences?

1. We found many interesting comments in the **back** issues of the newspaper.

   _____

2. He provided a substantial amount of financial **backing** for the candidate of his choice.

3. The politician told him to go to the **back** of the room and wait for him.

4. You can't take **back** your words once they are out of your mouth.

5. It would be fun to see a candidate laid **back** and hear his or her true opinions.

Selection 3.5: The Right Choice

Sometimes when you hire someone for a job, it's hard to know if you've made the **right** choice. Even though throughout the interview the person might have looked you **right** in the eye when you talked to him or her, you may still be unsure if that person will be all **right** for the job.

One of the ways you know if you selected the proper person is when issues come up that require objective responses. If the person responds from a **right**-wing or a left-wing perspective, you may feel that you are not getting the type of response that you need.

Another way you know if you hired the perfect person for the job is if he or she can respond when needed. If someone is off for the day, an emergency comes up, and you need for a person to come **right** away, the committed employee will find a way to get there as soon as possible. Even if the person doesn't live **right** in the same town, he or she will hop **right** in the car and come **right** up to the office.

When we interview people for a job, we use a form that has three columns. The column on the left is for positive attributes or favorable qualities. The column in the center is designed for neutral responses, and the one on the far **right** is for negative comments. The interviewee shouldn't have too many checks in the **right**-hand column if he or she wants to get the job.

When folks come in to interview for a job, they should wear the **right** attire, arrive **right** on time, and be **right** on the mark with their answers. If someone has a good personality and these other attributes are in place, there is a good chance that he or she is the **right** person for the job.

How would you sign the following sentences?

1. Sometimes there will be an emergency and you will need to come **right** away.

2. Please try to get as many check marks as you can in the **right**-hand column.

3. He looked **right** at her when he answered the questions.

4. It is important to arrive **right** on time for your job interview.

5. Are you feeling all **right** today? You look pale.

See, Take, Time, About, Raise

Selection 4.1: Needing Public Assistance

She was an older woman, and by the look of her clothes, her hair, and her over-all appearance, it was easy to **see** why she might need public assistance. When we had knocked on her door, we heard her call to someone inside, "Go to the door and **see** who it is." It was obvious that her eyesight wasn't good. When we showed her the papers from the court, she couldn't **see** the words clearly enough to make out what it said.

Her friend emerged from the kitchen and asked to talk with us in private. Once we went into another room, she told us she had been **seeing** to the care of the older woman. She asked us to please **see** that her friend would be taken care of. She was afraid that once she couldn't come by any more something awful would happen to her.

By the time we finished talking, it was getting late. We offered to **see** the older woman's friend home and told her we would be back in a few days to **see** how she was doing. Unfortunately, there are many people like her in the United States today. You **see** so often these individuals who live on a fixed income, and when unex-pected expenses come up, they don't have the resources to **see** to their basic needs.

She has been **seeing** a doctor, but when her medicine became too expensive, she stopped going. It was easy to **see** why she might be a good candidate for a nursing home. At least there they would **see** to it that she received the medicine she needed, had food to eat, and clean clothes to wear. We would have to **see** how we could help her achieve a better quality of life.

How would you sign the following sentences?

1. I can **see** why she probably needs public assistance.
   _____

2. She has been **seeing** a doctor for weeks but her condition hasn't improved.
   _____

3. We told her we would be back in a few days to **see** how she's doing.
   _____

4. Please go **see** who is at the door.
   _____

5. Looking at her clothes, it was easy to **see** that they had **seen** better days.
   _____

Selection 4.2: What's Your Take on It?

Andrew and Tara had a fight. She was so angry that she told him to **take** a hike. Instead, he followed her to McDonald's where she was ordering some **take**out food. He started to holler at her across the parking lot. She was trying to **take** in what he said, but she couldn't make sense out of a lot of it. He was saying some-thing to the effect that he didn't **take** her for granted, but she had heard the same song and dance before, and she was tired of it.

She decided to **take** her food home and eat it there. She didn't think she could **take** listening to him any longer. Once she got home and finished eating her salad, she decided she would go to her yoga class. She had **taken** up yoga six months ago when they first started having problems, and today would be a good day to **take** a drive over there and go to class.

She decided to **take** the back roads to get to her class, as this time of the day the interstate would be backed up. It was on one of the back roads that she saw the man **take** the woman's purse and run down the street. She tried to follow him in her car while she called 911, but he ran behind a couple of houses and she lost him. She went back to tell the woman she hadn't been successful, and she **took** the news very well.

Once the police arrived, they **took** down all of the information and said they'd be on the lookout for the man. At this point the woman had **taken** as much as she could; she started to cry and asked if someone could **take** her home. She thought she would **take** a nap, thinking that everything would look better when she'd had some rest.

You know, when things like this happen, I always wonder what the thief's motives are. Do you think it's for money, drugs, or just for the thrill of seeing if he can get away with it? Why do you think thieves do it? What's your **take** on it?

How would you sign the following sentences?

1. She got mad at her boyfriend and told him to **take** a hike.

   _____

2. She was tired of his thinking he could just **take** her for granted.

   _____

3. The officers **took** down all of the information.

   _____

4. She decided to **take** up yoga six months ago.

   _____

5. What's your **take** on the situation?

   _____

Selection 4.3: The Time of Our Lives

From **time** to **time** we have experiences that stand out as being exceptionally good or exceptionally bad. These experiences leave an indelible impression on our memories but with the passage of **time** will sometimes be forgotten. For some, the good experiences stand out as being the most memorable; others cling to experiences that were not as positive. I suppose that is why we have people who view the world negatively and those who are real upbeat and positive.

My aunt Peggy was one of those positive people; she always took **time** out to enjoy life. I remember the **time** when she was busy working, raising her children, and trying to make ends meet. She still managed to arrange **time** to play with her girls, read them books, and make sure they felt they were important.

She always kept a **time** out chair in the corner for when the girls forgot how to share, or when they decided their ideas were better than their mom's. It didn't happen often, but it was a good reminder for the girls to follow the Golden Rule.

One of the most memorable **times** we shared was when we took the girls to Disney World. They had the **time** of their lives. I think they went on all of the rides at least twice and sampled most of the goodies found in the park.

Another **time** that stands out in my memory was when the girls got older and we took them whitewater rafting. What a **time** we had going through the rapids! Wow! That was such an exciting experience, one that I will always cherish.

204

PART III
....
Multiple-Meaning
Words, Idioms, and
Vocabulary Building

Now **times** have changed. Several years after the rafting experience, my aunt Peggy became sick with cancer and passed away. I will always remember the good **times** we shared and the fun we had. It's **time** for the rest of us to follow her example, enjoy life, and make **time** for the things that are important. From **time to time** I think fondly of my Aunt Peggy.

How would you sign the following sentences?

1. We had the **time** of our lives.

   _____

2. She had a **time** out chair in the corner of her room for when the girls forgot to share.

   _____

3. From **time** to **time** we meet someone or have an experience that we will never forget.

   _____

4. My aunt Peggy used to say, "Take **time** to smell the roses."

   _____

5. What a **time** we had going through the rapids!

   _____

Selection 4.4: Character Education

Do any of the schools in your town have a Character Education program? You know, programs that focus on the values inherent in U.S. society. All of the schools in Georgia initiated a character education program **about** six years ago. Each school district follows a curriculum that focuses on topics such as respect, honesty, and fairness.

Some of the lessons are **about** famous people. Others talk **about** people the students know or would be likely to meet on a daily basis. I remember one story described a man who couldn't get **about** any longer. It focused on caring and how his family members took care of him and made sure all of his needs were met.

Another story talked **about** a girl who was caught cheating in class. She so wanted to be at the top of her class that she would do anything to get there. Within this short story, you got to hear the teacher's perspective. She said she was not **about** to give the girl a passing grade and reward her for her actions.

A teacher in another state heard about the program, called, and asked me **about** it. She wanted to know if she could borrow the curriculum. I told her I'd look **about** my office for it, see if I could find it, and then get it copied for her. I was **about** to start looking for it when the phone rang and I was reminded of a meeting I had to go to—so I left it for a task to complete later.

I'm all **about** sharing it with her. The content is good, the activities are a lot of fun, and the students seem to enjoy it. The whole curriculum is **about** 350 pages long, but it is well written. I know she'll be excited **about** receiving it. I hope when she implements it her students will enjoy it as much as ours have.

How would you sign the following sentences?

1. I'm all **about** sharing it with her.

   _____

2. She said she was not **about** to give the girl a passing grade.

   _____

3. I told her I'd look **about** my office for the book.

   _____

205

CHAPTER 4
See, Take, Time,
About, Raise

PART I

PART II

PART III

PART IV

4. The man hurt his back and couldn't get **about** any longer.

_____

5. I was **about** to start looking for it when it started to rain.

_____

Selection 4.5: Raise the Bar

The Club for the Deaf in Shreveport is always **raising** the bar to do bigger and better things. During the past several years, it has sponsored many students from the Louisiana School for the Deaf to attend summer camps and go to Gallaudet for Summer Learning vacations.

This year they are scheduling several fund **raising** activities so they can fund two scholarships and help worthy students attend one of the colleges or universities in Louisiana. They really are involved in worthwhile projects.

Last week I attended the meeting at its club house on the lake. People had to **raise** all of the windows in the building because the air conditioning had gone out. It really wasn't too bad in there. It was fun to go to the meeting. I got to see some children that I had all but helped **raise**. John and Suzie had worked at the Center when I was there, and I frequently took care of their children while they were out fund raising.

I remember a few years ago that building almost needed to be razed due to the antiquated electrical wiring. Luckily the club **raised** enough money to have the wiring replaced. It would have been sad if they had lost the building; it's a real beauty!

The next event that is scheduled is a spaghetti dinner. The group wanted to serve steak and potatoes, but the stores have **raised** the prices on beef again so they really can't afford to buy it. If they did, they'd have to charge more money for the tickets, and several members **raised** objections to that idea. Someone laughed and said if they wanted to serve steak they should start **raising** their own beef. We all thought that was pretty funny.

A couple of the members **raised** questions regarding the possibility of bringing in a famous Deaf professional to do a workshop. They thought people would pay to hear someone like I. King Jordan or Roz Rozen. It is something the club will explore throughout the year. All in all, it was a good meeting and very productive.

How would you sign the following sentences?

1. The Club for the Deaf in Shreveport knows how to **raise** the bar.

_____

2. The stores continue to **raise** the price of groceries, making it difficult to shop.

_____

3. A couple of members **raised** the question about bringing in a famous Deaf professional.

_____

4. Someone in the group **raised** an objection to **raising** the cost of the tickets.

_____

5. I **raised** my hand and asked a question about the Deaf professional.

_____

Short, Bank, Fall, Get Out, Line

Selection 5.1: Miss Deaf America

Have you ever been to a Miss Deaf America Pageant? Young women from all over the United States come and compete. When this event happens, they are never **short** on talent. It seems that only the brightest and the most talented make it to the stage.

Unlike the Miss America Pageant, you do not necessarily have to be tall to compete. Through the years several **short** women have participated in the event, and oftentimes the winner is between five feet and five foot four.

This year when the program planners were organizing the event they realized that they were one girl **short** of having an even number. This affected how the dance routines were choreographed. They had originally had an even number, but one girl's funding fell **short**. She didn't have enough funds to make it to the competition.

The program this year will include both a **short** and a long program. The **short** program will focus on the evening gown competition, the interview, and the talent competition. The long program will include those parts, as well as the sportswear, the commentary on community service, and how the young woman plans to spend her year as the winner.

Some of the girls make the mistake of giving **short** answers. They don't realize that the judges are looking for them to expand on their ideas, and by doing so some of them stop **short** of really getting to the meat of the discussion. Sometimes, when a contestant is unsure of an answer, she tends to respond with a **short** "yes" or "no." This will often make her come up **short** on points.

I look forward to this event every year. I prefer watching the long program over the **short** one. It is so refreshing to see all of the talent in the Deaf community.

How would you sign the following sentences?

1. Some of the girls make the mistake of giving **short** answers.

   _____

2. This year they are one girl **short** of having an even number for the dance routines.

   _____

3. The one contestant couldn't come because her funding fell **short**.

   _____

4. Even the girls who are **short** can compete in the event and oftentimes win.

   _____

5. This year they will only record the **short** program, not the long one.

   _____

207

CHAPTER 5

Short, Bank, Fall,
Get Out, Line

PART I

PART II

PART III

PART IV

Selection 5.2: Online Dating

Have you ever done any online dating? For individuals who don't have time to go out and socialize on a daily basis, this is becoming a popular way to meet people. Although it's not for everyone, if you use common sense it can be a way to meet some very interesting people.

Most online dating services keep a **bank** of names in their database. They charge a fee for you to access people's personality traits, but the fee that they charge is nominal and won't break the **bank**. You can usually find several people with interests that are similar to your own.

One time my friend Sarah met an IT specialist online. He lived in the northeast and would tell her stories about driving in the snow. It seems as if he worked in a **bank** and had to travel through the mountains in order to get to work. One day he was driving on slippery roads—the road **banked** to the left, and before he knew it he had ended up in a snow **bank.** At first he didn't call anyone for help because he **banked** on the fact that someone would see him and help him out.

However, after waiting for thirty minutes he realized that wasn't going to happen and he needed to call someone for help. At first he looked through the **bank** of numbers stored in his cell phone. After getting the answering machine on a few calls, he decided he better call 9-1-1.

It didn't take too long before a tow truck arrived on the scene and pulled him out of the snow **bank**. He really learned his lesson that day. He drove far more cautiously after that when he was in inclement weather.

Although my friend enjoyed visiting with him online, she realized that she could not live in the Northeast, so they remained good cyberfriends and nothing more than that.

How would you sign the following sentences?

1. He had a **bank** of numbers in his cell phone.

    _____

2. He was **banking** on the fact that someone would see he was in distress and stop and help him.

    _____

3. He lost control of the car and ended up in a snow **bank.**

    _____

4. The road **banked** to the left.

    _____

5. He worked at a **bank** in the Northeast.

    _____

Selection 5.3: Fall Festival

Do you have a **fall** festival in your town? We have one every year, and it's become so popular that people drive from all around just to participate. During that time, a lot of merchants set up booths, and you have to be careful not to trip and **fall** over any of the cords that are used by the vendors.

In my part of the country, the festival takes place when the weather is still warm. You don't have to worry about early snows happening, but you do have to watch for sudden showers that can bring torrents of rain **falling** from the clouds. And, the temperature might **fall** after the rain.

208

PART III
....
Multiple-Meaning
Words, Idioms, and
Vocabulary Building

There are always so many activities at the festival that you don't have to worry about anyone **falling** asleep. Even older folks who are in that habit of taking afternoon naps manage to stay awake during the daily activities. People have been known to **fall** in love with some of the crafts that they see and end up purchasing probably more treasures than they ever thought they would buy.

One year my cousins had a **falling** out with each other. Neither of them wanted to see the other one at the festival, so they both ended up staying home. I thought that was rather foolish, but sometimes you can't reason with anger.

Another year a friend of mine got suckered into buying something that wasn't worth the material it was made of. When the merchant started to describe the struggles she had endured making her trinkets, my friend **fell** for it and bought her sob story hook, line, and sinker. It was only later when my friend saw the same kind of trinkets in the store that she realized she'd been had.

I love the **fall** festival! I love visiting with old friends, making new friends, and just being out in the warm weather. It is the last chance to really have a good time before football season begins. Once that happens, there are no quiet weekends until Christmas.

How would you sign the following sentences?

1. One year my cousins had a **falling** out with each other.

   _____

2. Sometimes people **fall** in love with the crafts the merchants bring.

   _____

3. She was so gullible that she **fell** for her story and bought it hook, line, and sinker.

   _____

4. Sometimes during the festival torrents of rain **fall** from the clouds.

   _____

5. You have to watch the cords so you don't **fall** over them and get hurt.

   _____

Selection 5.4: The Graduation Party

I've been invited to Erika's graduation party, and I really don't want to go. It's being held in a noisy restaurant, and I won't know half of the people. I'm going to see if I can **get out** of going. Besides, what would I wear? I **got** something on my favorite pants and I can't seem to **get out** the stain. If I really have to go, I'll have to stop by the bank first and **get out** some money. Otherwise, I won't be able to **get** anything to eat or drink if I don't like what they're serving.

Erika and I met when we were both in college. We were riding an elevator to the third floor when the doors refused to open, and we couldn't **get out**. We were both so embarrassed when help finally came and we realized that it was the strap on my book bag that had gotten lodged between the two doors. That's why they refused to open.

We tried to keep quiet about what had happened, but eventually it **got out**, and people would stop and ask me about my famous door-jamming book bag. The story **got** old in a hurry. After that Erika and I became fast friends, and regardless what we did together, it always seemed to spell disaster.

One time we were in the cafeteria when a runaway cart was headed right toward us. We couldn't **get out** of the way fast enough. Before we knew it, we were both sprawled out on the floor. When we tried to explain what had happened, the cafeteria supervisor walked away before we could **get out** a word. We thought that was rude at the time but then realized she had just gone to **get** help, as she honestly thought we were hurt.

I guess I better **get out** of here and go to the party. The more I think of the things we've been through, the more I realize that it would be wrong of me if I didn't show up. Besides, I would want Erika to do the same for me. She's really been a great friend, and she's always been there to **get** me out of trouble when I couldn't **get out** of it by myself.

How would you sign the following sentences?

1. We couldn't **get out** of the way of the moving cart fast enough to avoid being hurt.

   _____

2. Maybe I can **get out** of going to the party.

   _____

3. I couldn't **get out** the stain on my pants.

   _____

4. She walked away before I could **get out** a word.

   _____

5. I'll go to the bank tomorrow and **get out** some money.

   _____

Selection 5.5: The Great Depression

Many of your grandparents or great-grandparents may have experienced the Great Depression. It was a time during the history of this country when the stock market crashed. Thousands of people lost money when the banks failed; businesses failed, and thousands of people were out of work. It didn't matter what **line** of work you were in, jobs just weren't available.

During that time, there were long **lines** of people waiting to get food and help so they could survive. The **lines** of cars that had previously **lined** the streets were nonexistent, as people couldn't afford to buy the gas. Those lucky enough to keep a job often had to rely on the bus **line** to transport them back and forth to work.

Those were the years when the banks didn't have any money. It didn't matter what your previous **line** of credit had been—there just wasn't any money to give out. Many people became desperate and turned to violence. That's where the government drew the **line.** The authorities said they were willing to help anyone but would not tolerate disobedience. It seemed like on a daily basis there was a **line** up at the police station where would-be offenders stood in a row waiting to be identified and later prosecuted. Sometimes the **lines** people used to declare their innocence would have almost been funny if the times hadn't been so hard.

Those who needed food were asked to sign their names or make an X on the **line** stating that they agreed to pay back the money once jobs were available again. It was a stressful time for everyone. People who lived during that time have no desire to experience it again.

210

PART III
....
Multiple-Meaning
Words, Idioms, and
Vocabulary Building

I can remember going into my great uncle's house. He had lived through the Depression and placed his canned goods all **lined** up in perfect rows on his pantry shelves. He said he never wanted to be hungry again, and he was preparing for the worst. It was indeed a dark time in U.S. history.

How would you sign the following sentences?

1. The government drew the **line** at violence; the authorities would not tolerate disobedience.

    _____

2. It didn't matter what **line** of work you were in, jobs were still scarce.

    _____

3. The bus **line** was used to take people back and forth to work.

    _____

4. It didn't matter what your former **line** of credit had been; there just wasn't any money.

    _____

5. The cars no longer **lined** the streets, as there was a shortage of fuel.

    _____

CHAPTER 6

Put, Pass, Shake, Pick, On

Selection 6.1: Getting a New Job

Justin was recently fired from his job, and it was right after he **put** in for a raise. Although he's **putting** up a good front, I know it bothers him. He had worked for a real jerk and finally decided he couldn't **put** up with his behavior any more. He knew his boss didn't like him either, and he finally **put** two and two together and decided he should look for a new job. But, before he had a chance to resign, he was fired. I've **put** in a good word for him at work, but so far there haven't been any openings. He **put** in for unemployment, but when they asked him to **put** down his address, he wasn't sure what to **put**, as he knew he'd have to move out of his apartment soon. In the meantime he has been helping his girlfriend **put** up curtains in her new apartment and **put** away boxes. With his free time he has discovered that he can **put** together a pretty good dinner.

Being fired can be a real **put** down. When someone says things that hurt your feelings or make you mad, you want to say something back and **put** them in their place. It's no fun. I hope that he'll find a new job soon so he can **put** all of this behind him.

How would you sign the following sentences?

1. Although he's **putting** up a good front, I know it bothers him.

   _____

2. He decided he couldn't **put** up with his behavior any more.

   _____

3. He **put** in for unemployment, but he didn't know what to **put** down for his address.

   _____

4. Being fired can be a real **put** down.

   _____

5. I hope that he'll find a new job soon so he can **put** all of this behind him.

   _____

 ### Selection 6.2: The Cute Graduate Assistant

What is the name of that cute graduate assistant who works with Dr. Phillips? He was **passing** out papers the other day, and I swear he made a **pass** at me. I have only spoken to him in **passing**, but I think he's really cool! I'm really not sure if he was flirting with me or not, but if so, that would be ok. He could **pass** for a movie star. He looks just like one—you know, tall, dark, handsome, and very athletic. I think his grandparents came from Italy, and his good looks have proba-bly been **passed** down from one generation to another.

I **passed** by him the other day in the library, but we were both in a hurry so neither of us slowed down to talk. Then, this morning he **passed** me in his car, honked and waved like we were old friends. I really think he's trying to get to know me. I hope he's not just being nice because he helps with the class that I'm taking. I'd hate to be **passed** over for someone who's cuter or smarter.

Sometimes I find myself dreaming about him. The other day I dreamed that I had **passed** out and he rescued me. He didn't **pass** the buck and ask someone else to take care of me. Instead, he did it himself. It was a great dream. Maybe I should try talking to him instead of just dreaming about him. I sure don't want life to **pass** me by. Who knows? He could be "Mr. Right."

How would you sign the following sentences?

1. I swear he made a **pass** at me.

   _____

2. I've only spoken to him in **passing**.

   _____

3. I **passed** by him in the library the other day, but we didn't have time to talk.

   _____

4. I had a dream that I **passed** out and he rescued me.

   _____

5. I don't want life to **pass** me by.

   _____

Selection 6.3: Working for an Independent Company

My dad works for an independent company. Last week they had a **shake** up at work. Apparently someone had been involved in some pretty shady deals, and when he got caught, he was on pretty **shaky** ground. As a matter of fact, he did-n't have any ground to stand on at all. Although he claimed he didn't get a fair **shake**, he's lucky that he didn't end up in jail. Everyone at work was pretty **shaken** by the whole ordeal. I don't know what possessed the man to get involved with such disreputable characters. I guess he just wasn't thinking.

Now everyone who works there is wondering what will **shake** down from the top. They don't know if security will be tightened, if new rules will be imposed, or if business will just continue as usual. The last time something like this hap-pened, the parties involved decided to air their differences, reach a conclusion, and end the discussion with a hand**shake.** No one knows if it will end the same way this time. It just makes you feel all **shaky** inside thinking about what might hap-pen next. My dad said he was just glad this kind of thing doesn't happen often. If it did, I think he'd have to look for a new job. He pretty much likes the status quo and doesn't like working in a **shaky** environment.

How would you sign the following sentences?

1. Everyone at work was pretty **shaken** up by the whole ordeal.

   _____

2. Although he didn't feel like he got a fair **shake**, he is lucky he didn't get put in jail.

3. It just makes you feel all **shaky** inside wondering what will happen next.

4. Last week they had a **shake** up at work.

5. Now folks are wondering what will **shake** down from the top.

Selection 6.4: Playing on the Dodgeball Team

Did you hear that Reid and Davis got **picked** to play on the national dodgeball team? The manager of the team called them and told them to **pick** a time when they could come by, sign the papers, and **pick** up their gear. Neither of them could believe they made the team.

Reid called Davis and told him he could **pick** him up around 3:30 on Wednesday, and they could go by the field house to get their gear. They want to get there early before everything is too **picked** over. Davis said that time would work fine for him—he didn't have anything planned for Wednesday anyway. Reid told him if he wanted they could stop by and **pick** up a bite to eat on the way, as he would have to work until around 3:00.

Davis said that was fine and asked Reid if he knew where he wanted to eat. He knew that Reid was a **picky** eater and that any place he might suggest wouldn't be quite what he wanted. He also knew that Reid would need a **pick** me up after working out in the sun all day.

Reid said he would **pick** between two places and would let Davis make the final choice when he arrived. He said he'd be driving his brother's old **pickup** when he came to get him because his car was in the shop being fixed.

My friend Joe said he hoped they knew what they were in for. Three of his friends had gotten hurt playing dodgeball. One had to have ten stitches taken in his chin, another broke his arm, and a third ended up **picking** up his teeth off the field. I do hope they will fare better than Joe's friends.

How would you sign the following sentences?

1. They want to select their gear before it gets too **picked** over.

2. Reid is a very **picky** eater. It is hard to find a place where he likes to eat.

3. Davis will need a **pick** me up after working all day in the sun.

4. Reid and Davis were **picked** for the dodgeball team.

5. He said he would **pick** you up in the old **pickup**, as his car is in the shop.

Selection 6.5: What's the Name of That Book?

What is the name of that book that everyone's been talking about? You know, the one that was **on** the *New York Times* bestseller list for months last summer? It

214

PART III
....
Multiple-Meaning
Words, Idioms, and
Vocabulary Building

focuses **on** how to get ahead financially, and it was **on** display at our local bookstore for weeks. We left **on** vacation before I could get a copy of it, and now it doesn't seem to be **on** any of the shelves.

The neat thing about the book is that it is supposed to give you pointers, not just go **on** and **on** with worthless information. I got turned **on** to reading books on finance after I took a basic course in economics. Now that I'm **on** to some of the secrets, I can't seem to get enough of the books.

I like to spend my Saturday mornings **on** the river just reading. It's so relaxing and so much better than just staying at home, turning **on** the TV and watching cartoons. I don't mind turning **on** sports in the afternoon, but I do enjoy the tranquility that the water provides early in the morning. Then, in the afternoon when all of the boaters get **on** the lake, it is so noisy that it loses some of its appeal for me.

On Saturday, I plan to go to the local bookstores in Atlanta. I figure that where it is a bigger city, surely a bookstore there will have it. If not, I can always request that the library get it through interlibrary loan. Or I could go **on** the Internet and try to find it there. I'll call you **on** Monday and let you know if I find it—if not, perhaps you can get **on** it and help me.

How would you sign the following sentences?

1. The book does not go **on** and **on** with worthless information.

   _____

2. I got turned **on** to finance after I took a basic course in economics.

   _____

3. I love to take my book, get in a boat **on** the river, and just read.

   _____

4. The book was **on** the bestseller list for weeks.

   _____

5. Now that I'm **on**to some of the secrets, I can't read enough of the books.

   _____

CHAPTER 7

After, Bare, Cool, Draw, Meet

Selection 7.1: Babies, Baseball, and Bob

After high school, Bob stayed home to look **after** his mom. His dad had been killed in a car accident during his senior year, and his mom wasn't doing well. He decided he needed to stay with her as she made the transition from being a married woman to being a widow. **After** a couple of years, she seemed so much better that Bob decided he could get on with his life.

He had played baseball in high school and had been recruited by a college near his home. The coach had told him that **after** he reached a point at which he could leave his mom, he would like to have him play. You see, he took **after** his dad, the famous Braves pitcher. He arrived at the field **after** the regularly scheduled practices had started, but the coach told him to suit up and come onto the field.

The team practiced late in the day **after** classes were over. Even **after** weeks of practice, the team was looking pretty ragged, and the coach was worried about the first game. Much to his surprise, they won! They went on to take the state championship **after** they captured the district and the region.

Shortly **after** the championship, Bob meet Betty and they started dating. Within the year they were married. Now they have two children—their first daughter looks like Betty and the second one takes **after** Bob. I wonder if she'll become a softball player and live happily ever **after** on the baseball diamond like her dad.

How would you sign the following sentences?

1. **After** his dad died, he stayed home and looked **after** his mother.

   _____

2. The team practiced late in the day **after** classes were over.

   _____

3. He takes **after** his dad; he is a true athlete.

   _____

4. She is petite with blue eyes and blonde hair; she takes **after** her mom.

   _____

5. In most fairy tales the couple lives happily ever **after**.

   _____

Selection 7.2: Old Mother Snodgrass

All of you have heard the story about Old Mother Hubbard. You know the woman who had no food—her cupboards were **bare**, her refrigerator was **bare**, and there was nothing in the house for her or her dog to eat. Well, Old Mother Snodgrass was pretty much just like her. She lived in a **barren** part of the country—almost like the desert. There were no homes for miles, and nothing would grow on her land.

She wore thread**bare** clothes, walked **bare**footed around the house, and **barely** had enough to eat. Actually, when you looked around her house, you realized that she had just the **bare** essentials she needed just to stay alive. She had running water, and one shelf in her pantry was full of soup. All the other shelves were **bare**.

Some days it seemed like she could **barely** get out of bed, let alone get dressed. Even though a lot of people were worried about her, most of them stopped checking on her because they were afraid of the wild dogs who roamed around her property. Most of the time when people would drive up and try to get out of their cars, the dogs would **bare** their teeth at them and bark. People were afraid of what might happen if they tried to approach the house. Most folks never made it out of their cars, let alone in her front door, but those who did said her walls were **bare**. What's more, in the winter they said there was **barely** enough heat to keep her warm, let alone comfortable.

I've often wondered what ever became of Old Mother Snodgrass. Even though I **barely** knew her, I wanted something better for her. I wanted life to be kinder to her and provide her with more than just the **bare** necessities.

How would you sign the following sentences?

1. Her shelves were almost empty and she **barely** had enough to eat.

   _____

2. The dogs were mean and would **bare** their teeth at passersby.

   _____

3. She lived in a very **barren** part of the country.

   _____

4. In the winter, there was **barely** enough heat to keep her warm.

   _____

5. She had the **bare** essentials to eke out a living.

   _____

 Selection 7.3: Cookout at the Club for the Deaf

Last Saturday was the cookout at the Metro Club for the Deaf. Jason was in charge of all of the preparations, and it seemed as if the cookout was doomed before it ever got started. It all started when Jason asked Todd to put the meat in the **cooler**. Well, you guessed it, Todd forgot. About two hours later, Jason realized the meat was still on the counter. He was about to lose his **cool** when he realized the meat was still partially frozen and not ruined.

Next Jason went to check on the grill. He forgot that he had turned it on high to preheat it, and when he went back to check on it, he realized that he would have to let it **cool** down before he could cook anything on it. That would mean that he would be late starting the steaks. At that point, he decided it was too hot to stay outside and that he needed to **cool** off in the clubhouse.

That is when the real trouble started. Pete was in there, running his mouth making cracks about Jason. Usually, Pete is a pretty **cool** dude, but he'd had a few too many beers, and he was wagging his tongue just to hear himself talk. He said Jason shouldn't have been in charge of the cookout and that at the rate he was going they'd never get to eat. Jason decided he needed to keep his **cool**, and **cool** off before he flew off the handle at Pete.

Between the meat, the grill, and Pete, Jason wasn't having a good day. Then it hit him that he had forgotten to ask anyone to pick up the beans from the deli and the cake from the bakery. This was not **cool**. Now he didn't know what he was going to do to salvage the cookout. All he could to was text message his buddy and ask him to pick up the rest of the stuff and bring it on his way to the club house. He sure hoped he could reach him.

How would you sign the following sentences?

1. Pete is usually a pretty **cool** guy.

   _____

2. He decided he'd better **cool** off before he flew off the handle at him.

   _____

3. Jason went in the clubhouse so he could **cool** off.

   _____

4. He needed to let the grill **cool** down before he could cook on it.

   _____

5. It wouldn't be **cool** if everyone found out he forgot to pick up the beans and the cake.

   _____

Selection 7.4: Studying Drafting at NTID

Did you know that NTID has an excellent drafting program? It teaches its students how to **draw** using CAD—a computer-aided drafting program. Talented students from all over the country are **drawn** to that program. It prepares them to be highly competitive and marketable. Not only do they take several academic classes but a number of skills courses as well.

During the semester they participate in several projects. For one of them, they **draw** names and are put in groups of three to complete a challenging design. Then they have to **draw** on all of their previous experience to develop the best design possible. The winning team is awarded a thousand dollars and a really neat plaque. Last year the competitors were so talented that the competition ended in a **draw**. The judges honestly couldn't make a decision about which team had the better design.

When the **drawings** were put on display, they **drew** accolades from all who saw them due to the technical ability exhibited by the students. Their work in general was incredible. The reputation for the contest has spread across campus, and now the exhibition **draws** big crowds. Once the calendar for the academic year is **drawn** up and students and faculty know when the event is going to be, many make sure well in advance that they will have time to go by and admire the work. It has been a great way to showcase the students' abilities and talents.

How would you sign the following sentences?

1. Last year the competition was so stiff it ended in a **draw**.

   _____

2. Students from all over the country are **drawn** to that program.

   _____

218

PART III
....
Multiple-Meaning
Words, Idioms, and
Vocabulary Building

3. The exhibition displaying the students' work **draws** big crowds.

_____

4. The academic calendar is **drawn** up early in the summer.

_____

5. We **drew** names to determine who our **drawing** partners would be.

_____

Selection 7.5: The Swimming Meet

Sheryl and her twin sister Sam both compete on the swimming team. Last week they had a **meeting** after school to discuss the upcoming **meet.** The coach told them which teams would be competing, which events they would participate in, and what time they needed to show up.

He told them if anyone wasn't planning on coming they needed to let him know by Friday so he could **meet** the deadline and only register those who were planning to compete. The registration fee for each swimmer was $25.00, and he didn't want to pay for anyone who knew they couldn't attend.

After the **meeting** Sheryl told Sam she needed to **meet** with one of her teachers because she needed to redo a paper. Apparently, what she had written didn't **meet** the teacher's expectations, and she was going to have to do it over. She didn't want to risk a bad grade and get thrown off the team. She didn't know if the teacher would **meet** her halfway and just let her rewrite part of it or if she'd have to redo the whole thing. She was hoping that's what she'd do. She told Sam to go ahead and she'd **meet** up with her later at the house.

How would you sign the following sentences?

1. The paper that Sam wrote didn't **meet** the teacher's expectations.

_____

2. The swimming **meet** was scheduled for a week from Saturday.

_____

3. We've got to submit our registrations today if we want to **meet** the deadline.

_____

4. I'll **meet** up with you after I finish what I'm doing.

_____

5. Do you think she will **meet** me halfway and accept what I've done?

_____

CHAPTER 8

Box, Ring, Jump

Selection 8.1: Taking on a New Meaning

Let me tell you about the word **box**. It has taken on several different meanings over the past decades. We all know that we can use a **box** to put our things in and that **box** can mean to fight. I remember my dad watching **boxing** matches on TV every Friday night when I was growing up.

I'm sure you've heard the expression, "I will **box** your ears if you do that again." Of course, this means that if you keep doing something inappropriate, it will not fare well for you. We have also heard the expression that you need to think outside the **box.** When **box** is used in this way, it means that you should look for alternate solutions to a problem.

However, how many of you have heard the expression, "he's **box**," meaning that he is a special needs student? Apparently, the expression was developed when special education students received all of their instruction in one room rather than being included in other classrooms. The phrase then was extended to "quit acting **box**," meaning that the person was acting crazy.

These expressions have given a whole new meaning to the word **"box."**

How would you sign the following sentences?

1. My dad used to watch **boxing** on TV every Friday night when I was growing up.

   _____

2. Do you have a **box** that I can put the sweater in so I can mail it back?

   _____

3. I'm going to **box** your ears in if you don't stop doing that.

   _____

4. Quit acting **box**—I don't like it.

   _____

5. What does the word **box** mean to you? What do you think of when you hear it?

   _____

Selection 8.2: Expressions That Include "Ring"

Have you heard people from England say "**Ring** me up when you're ready to go" or the expression "**ring** my chimes"? These expressions use the word "**ring**" in different contexts than many people are used to hearing.

220

PART III
....
Multiple-Meaning
Words, Idioms, and
Vocabulary Building

For many of us when we hear the word **ring**, we think of a piece of jewelry or a **ring** around the bathtub. Some think of the **ring** where boxing matches take place while others think of a celebration, as in "**ring** in the New Year." Pre-K teachers tell children they will play **Ring**-around-the-Rosy, and on field day they will have a **ring** toss.

My mom used to say she'd **wring** my neck if I did something wrong, and my brother says his son is a dead **ringer** for Uncle Ralph. Some words just have a nice **ring** to them, while others we wish we would never hear repeated.

How would you sign the following sentences?

1. Some think of the **ring** where boxing matches take place.

   _____

2. Let's all get together on December 31st and **ring** in the New Year.

   _____

3. I need to clean my bathtub; it has a dark **ring** around it.

   _____

4. **Ring** me up when you want to go.

   _____

5. She is a dead **ringer** for my Aunt Kate.

   _____

Selection 8.3: Thinking Before You Leap

Why do some people **jump** the gun and form conclusions that aren't accurate? Like the time I had to have someone **jump** start my car, and he assumed I had left my lights on, when in fact I needed a new alternator. It's like people don't have the full picture before they react.

Some people just get **jumpy** when they are anxious or are under a lot of stress and respond without thinking. Other times people quickly **jump** for joy without realizing that their response was premature. Then they're in for a huge disappointment when the reality of the situation hits them. Other times people **jump** into situations with both feet before they realize what they've done. Then they have to **jump** through a number of hoops to get out of the mess they've created.

We've all been guilty of **jumping** on the bandwagon before we have a clear picture of what or who we're supporting. Then we have to find a graceful way to disassociate ourselves from the situation before we suffer further embarrassment.

The bottom line is that we should all think before we leap and find ourselves in situations we didn't bargain for only because we **jumped** on something too quickly.

How would you sign the following sentences?

1. Sam **jumped** the gun and bought the drinks for the party before it was scheduled.

   _____

2. When I found out I had passed the class, I **jumped** for joy.

   _____

3. How many hoops did you have to **jump** through to get the idea approved?

_____

4. Will you **jump** on the bandwagon and support that cause?

_____

5. Can you try **jump** starting my car? It won't start.

_____

CHAPTER 9

Out, Use, Over, Kick, Mind

Selection 9.1: The Outing

I'm going **out** of town this weekend to see my best friend. I haven't seen him for months, and I'm really looking forward to it. He lives in Atlanta and is a huge Braves fan. He said while I was there he'd take me **out** to a ballgame. That would be great! The last time I visited him, we went to a game, and I can still remember it.

It was a close game, and during the ninth inning the bases were loaded and there were two **outs**. The score was tied, and the Braves were depending on the next run to win the game. The batter hit the ball **out** into the **out**field, where it was caught, and the score remained tied. The game continued for six more innings before the Braves finally got a run and won the game. Some of the fans from Cleveland were so angry they got **out** of control. They started throwing bottles and protesting and got thrown **out** of the stadium by the police. They were really **out** of line.

I don't know what people get **out** of acting that way. It doesn't change anything and if anything just sets a bad example for kids. People who act that way should be banned from the stadium. It just takes a lot of fun **out** of going to the games. By the time we left the game I was worn **out** from all the excitement.

How would you sign the following sentences?

1. The fans were throwing bottles so the police threw them **out** of the stadium.

    _____

2. Sometimes people talk or behave in a way that is way **out** of line.

    _____

3. I don't know what people get **out** of acting that way.

    _____

4. He said he'd take me **out** to a ballgame.

    _____

5. I was worn **out** from all the excitement.

    _____

Selection 9.2: The Old Junker

Justin has had his old junker of a car for years. It **uses** so much gas; every time you turn around he's filling it up again. It must be almost fifteen years old. Back in its day, it **used** to be a good car, but now it needs more repairs than it's probably worth.

For some reason Justin just won't part with it. I don't know what's wrong with him. He just isn't **using** his head. He should be able to see that it's not worth much any more. I've talked to him about it until I'm blue in the face, but it's no **use.** He just refuses to buy a new one. Instead, what does he do? Every time his car ends up in the shop, he asks if he can **use** mine. I only **use** mine once or twice a month, so it doesn't have many miles on it, but that's not the point. He needs to buy a new one.

It's not like he doesn't have any money—and besides, if he doesn't want payments he could buy a **used** one. I think he's pretty tight. He would want to get money for his old car if he traded it in, and I don't know anyone who would have a **use** for his old one. It would be different if he didn't **use** it everyday. He lives thirty miles from work and depends on it to get him back and forth. I've **used** up all my energy talking to him about it. He'll just have to come to the realization that he needs a new car on his own.

How would you sign the following sentences?

1. Back in its day, it **used** to be a really good car.

   _____

2. He needs to **use** his head and figure out how much the old junker is costing him.

   _____

3. He **uses** my car every time his is in the shop.

   _____

4. Would you have a **use** for an old junker? I wouldn't.

   _____

5. I've **used** up all of my energy trying to convince him to buy a new car.

   _____

Selection 9.3: Planning the Fall Festival

Who's in charge of the fall festival this year? Remember last year when that crazy lady was in charge? She was really in **over** her head. She was so afraid that someone would try to put something **over** on her that she made us look **over** the budget a million times. She was so sure she would **over**look something and then we would blame her if it wasn't a success.

She was so scatterbrained and uptight that we all knew if the slightest thing went wrong, it would push her **over** the edge. It was as if she made the slightest mistake it would take her forever to get **over** it. I know all of us used to be so glad when her meetings were **over**. We just got so tired of sitting and listening to the same information **over** and **over** again. I think if I had had to go to too many more meetings it would have pushed me **over** the top. She would say that the meetings would be **over** by three but invariably they would continue until five or six.

One time she totally lost it. Someone had jumped **over** one of the items on the agenda. When she realized it, she went off on a tirade of how we should be paying better attention. Someone finally told her she needed to get **over** it. Wow! I'm not sure how we got stuck with her last year, but this year we have to have a better chairperson. If not, I'm going to resign at the end of the first meeting. I can't go through this again two years in a row.

How would you sign the following sentences?

1. This is a demanding project and she is in way **over** her head.

   _____

2. Someone jumped **over** one of the agenda items, and it really made her mad.

   _____

3. We told her that she needed to get **over** it and quit ranting.

   _____

4. She asked us to look **over** the budget to make sure there wasn't a mistake.

   _____

5. She was so afraid that someone would put something **over** on her.

   _____

Selection 9.4: Paint Ball Wars

Have you ever gone anywhere where you can have a paint ball war? You know, where you dress up in painter's clothes and then shoot paint balls at each other? It's a real **kick.** We used to go and play every Saturday until we got **kicked** out of the place where you could go and play. It's all because Kelly **kicked** one of the balls instead of throwing it and in the process tore up the grass. It was pretty funny, but the manager didn't think so.

He told us we could either chip in and pay for the damage, or we couldn't come back. Kelly **kicked** up a fuss at that idea, so we've lost our favorite place to play. And what makes it worse is that we haven't found another place in town that has paint ball. We've found places that play **kick**ball, but that really isn't what we're looking for. I guess we're just going to have to **kick** the habit and find a new sport.

What made it so much fun for me was going with Kelly. He has been my side**kick** for years, and we've had a lot of good **kicks** together. Now, we'll have to look for another way to have some fun.

How would you sign the following sentences?

1. I guess we're just going to have to **kick** the habit.

   _____

2. He has been my side**kick** for years.

   _____

3. We got **kicked** out of the park for being rowdy.

   _____

4. He really **kicked** at the idea of having to pay for the damage.

   _____

5. Kelly is such a **kick.** I like doing things with him.

   _____

Selection 9.5: Terrible Twos

I know you've all heard of the terrible twos, that wonderful age when little people seem to have **minds** of their own. At this delightful stage, they like to use the word "no" and oftentimes won't **mind** their parents. They are curious little toddlers who like to explore and frequently look for ways to venture into new territory.

My friend Joe doesn't **mind** if they are adventuresome and curious as long as they **mind** their own business. I asked him one time if he would **mind** looking after my 2-year-old, and he said he wouldn't **mind** taking care of him if I would promise to be back on time. While he was **minding** my son, I took advantage of the time to do some Christmas shopping. **Mind** you, when I returned, I found Joe and my son playing together on the floor. They were engaged in a **mind**-bending exercise that only Joe could come up with.

I had a **mind** to remind Joe that he said he would take care of him as long as it didn't require any extra effort on his part. You would have never guessed how engaged he would get with this little person. Sometimes I don't think we know our own **minds** and surprise ourselves when we are given the opportunity to do things we didn't think we'd enjoy in the first place.

How would you sign the following sentences?

1. Two-year-olds can have **minds** of their own.

   _____

2. Do you **mind** watching him for me while I do some Christmas shopping?

   _____

3. **Mind** you, when I returned, the two of them were playing on the floor.

   _____

4. You need to make up your **mind** if you're going to go or stay.

   _____

5. Sometimes we need to **mind** our own business so we won't get in trouble.

   _____

Bone, Miss, Low, Cut, Point

Selection 10.1: Studying for the Test

Have you ever had a professor schedule a test right after Thanksgiving? I have. Last year my anatomy teacher scheduled her test on **bones** for the day after we got back from Thanksgiving break. So, after eating dinner, my mom said she would **bone** the turkey while I went off to study. I thanked her for cleaning up for us and didn't stay to help, as I knew I had a lot to learn before the big test.

While I went into my room to **bone** up on the material, my mom started working on the turkey. I was about halfway through learning all of the **bones** in the body when my brother came in and said he had a **bone** to pick with me. I could tell that he was really ticked off. He started ranting and raving, and it took me a few minutes to realize what he was upset about.

Then I got it. He thought I had given the dog a turkey **bone** to chew on. What a **bone**head, like I would do something like that! I told him that I hadn't done any such thing, that the dog had probably gotten in the trash and pulled one out. For some reason, it never occurred to him that the dog could have done it on his own. After he left, it took me a good thirty minutes to get back on track.

How would you sign the following sentences?

1. Mom told me that she would **bone** the turkey while I went to study.

   _____

2. My brother told me that he had a **bone** to pick with me.

   _____

3. I went into my room to **bone** up on the material.

   _____

4. The test was going to cover all of the **bones** in the human body.

   _____

5. Why would anyone give a dog a turkey **bone** unless he just didn't know any better?

   _____

Selection 10.2: Missing Miss Brooks

I really **miss Miss** Brooks. She worked here for over ten years and took such great care of all of us. Now that she's gone, we've been interviewing people almost daily trying to fill her position. The last woman who applied has **missed** three appointments, and we've yet to interview her. She seems to have the best qualifications, but she just can't seem to get here.

227

CHAPTER 10
Bone, Miss, Low,
Cut, Point

PART I

PART II

PART III

PART IV

Last week she called and said she had just **missed** hitting a car on her way to the interview and was so rattled that she decided she couldn't come that day. Then she decided to ride the Metro to the interview, but she **missed** getting on the train, so that was another interview that had to be canceled. Maybe I **misled** her when I told her we were a flexible company. Maybe she didn't realize how critical it was to show up for the interviews. She doesn't seem to have any remorse when she doesn't make it.

She has already **missed** the deadline to get all of her paperwork in. It's like she's **missed** the point of how critical it is that we find someone to take Miss Brooks's place. Somewhere along the way she must have **missed** the boat when it comes to common sense and courtesy. Maybe she isn't the person we're looking for after all. What a shame to have all of those credentials and no common sense!

How would you sign the following sentences?

1. I really **miss Miss** Brooks, don't you?

   _____

2. On her way to the interview, she was putting on makeup and just **missed** hitting a car.

   _____

3. She tried to ride the Metro but **missed** her connection.

   _____

4. She **missed** the deadline and didn't get all of her paperwork in.

   _____

5. I don't want to **mislead** her by giving her one extension after another.

   _____

Selection 10.3: The Lowdown on Millie

Millie lives in the **low**-rise apartment on Eisenhower Street. She's on a fixed income and does anything she can to save money. In the winter she **lowers** the temperature in her apartment so she can save on energy costs. She looks for the **lowest** priced items to eat in the grocery store, often depending on things that aren't good for her just so she can save money. Oftentimes, what she buys isn't the best, and as a result she ends up functioning at a very **low** energy level.

One time I tried to call her on her cell phone for a week to check on her and see how she was doing. I couldn't figure out why I couldn't get her to answer. Only later did she let me know that her battery was **low** on her cell phone, and she had turned it off until she could buy a new charger. Sometimes the stories she tells about her financial situation really make me feel **low**. She never feels sorry for herself and never complains. Maybe it's her upbeat attitude that makes me feel so bad.

One time I was going on and on about my **low**-rise jeans, how they weren't in style any more, and how I needed to buy some more fashionable clothes. She just smiled and nodded and didn't say a word. Later I really felt like a louse. There I was giving her the **low**down on fashion when she didn't even have enough money to go shopping, let alone buy new clothes. Millie always says that someone else is always worse off than she is. What a positive person she is!

How would you sign the following sentences?

1. I felt so **low** after I had given her the **low**down on jeans and what was in style.

   _____

2. The battery on her cell phone was so **low** that she couldn't receive calls.

_____

3. She is always **lowering** the temperature in her apartment to save on fuel costs.

_____

4. Sit down and let me give you the **low**down on Millie.

_____

5. If you would eat more carbohydrates, you wouldn't function at such a **low** energy level.

_____

Selection 10.4: Auditions for the Play

Steve has always been actively involved with drama. In high school, he was the president of the Thespian Club and set his sights on Broadway after graduating from college. When he moved to New York, he wasn't sure he'd make the **cut** and be asked to join one of the local acting guilds. He had heard about other guys trying out and all of the **cutting** remarks that the agents made after they would read lines from the script.

One time one of the agents was talking nonstop, and Steve felt compelled to **cut** in and ask a quick question. That was the only way he'd know if he should stay for the audition or **cut** across the lot to audition for another show instead of that one. It seemed as if his whole life was starting to center around **cutting** calls for auditions out of the paper with the hope of making it.

Some of his friends were very supportive of what he was trying to do, while others said he should just **cut** to the chase, ask his agent if he would ever make the **cut**, and then go from there. Others just told him he was doomed to bit parts that wouldn't amount to anything. He really tried to avoid those comments.

Then one day when he was **cutting** up, waiting for an audition, a talent agent heard him and thought he'd be great for comedy. He finally got his big break. His buddies were so excited they got a cake that said "Congratulations" and told him to **cut** it. He was really touched. He told the guys to **cut** it out and stop bragging on him, but secretly he was glad that they cared enough to talk about him.

How would you sign the following sentences?

1. I hate talking to her; she always makes such **cutting** remarks.

_____

2. Poor Steve was really having trouble making the **cut.**

_____

3. Do you want to **cut** the cake or do you want me to?

_____

4. I started to **cut** across the lawn when I realized there was a big dog hiding in the bushes.

_____

5. You need to **cut** it out and stop playing around before someone gets hurt.

_____

Selection 10.5: She Lacks a Sense of Direction

Marie has her mother's genes, which means although she is cute and funny, she also has no sense of direction. Her dad has tried for years to help her master the art of following maps, but it's **pointless.** She just can't get it. What's the **point** of giving someone directions when she can't even find north on a map?

The other day her dad said, "Let me give you some **pointers.**" With that he went on to explain how she could use the sun and the mountains as her guide. He said at the **point** where the roads cross, you know you're always going south. But, Marie still didn't get it.

She told her dad that if he could just **point** her in the right direction, she would look for landmarks along the way, and she'd be able to find her way back. She said she was accustomed to looking for the green house and the bank on the corner. Those were the kind of directions she could follow. She just didn't have a sense for compass directions.

Her dad was about to ask her a **pointed** question and ask her what was wrong with her when she reminded him that she was just like her mom. She **pointed** out that for years her mom had managed to get around just fine by locating her own landmarks. With that, he gave up and told her to approach driving and finding things in a way that she would be most comfortable with. He realized that the **points** he was trying to make were way beyond his daughter's level of comprehension.

How would you sign the following sentences?

1. What's the **point** of continuing this conversation if your mind is already made up?

   _____

2. Please **point** me in the right direction, and I'll be on my way.

   _____

3. Up to a **point** I agree with you, but after that we're on different pages.

   _____

4. May I ask you a rather **pointed** question?

   _____

5. He made three **points** that were critical to making a decision.

   _____

PART I

PART II

PART III

PART IV

Idioms

The English language is comprised of a number of words, phrases, and expressions that when conveyed can be intended to have either a literal or an idiomatic meaning. When a speaker intends for his words to be taken literally, as in "Don't count your chickens before they hatch," he is referring to the fact that you won't have a final count of the number of chickens you actually have until they all hatch out of the eggs. On the other hand, if he is using the phrase idiomatically, he means, don't count on a profit before you have the money in hand, or don't base your plans or something that may or may not happen.

According to Webster's *New Universal Unabridged Dictionary*, an idiom is "an accepted phrase, construction, or expression contrary to the usual patterns of the language or having a meaning different from the literal" (McKechnie, 1993). In this respect words, phrases, or expressions are used to express a thought or idea that cannot be derived from a literal interpretation of the individual words. Makkai, Boatner, and Gates (2004) identify idioms by parts of speech, i.e., verbs as in *"get up, work out,* and *turn in,* or nominal idioms as in *hot dog* and *cool cat."* They further group idioms as adjectival as in *"salt and pepper"* or adverbial as in *"like the breeze"* (p. vii).

There is a large group of idioms that are comprised of entire clauses as in *"seize the bull by the horns"* or *"caught between a rock and a hard place."* Many of these idiomatic phrases indicate that you have to choose between two equally unpleasant alternatives. These idioms have been referred to as *tournures.* The word is taken from the French and means "turn of phrase" or "phraseological idioms."

What is important to note is that all idioms share a common characteristic in that none of them correlate with a given grammatical part of speech and all of them require a paraphrase longer than a word to explain what they mean (Makkai, Boatner, & Gates, 2004, p. vii).

There are two large classes of idioms: phraseological idioms and those that are comprised of established sayings and proverbs. The origins of many of these sayings and proverbs have been passed down from our early ancestors or can be found in well-known literary resources. Phrases such as *"Don't count your chickens before they hatch"* and *"Get by by the skin of your teeth"* are representative of these types of idioms (Makkai, Boatner, & Gates, 2004, p. vii).

Idioms can be very challenging for English language learners as well as sign language interpreters. Below are several selections that contain idioms and idiomatic phrases. The selections include statements that one might use in everyday conversation.

Selection 11.1: Adjusting to the College Team

Zane played a lot of football at the Washington School for the Deaf. As a matter of fact, he was the star quarterback for the team. Then he graduated from a place where he had been a **big fish in a little pond** and went on to play college ball.

Like most kids right out of school, he had a big ego and thought he could do anything. He was used to **getting all the breaks**, and then his luck seemed to change.

He didn't realize what it would be like to be the **low man on the totem pole** and how he'd really have to **buckle down** and work if he wanted to get some play time. He knew that **everybody and his dog** would be coming to the first game, and he wanted to make sure that he would **make a good showing** on the field. He wanted all of the fans from his former high school to **sit up and take notice** that he really did have what it takes to play college ball.

So for weeks he showed up for practice early, worked hard, and listened to what the coach said. All of his hard work paid off. He **made the cut** and was ready for the first home game. Now if he could just **put his money where his mouth was** and deliver, he would still be regarded as the school hero.

How would you sign the following sentences?

1. He was used to being a **big fish in a little pond.**

   _____

2. He decided he'd have to **buckle down** and really work if he wanted to play.

   _____

3. He knew that **everybody and his dog** would be coming to the game.

   _____

4. He wanted **make a good showing** on the field.

   _____

5. He wanted all of his fans **to sit up and take notice** when he played in his first game.

   _____

Selection 11.2: The Road Trip

When Marie and Todd started off on their road trip to drive from Colorado to California, they had no idea what they'd be in for. Two hours into the drive they hit a thunderstorm, and it started to **rain cats and dogs**. They didn't know whether they should pull off the road or keep going. They couldn't tell if they'd drive out of it or if it would just get worse. Todd said they'd just **play it by ear** and keep driving.

They kept **inching their way along** when Marie noticed a break in the clouds up ahead. They were both relieved when they finally got out of the torrent of rain. They thought the worst of it was over when they seemed to drive into it again, and then they got a flat tire. Todd got out and changed it, and just as they got back on the road another car **cut in** front of them causing Todd to lose control and swerve off the road into a tree.

As they sat waiting for the tow truck, Marie tried to remain positive. She reminded Todd of the old saying that **"Every cloud has a silver lining."** Somehow Todd didn't see it that way. He told her that the whole trip had **started off on the wrong foot** and that they just should have stayed home. Marie told him then that he better decide if he wanted to turn back toward home or have the tow truck take them to the next town.

By the time the tow truck arrived, Todd had **cooled off** and decided they should continue on their way. Todd said later that this was **par for the course** based on some of their previous trips. By the time they arrived in the next town it was almost dark. Todd knew that after a good night's sleep they'd both be **good to go**.

232

PART III
....
Multiple-Meaning
Words, Idioms, and
Vocabulary Building

How would you sign the following sentences?

1. After a short time on the road, it started **raining cats and dogs.**

   _____

2. Todd said that the whole trip had **started off on the wrong foot.**

   _____

3. Marie reminded Todd of the saying: **Every cloud has a silver lining.**

   _____

4. They were driving along when another car came out of nowhere and **cut them off**.

   _____

5. Todd said that their experience was **par for the course.**

   _____

 Selection 11.3: Mean Girls

You've all heard stories about mean girls—you know, the ones that will **stab you in the back** for no good reason. We've all met girls like that or have heard others talk about them. They pretend like they're your friends, and then when you think you're **getting in good** with them, they will **brush you off** without giving you a second thought.

One of my friends got in with the wrong crowd. We told her she better **watch her step** because the group she was choosing to hang with were all **wrapped up** in their own little world. If you couldn't compete with their money or style, they would eventually ostracize you and make very **cutting** remarks. My friend refused to listen, and when they started making fun of her, she was reduced to tears.

It always **boggles my mind** how cruel girls can be to each other. You don't seem to see that with guys. Guys usually couldn't care less about what someone says, and when they do have a **falling out** with someone, they are more inclined to settle the **beef** by talking or **throwing a punch** if it really gets out of hand. In this respect, it's too bad girls can't be more like guys. They seem to spend far less time being **full of themselves** and more time just being one of the guys.

How would you sign the following sentences?

1. It always **boggles my mind** how cruel girls can be to each other.

   _____

2. Guys seem to settle a **beef** by talking or **throwing a punch.**

   _____

3. She had a **falling out** with the group after they made fun of her.

   _____

4. You need to **watch your step** when you try and then finally succeed in getting into some groups.

   _____

5. Zoe had a bad habit of making **cutting** remarks when she didn't like something.

   _____

233

CHAPTER 11
....
Idioms

PART I

PART II

PART III

PART IV

Selection 11.4: Being Frugal

Have you ever heard the expression, "You need to **save your money for a rainy day**?" I think my dad and his ancestors created the expression. I have never seen such a **penny pincher** in my whole life. He is so **tight his shoes squeak.** He refuses to buy anything unless it's on sale, and once he makes a purchase he expects it to last for an eternity.

One time he bought a jacket and wore it for fifteen years. When it finally **bit the dust** and he had to buy a new one, he **went off** on a tangent about how they don't make things like they used to. He bought his next jacket **on the cheap** and then wondered by it didn't **hold up** at all. My mom could never **get it through his head** that you get what you pay for. Regardless of what she would say, her advice always rolled off my dad like **water off a duck's back**.

Now that I'm an adult, I've taken what he said **with a grain of salt**. Whenever he wants to give me advice, I let it **go in one ear and out the other**. I try to save money where I can, but I use my sister's advice when it comes to buying clothes. I figure out the cost and divide it by the number of times I think I'll wear the item. This formula has seemed to work for me.

How would you sign the following sentences?

1. My dad is **so tight his shoes squeak.**

   _____

2. When my mom tries to give my dad advice, it is like **water off a duck's back**.

   _____

3. I take what my parents say **with a grain of salt.**

   _____

4. My grandfather always said "**save your money for a rainy day.**"

   _____

5. Regardless what we tell him, we can't seem to get the point **through his head.**

   _____

Selection 11.5: Jen's Boss

Have you ever met Jen's boss? He works on the third floor and is the head of the accounting department. He never smiles and always seems gruff when you try to talk with him. I asked Jen about him one time and she said **his bark was worse than his bite.** She said he always **talks big**, but when it comes right down to it he's a softie at heart.

Jen said he's always been an overachiever and that some of his ideas would just **blow your mind**. He has come up with some awesome ideas of how to help the company save money. He has never been one to **put all of his eggs in one basket** and has encouraged others to spread out their investments among a variety of companies.

One time, one of the other associates tried to tell him that his approach to investments was all wrong. Instead of changing how he did things, he **dug in his heels** and **stuck to his guns.** He has always said it is a **dog eat dog** world out there, and consumers should have someone who always **plays it safe** when they are looking at investing their money and saving for retirement.

I have never dealt with her boss before. I've only seen him from a distance, but I trust Jen, and I'm trying to take her words to heart when she said, you **can't**

judge a book by its cover. I guess in the future if I ever need financial advice, I'll make an appointment to see him.

How would you sign the following sentences?

1. Some of her boss's ideas are phenomenal; they would **blow your mind.**

_____

2. When the others disagreed with him, he **dug in his heels** and held his ground.

_____

3. It can be a **dog eat dog** world out there.

_____

4. We all know that you **can't judge a book by its cover.**

_____

5. Jason's **bark is worse than his bite.**

_____

Additional Work with Idioms I

 Selection 12.1: Advanced Calculus Class

Shontavia thought the advanced calculus class would **be a breeze**. Little did she know that she'd be **over her head** before the class really got **off the ground**. She had taken calculus at CSUN and had a dynamite interpreter. She just assumed that she was in for a similar experience. Little did she know that this class would move at such a quick pace that she would soon find herself working double time just so she could **keep up.**

The first day of class the teacher put everyone **on the spot**. She asked each of them to come up to the board and solve a problem. Shontavia was stuck. She didn't have a clue what she should do first. She just wanted to get out of the class and **bury her head in the sand**; she was so embarrassed. Needless to say, the whole experience **left a bad taste in her mouth.**

That evening she called one of her friends from CSUN. She knew that he was taking a similar class at Gallaudet. She wanted to get his **take** on what she should do. After she described the class and what had happened, he asked her a bunch of questions. The more she talked, the more she realized she needed the class for her major. She decided she should **hang in there,** get a tutor, and try to **make the best of it.** If not, she knew she'd have to repeat the class and VR wouldn't pay for it.

How would you sign the following sentences?

1. She had no idea she'd be **over her head** before the class really got started.

   _____

2. The whole experience left a **bad taste in her mouth.**

   _____

3. She called her friend at Gallaudet to get his **take** on what she should do.

   _____

4. She decided she should just **hang in there**; she didn't have another choice.

   _____

5. She decided to get a tutor and try to **make the best of it.**

   _____

Selection 12.2: Coaching Little League

Have you ever coached a little league team? Well, let me tell you, I have, and it has its **ups and downs.** The kids are great and they're so much fun to be with,

236

PART III
....
Multiple-Meaning
Words, Idioms, and
Vocabulary Building

but the parents can be a real **pain in the neck**. They all think their kids are star athletes and that they shouldn't have to do any bench time. But when you have twenty kids on the team and only nine can play at a time, somebody has to sit on the bench.

Last week was our first game. Let me just **paint you a picture** of what happened. I was busy talking with the team, laying out the **ground rules**, when one of the parents decided he would come over and throw in his **two cents' worth**. What he was saying was in direct opposition to what I'd been telling them. When he finished his diatribe, they all looked at me in confusion.

I wanted to **read the riot act** to the parent, but instead I **let it go** and continued with my last-minute instructions. Once the game got started, it was fun to see the kids having a good time. When they were at bat, they tried so hard to hit the ball, and when they were out in the field, they ran until I thought they'd drop from total exhaustion. They really have come together as a team this year and have turned out to be pretty good **eggs**. If asked to coach the team again next year, I would probably say, "Yes."

How would you sign the following sentences?

1. Coaching the little league team has had some real **ups and downs**.

   _____

2. Some of the parents can be a real **pain in the neck.**

   _____

3. Let me **paint you a picture** of how the pre-game activities usually go.

   _____

4. I wanted to **read him the riot act**, but I decided it wouldn't be worth it.

   _____

5. I have some pretty good **eggs** on my team.

   _____

Selection 12.3: The Hypochondriac

Have you ever met or known a hypochondriac? You know someone who complains all the time about how he feels. I knew a guy one time who was one. No one ever wanted to ask Marv how he was doing because all he did was complain. You'd think by talking to him that he was on his **last legs**.

He was a master of **one-upmanship.** It didn't matter how you felt, or what was wrong with you, he always felt worse. No one enjoyed being around him. I often wondered why he **turned out** that way. No one else in his family was like him, and they didn't enjoy listening to him either. He always sounded like he had **one foot in the grave.**

I remember one time a group of our friends decided to play a trick on him. It was all meant to be **good clean fun.** They bought a bunch of bandages and wrapped up one of the girls to make her look like she'd been in a terrible accident. They wanted to let him see **in a big way** how he sounded when someone asked him how he was doing.

After they had Katie all bandaged up, they called Marv over and told him she'd had a terrible accident. She started to describe her ailments. Much to their surprise he didn't say a word. They had definitely **pulled the wool over his eyes.** Later, when Marv found out it was a joke, he **blew a gasket**. Maybe it wasn't a good idea in the end, but at least for a short time, he quit complaining.

237

CHAPTER 12
....
Additional Work
with Idioms I

PART I

PART II

PART III

PART IV

How would you sign the following sentences?

1. Marv always makes it sound like he has **one foot in the grave.**

   _____

2. When you describe how you feel, it's like he's practicing **one-upmanship** with his list of complaints.

   _____

3. A group of us got together and decided to have some **good clean fun.**

   _____

4. Their masquerade was so successful that they succeeded in **pulling the wool over his eyes.**

   _____

5. Marv **blew a gasket** when he realized that the joke was on him.

   _____

Selection 12.4: The CEO

Ryan is the CEO of the newest video phone company in Seattle. He's really the **top dog**. He didn't start out that way—not at all. Actually, he started working for another company when he was **fresh out** of college. He started his career in sales, and after a few years of traveling around the country he was given a desk job. Basically, he started **from the ground up** learning the rules from sales to supervision of how a video phone company is run.

Then about a year ago he heard that a new company was coming to town and that they were advertising for a CEO. Ryan realized that although he was **on the fast track** within his company, the CEO wasn't going anywhere, and he would never have that position. It was time to **branch out** and apply for something new.

He was convinced that he **had a good head** for business and that it was time to apply for the job and see what would happen. So, **on the QT** he mailed in his application and was very happy when he was asked to come for an interview.

Throughout the interview, Ryan felt that the job was **made for him.** After he was hired, he **dug in** and has been largely responsible for turning the company into the successful business that it is today.

How would you sign the following sentences?

1. Ryan is the **top dog** of the new video phone company.

   _____

2. He has learned the business **from the ground up.**

   _____

3. He was **on the fast track** to becoming the new CEO of the company.

   _____

4. He applied for the new job **on the QT.**

   _____

5. Ryan has a **good head on his shoulders** and would be great at any job he was given.

   _____

Selection 12.5: Getting Fit

One of these days I'm going to get in shape. How many times have you made this statement? All of us who are **couch potatoes** have made comments like this when we've tried to play ball, run a race, or do something that makes us realize how out of shape we really are. That's when we head to the gym to **work out** and **pump iron.**

That's when we **cut out** eating all of our favorite foods and try to lose those extra pounds. For most of us this dedication is **short lived.** We realize that getting in shape is usually **easier said than done** and that it requires **buckling down** and really working hard. Sometimes it doesn't seem like the effort is worth it.

For those **dyed in the wool diehards** who religiously stick with their exercise programs, the rewards are great. After a few short weeks of going to the gym, they generally feel better and have more energy. By the time they've shed about ten pounds, they notice a real change in how their clothes fit and it all seems to be worth it.

How would you sign the following sentences?

1. If I really want to lose weight, I'm going to have to **cut out** all of my favorite foods.

   _____

2. Many of us who are **couch potatoes** realize we've gained a few pounds and don't have much energy.

   _____

3. That's when we decide we've got to **buckle down** and do something about our weight problem.

   _____

4. Only the true **diehards** remain faithful to their exercise routines.

   _____

5. **One of these days** I'm going to sign up for an exercise program at the gym.

   _____

6. He is a **dyed in the wool** procrastinator when it comes to exercise.

   _____

Additional Work with Idioms II

Selection 13.1: Winter Weather

It's almost November; the days are getting shorter and the temperature is starting to drop. Soon the warm days will be **few and far between**. That means I need to start getting our house ready for winter. It's time to bring in some of the plants and make sure we have enough firewood to last us for the next few months.

I've been meaning to cut some wood for the past few weeks, but it seems as if I never have enough time to **get around** to doing it. It's not that I mind using the log splitter, but with all the other things that need to be done, it seems that chopping wood always gets put on the **back burner**. Time is **getting short.**

Josh told me I wouldn't need so much wood this winter if I'd just **cut back** on how warm I keep my house. He doesn't seem to understand that some of us feel the cold more than others and that you can only drink so much hot chocolate. He told me I should just bundle up and I could **get by** with a lot less wood. I told him I didn't mind spending the time or the money on firewood. I'd rather **cut corners** somewhere else and have the money to spend on heat.

I really love living in the mountains. I like to see it snow in the wintertime and watch ice form on the lake. I just wish it didn't get so cold. Josh said I **can't have it both ways**. He suggested I either move to a warm climate and forget the snow or stop my bellyaching and bundle up more. I know he's right, but I'd hate to give up the beauty of winter in the mountains. It has a charm all of its own.

How would you sign the following sentences?

1. The warm days are **few and far between** during the winter.

   _____

2. I just haven't **gotten around** to chopping wood for the fireplace.

   _____

3. I would rather **cut corners** and eat soup every day than give up my heat.

   _____

4. Josh suggested I bundle up and **cut back** on the heat.

   _____

5. I wish I could have warm weather and snow at the same time, but I know I **can't have it both ways.**

   _____

Selection 13.2: Cassie Interviews for a New Job

Did you hear about Cassie's job interview? She's been unhappy for the past few months where she's been working and decided she'd start applying at other firms. There was one company she went to that didn't seem very promising from its website and from the information it sent her. But once she went for the interview, she realized that there was **more there than meets the eye.**

Once the interview started, she really **hit it off** with the unit supervisor. She realized that they could sit and **talk shop** for a long time. Their backgrounds were so similar, and they enjoyed working on the same kinds of projects. She was really **a breath of fresh air** compared to some of the people at the company where she worked. It was nice to be able to focus on projects rather than on people.

When the interview was over, she thanked the woman for taking time to meet with her. The woman told her that she had exceptional skills. Cassie really hoped that she meant it and wasn't just paying her **lip service.** She really hoped she'd **stand out** and that when she left, she'd be seriously considered for the job. Too many times, she's had a good interview and then realized that once **out of sight, out of mind.** She sure hoped that wouldn't happen this time. It seemed like such a good fit.

How would you sign the following sentences?

1. At first glance she didn't think they had much to offer, but she quickly realized there was **more there than meets the eye**.

2. When they started to talk, they really **hit it off**.

3. Cassie had so much fun **talking shop** with the unit supervisor.

4. She was hoping she just wasn't paying her **lip service** when she told her she had excellent qualities.

5. You know what they say, "**out of sight, out of mind**." She hoped that wouldn't happen this time.

Selection 13.3: Brutus the Overgrown Puppy

Brutus is an eight-month-old mutt. He's oversized, weighing about eighty-five pounds, and he has more energy than he knows what to do with. At first he appears docile but once he has a **lay of the land**, he takes off running like a **ball of fire**. It's as if he has all of this pent-up energy just waiting for the right minute to release it.

It wouldn't be so bad if he didn't still have so many puppy characteristics. He is just like a **bull in a china shop.** He is constantly knocking things over as he runs through the house, and when he gets excited and starts wagging his tail, it will **beat you to death**. What's more, he's one of the most curious puppies I've ever seen. He has his nose into everything, and you have to **watch him like a hawk.**

I told his master that he needed to take him to obedience school to train him. That is the only way he'll be a fun dog to be around. I told him if he didn't **take the bull by the horns** soon and get the dog trained, his mutt would never know who was in control. He said he was pretty well trained already, but I told him he was **far from it**.

241

CHAPTER 13

Additional Work
with Idioms II

PART I

PART II

PART III

PART IV

Any dog that jumps on you, runs through the house barking, and makes confetti out of newspaper is not well trained. I think Brutus's owner needs to **bite the bullet**, admit that the dog is not well trained, and find a good obedience school for them to go to. That is the only way he'll be a dog people will want to be around. Otherwise, I'm afraid as Brutus gets older he's going to **drive away** all of his master's friends.

How would you sign the following sentences?

1. Brutus is like a **bull in a china shop**; he needs some kind of training.

   _____

2. When you turn him loose in the house, you have to **watch him like a hawk.**

   _____

3. He's such a nosy dog; he doesn't **miss a trick.**

   _____

4. When he gets out of his crate at the end of the day, he runs through the house like a **ball of fire.**

   _____

5. My friend thinks his dog is well trained, but he is **far from it.**

   _____

Selection 13.4: The 5K Run

The Metro Club for the Deaf is hosting a 5K run next weekend to raise funds for their Deaf softball team. They want to play in the northeast conference, which means they'll have to travel a lot next year. They probably don't have a **ghost of a chance** at winning, but they'd still like to meet some of the players on the other teams.

Once they **made up their minds** that they wanted to do this, they started talking about how they could raise money. They thought about hosting a bake sale, but then they weren't sure how many people would come. They also considered having a raffle, but that involved a lot of work. Then they **hit on** the idea of the 5K run. They knew that a number of people liked to run and the **sky was the limit.** They could set a $15.00 registration fee and hope that dozens of people would sign up. No telling how much money they could raise.

They knew they'd have to hurry and start advertising for their event if they wanted to earn enough money before the conference registration fee was due. They printed up flyers and organized the route for the run. They had it planned **down to the last detail.** A month before the race, they contacted the police to make sure the roads could be blocked off and that they'd be there for assistance.

Word of the race **spread like wildfire** and it quickly became the **talk of the town.** Over 500 people signed up to run and others volunteered to help. Club members were overwhelmed with the amount of community support they received. They knew that the person who came up with the idea to host a 5K deserved a **pat on the back.**

How would you sign the following sentences?

1. They didn't have a **ghost of a chance** at winning the tournament, but they wanted to meet some of the other players.

   _____

242

PART III
....
Multiple-Meaning
Words, Idioms, and
Vocabulary Building

2. The race that the Metro Deaf Club was sponsoring became the **talk of the town.**

_____

3. Word of the race **spread like wildfire** within in the community.

_____

4. They couldn't think of any good fundraisers until they **hit on** the idea of sponsoring a 5K.

_____

5. They knew with that type of a fundraiser, the **sky was the limit.**

_____

Selection 13.5: Pen Pal

When you were growing up did you ever have a **pen pal**? I had one when I was in high school. He lived in Japan, and we exchanged several letters. He would tell me all about his family and where he went to school, and I shared similar information. One time he wrote in a letter that he had heard someone use the expression "**pay through the nose**," and he wondered if I could explain it. I told him I could, but I wouldn't be able to explain its origin. It was fun to talk about one of our English idioms.

We wrote back and forth for about a year. His letters were always interesting and informative. I often thought while reading his letters that he would have been a fun person to **hang out** with. Anytime I would share my dreams with him, he never **put a damper on** any of my grandiose ideas. Likewise, I listened to his ideas with the same amount of enthusiasm.

Shortly before the end of my high school year, I received a letter from him saying that his father had **passed away** and that his whole world had been **turned upside down.** I know after that happened, he had to **grow up** quickly and take on the responsibility for his family. That was the last time I ever heard from him. I have often wondered what happened to him and what he's doing today.

How would you sign the following sentences?

1. Have you ever had a **pen pal**? I had one in high school.

_____

2. Do you know what it means to **pay through the nose**? I don't.

_____

3. He always sounded like he'd be a fun person to **hang out** with.

_____

4. His father **passed away** when he was a senior in high school.

_____

5. His whole world was **turned upside down** when his father died.

_____

CHAPTER 14

Additional Work with Idioms III

Selection 14.1: Not Our Year

This year our football team just hasn't been **up to par**. It doesn't seem to matter what they do, they just can't seem to win a game. The coach recruited a group of new players both for offense and defense, but so far it hasn't seemed to make a difference. We all thought this season would be a **piece of cake**. Boy, have we been disappointed!

The team entered the season wanting to **settle a score** from last year. An unknown team scored a **shutout** against them, and it was a real embarrassment. They knew in order to **save face** they'd have to stage a **comeback** this season. But, how successful they'll be **remains to be seen**.

During the first several weeks of practice, several players suffered injuries and have been forced to sit on the bench. The star quarterback has been unable to play, and two of the wide receivers have been **out of commission**, too. Any one who's a sports fan knows you've got to have your starting players in **top shape** if you want to win a game. There are **no two ways about it.** I'm not sure what will happen to the coach if we have another losing season. He might be **sacked.**

I'd **give my right arm** to get the team back on the road to success. It's hard going to the games week after week and watching your team lose. Maybe our luck will change soon.

How would you sign the following sentences?

1. This year our football team hasn't been **up to par.**

   _____

2. I would **give my right arm** to see our team win some games.

   _____

3. We all thought with the new players that this season would be a **piece of cake.**

   _____

4. There are **no two ways about it;** it's hard to win when half of your players are injured.

   _____

5. We had a **score to settle** with another team even before the season started.

   _____

Selection 14.2: Health Insurance

How do you feel about your tax dollars going to help people who are **down on their luck** pay for health insurance? There seems to be a big controversy today about using tax dollars this way. There has been a **hot and heavy** debate in the senates in some states regarding if this is something local citizens should do.

Some public officials have **gone on record** stating that there aren't that many poor people who don't have insurance, and therefore tax dollars shouldn't be allocated for this cause. Opponents contend that those officials have their **heads in the sand**, and they don't have any idea what they're talking about. In the meantime, many poor people are living **hand to mouth**, wondering what they would do if they or one of their children got sick.

Someone wrote an editorial in the paper recently saying that those who are being **hard nosed** about not wanting to support the poor should go and **hang out** with them for a week or so. The author of the column stressed that experience would really **open up their eyes** to what it's like to be poor. I'm not so sure if they really did that they'd **see the light** and really get a **handle on the problem.**

I'm not sure where it will all end, but I can tell you honestly that I get a **lump in my throat** every time I see a homeless person or a child who has to do without because there isn't enough money to go around. It seems like in a country like the United States we should be able to take care of our nation's poor people.

How would you sign the following sentences?

1. There has been a **hot and heavy** debate in some states about how we should spend our tax dollars.

    _____

2. Some people in this country are living from **hand to mouth**.

    _____

3. Living the life of a poor person might **open one's eyes** to what they experience on a daily basis.

    _____

4. I wish our country could **get a handle** on the war on poverty.

    _____

5. I get a **lump in my throat** every time I see a homeless person.

    _____

Selection 14.3: A Good Song

Have you ever wondered why some people like some songs while others **can't stand** the same type of music? Take **bubble gum music** for example. Some teenage girls seem to **hang on** every word as if the ballad were written especially for them. Every time their favorite song comes on the radio they sit mesmerized, enjoying every beat until it ends.

While some teenagers seem to prefer that kind of music, adults seem to prefer a wider range of music. While some enjoy listening to country music, others consider it a **fate worse than death** if they are stuck in a car with a country music lover. It just **goes to show** that what one considers a nice sound another considers an annoying twang.

I've often wondered how record companies know a song will **be a hit**. I'm not sure if they just have a sense for what people like or if they're just lucky. Sometimes I think they're just making a **stab in the dark.** There are times I hear a song and I think **fat chance** that one will **make it**. Then I'm always surprised when I see it's made the top ten.

I know I could never **make it** as the head of a record company. My taste in music is too narrow, and I'm sure it only appeals to my own generation. I do admire those who have succeeded in that industry. **Hats off** to those who continue to provide us great songs for our listening enjoyment. We do appreciate it.

How would you sign the following sentences?

1. Some people consider it a **fate worse than death** if they have to listen to country music.

   _____

2. I wonder how record companies know that a song will **be a hit.**

   _____

3. Some teenage girls really prefer **bubble gum music.**

   _____

4. I'm sure some recording companies are making a **stab in the dark** with the potential success of some songs.

   _____

5. **Hats off** to those who continue to provide us with great music.

   _____

 Selection 14.4: The Weatherman

From time to time, a weatherman's job can seem to be one of the most stressful jobs on earth. Even with **state-of-the-art** equipment, it can be extremely difficult to predict storms and weather patterns. A storm may look like it's headed in one direction, and at the last minute it switches course.

Oftentimes weathermen wait to predict storms until **the eleventh hour.** Then they have to **cut into** current programming to let viewers know that severe weather is headed their way. This can be dreaded news for anyone but especially for someone who has experienced it and watched everything they own go **down the drain**. It is heartbreaking to watch those stories on TV and realize how quickly we can lose everything.

When you're not in the path of the storm, it's interesting to hear the weathermen give a **running commentary** on the weather and what they anticipate will happen. They provide viewers with **up-to-the-minute** information, telling them when to take shelter and when to evacuate.

My sister used to say that a weatherman had the only job in the world in which you could be wrong more than 50 percent of the time and still keep your job. She was probably right. But in all fairness, with **Mother Nature** being so unpredictable, I am always amazed that they are **on target** as much as they are.

How would you sign the following sentences?

1. When a storm is in progress, weathermen give us a **running commentary** on what's happening.

   _____

2. They frequently provide viewers with **up-to-the-minute** information.

   _____

246

PART III
....
Multiple-Meaning
Words, Idioms, and
Vocabulary Building

3. Most weather stations today have **state-of-the-art** equipment.

_____

4. Sometimes weathermen have to **cut into** programs to provide us with weather warnings.

_____

5. The path of the storm can be hard to predict, forcing weathermen to wait until **the eleventh hour** to predict the storm's path.

_____

Selection 14.5: Phrases That Include the Word "Dog"

Have you ever noticed how many idioms and proverbs have the word "dog" in them? It's really interesting. While some of the phrases are pretty commonplace, like the **dog days** of summer, others are less familiar like "**take the hair of the dog that bit you**." This phrase is frequently offered to someone who has had too much to drink the night before and is suffering from a hangover. This suggestion means that the person should have another drink.

While many of you have heard the expression "**the tail wags the dog**," perhaps a less popular expression is "**dog in the manger**." For those of you unfamiliar with this phrase, it generally refers to a person who refuses to share something that he or she has, even though that person has no use for it.

How many of you have heard the phrase "**see a man about a dog**"? It is an old proverb indicating that the person needs to excuse himself and find a restroom. All of us feel from time to time that we live in a **dog-eat-dog** world, and we sometimes yearn for a **dog's life**.

It's just fascinating to me how many sayings incorporate one three-letter word into them and how varied the meaning of the word becomes when used in these instances.

How would you sign the following sentences?

1. It can be a **dog-eat-dog** world out there.

_____

2. Sometimes don't you yearn for a **dog's life**?

_____

3. Tom told his host he needed to **see a man about a dog**.

_____

4. Shelly doesn't need all that room; why is she being a **dog in a manger**?

_____

5. Are you enjoying the **dog days** of summer?

_____

CHAPTER 15

Additional Work with Idioms IV

Selection 15.1: The Fire

Recently, a friend of mine received an email with some distressing news. She came running to see me, and it was obvious that she was **beside herself.** A friend of hers had been **working her fingers to the bone** trying to get her business up and going. She had finally succeeded and had been open for less than a week.

She'd opened a small French market and had vendors bring their goods from all over the state. It looked as if the business was going to **take off** and be a huge success. That's when disaster seemed to strike. During the night, a fire broke out in her store. It **spread like wildfire** before the firemen could get to the scene and put it out. Everything was lost.

She was just devastated. The fire inspectors told her that in their opinion that **without a doubt** someone had intentionally started the fire. She about **flipped out** when she heard that. Who in their **right mind** would do something like that? She couldn't begin to imagine who the arsonist might be. Who would hate her that much to do something like this?

After she **dropped the bombshell** on me, I, too, tried to think of who might do something like that. It's now been two weeks, and the police still don't have any leads. My friend has **picked up the pieces,** and she's going to rebuild. She's always been one to **hoe her own row** and I have no doubt that she will succeed.

How would you sign the following sentences?

1. My friend called me, and it was obvious that she was **beside herself**.

   _____

2. She has been **working her fingers to the bone** for weeks getting ready for the grand opening.

   _____

3. After she **dropped by bombshell** on me, I tried to think of who might have set the fire.

   _____

4. She has always been one to **hoe her own row**.

   _____

5. When things fall apart, she always **picks up the pieces** and goes on.

   _____

Selection 15.2: Running for Public Office

How do you feel about politics? Do you look forward to November when it's an election year? I always feel sorry for the candidates who have to do the **green bean and chicken** tour. They go from city to city or state to state **stumping** for votes. It seems like every other week there is a new **straw poll** as people try to predict who will win.

I think today in order to enter a race you need to have a **sterling character** because it seems that the media and the opponents go to **great lengths** to **dig up dirt** and broadcast it to the world. You've also got to have **thick skin** if you want to enter the race.

Campaigning can be very expensive. Those candidates who are born with a **silver spoon in their mouths** have a definite advantage over the **average Joe blow**. Advertisements alone can cost thousands of dollars. Sometimes I think it would be fun to **be a fly on the wall** and get the **lowdown** on how much candidates really spend and what they really believe.

How would you sign the following sentences?

1. Candidates have to go from city to city **stumping** for votes.

   _____

2. Some candidates are born with a **silver spoon in their mouths**.

   _____

3. I would like to **be a fly on the wall** and listen to the conversation.

   _____

4. To run for office today you need to have a **sterling character**.

   _____

5. Do you have the **lowdown** on the man running for mayor?

   _____

Selection 15.3: Jeremiah Needs a New Truck

Jeremiah has an old clunker of a truck. He's had it for over twenty years, and little by little it's starting to fall apart—literally. It's been repaired so many times that almost everything on it is new. Still it has trouble starting. Trying to keep it on the road has really **hit** Jeremiah **in the pocketbook.**

Last week I asked him why he didn't just **bite the bullet** and buy a new one. He said they weren't making cars like they used to, and he didn't want to get stuck with a **lemon.** He almost **bit my head off** when I told him it was time he got rid of his old junker. You would have thought I'd insulted an old friend.

You'd think he'd **give in** and at least start looking. He just doesn't have a dependable vehicle. I can't even begin to count the number of times his truck has left him **high and dry**. I really wish he'd have a **change of heart** and reconsider. I hate to think of him stranded some night on a country road with no one to come and get him. Sometimes he can be as **stubborn as a mule**.

I guess I better leave well enough alone if I want our friendship to remain intact. I really do value him as a friend and just worry sometimes about his choice of transportation.

How would you sign the following sentences?

1. The repairs on Jeremiah's truck have really **hit him in the pocketbook.**

   _____

2. He almost **bit my head off** when I told him he needed to get rid of his old truck.

_____

3. You'd think he'd **give in** and start looking.

_____

4. I don't want his truck to leave him **high and dry.**

_____

5. He can be as **stubborn** as a mule when it comes to buying a new car.

_____

Selection 15.4: Helping the Homeless

Someone once said that most of us are one paycheck away from being homeless. I wonder how we would view homeless people if the **shoe was on the other foot.** My friend Mary Sue has done a lot of work with homeless people. She has helped build houses for them, worked in the soup kitchen, and taken medicine to the shut ins. She never talks about it much.

I've always admired her and her work. She really shows a lot of compassion and is a true example of how **actions speak louder than words.** Whenever she is out working in the community, and the jobs are hard, she just **grins and bears it** and keeps working. She always has a smile on her face and is a joy to be around.

I'm not sure how long she's been working with people who are less fortunate than she is. I just know that she **always looks on the bright side** and stays positive even in the worst of situations. She's **easy going**, and nothing seems to get her down.

I wish there were more people like her in the world today. I can't help but think if there were, it would be a whole lot better place to live. I just **thank my lucky stars** that I know her and that I can call her my friend.

How would you sign the following sentences?

1. How would you feel if the **shoe was on the other foot**?

_____

2. She does so many charitable acts—she is a true example that **actions speak louder than words.**

_____

3. Regardless what the job entails, she just **grins and bears it.**

_____

4. Mary Sue always **looks on the bright side** regardless of the situation.

_____

5. I just **thank my lucky stars** that we're friends.

_____

Selection 15.5: Grandma's Philosophy

Grandma grew up in the backwoods of Kentucky. She was raised with hard work and long days. She was always told anything worth doing required **blood, sweat, and tears**, and she needed to **buckle down** and apply herself if she wanted to

250

PART III
....
Multiple-Meaning
Words, Idioms, and
Vocabulary Building

amount to anything. Her daddy never had any patience for people who had the **life of Riley**. He felt that hard work was what built character.

Grandma learned at an early age that you got in trouble if you **talked back**. She learned that you needed to respect people and be polite when answering questions. Grandma also learned the value of taking care of things. Her mamma used to always tell her that "**a stitch in time saves nine**." She always said that she never quite understood that until she got older.

When we would visit grandma, we were expected to **toe the line**. If we didn't, we'd get a real **dressing down.** She set high standards, and everyone who came to stay with her had to abide by her rules. She was probably the one responsible for a lot of our early moral development. And even though she was strict, she was also **generous to a fault**. I can't ever remember her not doing for others.

Grandma **passed away** a few years ago, and I miss her dearly. Her old adages helped shape my life, and I know a lot of what I do is a reflection of her beliefs. I know she is at rest after her many long hard years of work.

How would you sign the following sentences?

1. Some jobs are just harder than others—they require a lot of **blood, sweat, and tears.**

   _____

2. Grandma told us we needed to **buckle down** and do our work if we wanted to be successful.

   _____

3. One of her favorite sayings was "**a stitch in time saves nine.**"

   _____

4. If we didn't **toe the line**, we'd get a real **dressing down.**

   _____

5. Grandma was always **generous to a fault.**

   _____

CHAPTER 16

Vocabulary-Building Exercises

Selection 16.1: Unpleasant School Experiences

The dropout rate in the United States for high school students is staggering. Every year thousands of students opt for a life outside of school once they're old enough to make the choice. When asked why they drop out of school, they invariably cite unpleasant family or school experiences as the cause. Some have encountered many **impediments** along the way: drugs, divorce, and gang membership. Others have grown up in **abusive** homes and need to escape as quickly as possible.

Most arrive at adulthood **semiliterate**. They search for jobs only to discover that because they cannot read, they are **doomed** to minimum wage jobs with no hope for advancement. They **perceive** the world as being **condescending** and quickly become resentful because they have been passed through a system where they didn't learn a thing.

Struggling with their feelings of **inferiority**, some **instinctively** begin to look for ways to **alleviate** the problem. Others **harbor** feelings of resentment and begin engaging in **subversive** activities hoping to gain a sense of purpose for living. This **turbulent** lifestyle frequently leads them to a life of crime and a dead-end street. It is a sad reflection on our current educational system. It shows how **ill equipped** the schools are to deal with diverse populations.

How would you sign the following sentences?

1. Most arrive at adulthood **semiliterate.**

   _____

2. Others **harbor** feelings of resentment and engage in **subversive** activities.

   _____

3. This **turbulent** lifestyle frequently leads them to a life of crime.

   _____

4. The schools today are **ill equipped** to deal with diverse populations.

   _____

5. There are many **impediments** to accessing a quality education.

   _____

Selection 16.2: The Breadbasket of America

We often think of the Midwest as the "breadbasket of America" because that's where many of our nation's farms are. Farming today has become very **progressive**, and it's not at all what it used to be. However, when Mother Nature

252

PART III
....
Multiple-Meaning
Words, Idioms, and
Vocabulary Building

decides to rear her ugly head, farmers frequently find they are at the mercy of the weather.

Farmers today are **plagued** with insects, droughts, and unpredictable weather patterns. These are only some of the **culprits** that can determine the success or failure of a crop. **Ironically**, what can make a crop can also break it. **Unforeseen** hail storms can conceivably **render** a crop of beans worthless if they are too bruised by the hailstones to be sold.

Last year a group of farmers **convened** in Washington to meet with members of Congress about crop protection. They were **disillusioned** with the previous year's crops and wanted to see if they could get insurance against future storms. They stood outside in the **stifling** heat waiting to get an appointment with the Secretary of Agriculture.

My dad used to always say that you've got to have nerves of steel if you want to be a farmer. You never know from month to month if you'll have money in the bank at the end of the season or if you'll have to take out another loan. It would be tough to be a farmer, but I'm sure glad a number of people enjoy farming. Where would we be without them?

How would you sign the following sentences?

1. Farmers today are **plagued** with rain, hail, and insects.

   _____

2. **Ironically**, what can make a crop can also break a crop.

   _____

3. A group of farmers went to Washington to **convey** their opinions to government officials.

   _____

4. They stood in the **stifling** heat waiting for an appointment.

   _____

5. Farming today is far more **progressive** than it used to be.

   _____

Selection 16.3: Visit to the Oncologist

One of the things most of us dread is being told that we're being referred to an **oncologist** for treatment. I remember going with a friend to the doctor's office one time and watching her sit **transfixed** after an initial diagnosis and referral was made. She hadn't been feeling well for a long time, but the referral caught her totally off guard. She sat there feeling terrified and extremely **vulnerable**. What she thought had been a **benign** lump had turned into cancer.

After her initial diagnosis was made, she began reading up on cancer. She quickly realized that her condition was **graver** than she initially thought. The **fatality** estimate for this type of cancer was thirty times higher than what the AMA had **forecast** earlier. However, there were new treatments being offered that **conceivably** might **eradicate** her disease. She was told that it was **plausible** that after treatment she could live a very long and full life.

She listened intently to what she was told, opted for a very **aggressive** treatment plan, and took **meticulous** care to make sure that she participated in all of the procedures. Today I am happy to report that she is a healthy, vibrant woman who **radiates** beauty and self-confidence from the inside out.

How would you sign the following sentences?

1. She sat **transfixed** when she was told she needed to see an **oncologist.**

   _____

2. She soon realized that her condition was **graver** than she initially thought.

   _____

3. There was a treatment being offered that **conceivably** might **eradicate** her disease.

   _____

4. It was **plausible** that after treatment she could live a long and full life.

   _____

5. Today she **radiates** beauty from the inside out.

   _____

Selection 16.4: People Watchers

Are you a **fervent** people watcher? When you're stuck in between flights, do you like to sit and read, work on your laptop, or just spend the time watching people? People watching can be a lot of fun just to see how **ostentatious** some people can be. They walk through the terminal with their **flamboyant** clothes and accessories. People watchers can become **riveted** to them as they walk by. It's almost as if their **mantra** is, "Hey, look at me; look how much I'm worth!"

Other people are quite **unpretentious**. They might be worth millions, but you'd never know it. They don't **flaunt** anything, and their manner of dress certainly doesn't **compel** anyone to stare at them. Still, there is something about them that conveys **celebrity** status. Maybe it's in their manner of dress; perhaps it is just conveyed in their overall presence—how they walk and how they take command of the situation.

It is **inevitable** that if you spend enough time in airports, you will eventually see some very **ingenious** outfits that can be **dubbed** as either high style or as shabby chic. For those who are **bona fide** people watchers airports can provide a great form of entertainment.

How would you sign the following sentences?

1. I thought the clothes she picked were rather **ostentatious.**

   _____

2. Bob is very **unpretentious**. You'd never know he has a lot of money.

   _____

3. Shirley didn't **flaunt** her three-carat ring, but you couldn't help but notice it.

   _____

4. Elton John has always been a **flamboyant** character.

   _____

5. **Bona fide** people watchers can find airports very entertaining.

   _____

Selection 16.5: The Advertising Industry

Have you ever wondered how much **empirical** data is really behind the products that you buy? Advertising agencies spend millions of dollars promoting their products that **allegedly** cure any **malady**. Every day you can listen to or read a **barrage** of advertisements containing enough **hype** to confuse the average consumer.

Today ads can be very **savvy**, and it can be very difficult to **decipher** the facts from the amount of **bogus** information that is being spouted. People buy products hoping for a quick cure, only to discover that what they bought isn't any more effective than the last product that they invested in.

The American people are **inundated** with advertisements. They are everywhere you go, and everywhere you look. They're in magazines, on television and radio, and they have even **infiltrated** the Internet. Recently a columnist suggested that the government declare a **moratorium** on advertising agencies, preventing them from bombarding the general public with **ludicrous** information. That in itself was rather a **brash** statement, considering the fact that we live in a country that endorses the concept of free speech.

It is the consumers' **prerogative** whether they want to pay attention to the ads or buy the products. However, it seems like there should be some mechanism in place to help prevent consumers from being **disillusioned** with products that they have been told will yield specific results.

How would you sign the following sentences?

1. How much **empirical** data is actually collected on a product before it is sold?

   _____

2. The American people are **inundated** with a **barrage** of advertisements.

   _____

3. Ads are everywhere; they have even **infiltrated** the Internet with **ludicrous** information.

   _____

4. It is the consumers' **prerogative** if they do or don't pay attention to the media.

   _____

5. The columnist declared that the government should declare a **moratorium** on advertising agencies.

   _____

Additional Vocabulary-Building Activities I

 Selection 17.1: Charting New Territory

There are numerous historical accounts of pioneers who blazed trails into virgin territories to put down roots and begin new lives. Some of these pioneers started as immigrants from other countries, coming to the colonies so they could escape warlords and **feudalism.** Although many were intent on conquering new **vistas**, they had no concept of the harsh realities that would eventually confront them.

There is a **plethora** of information on how the early pioneers survived their first few years on the prairie after **forging** a path through the wilderness. Several were very **innovative** and quickly became accustomed to their new lifestyle, relying **solely** on the land for food and shelter. Others perished during the first winter due to a series of **maladies** that overcame them. From **predators** in the form of other inhabitants to shortages of food and **pestilence**, those who were not hearty did not survive.

One only has to visit places like Williamsburg today to gain insights into the hardships the early settlers endured. Reenactments of how the early settlers **foraged** for food and how they made candles and soap as well as other household items is a **phenomenon** worth viewing. It certainly paints an **evocative** picture of what this country was like during the pioneer days.

How would you sign the following sentences?

1. There is a **plethora** of information on how the early pioneers survived their first winter.

   _____

2. Many of the early pioneers **forged** a path through the wilderness **foraging** for food.

   _____

3. The early settlers explored many new **vistas**.

   _____

4. There were many **predators** on the prairie.

   _____

5. It certainly paints an **evocative** picture of what this country was like several hundred years ago.

   _____

Selection 17.2: Sports Heroes

When football made its **debut** in this country, it triggered a level of excitement that no one would have thought possible. Today millions of sports fans **converge** on stadiums or become glued to their television sets, **engrossed** in sporting events that occur on a weekly basis during the season. This **fervor** of excitement has **spawned** a whole new era of products as sponsors **extol** the virtues of their teams.

Teams that were once **virtually** unknown are now **ubiquitous** due to the number of novelties designed to promote team spirit. Advertising agencies never seem to **skimp** on the latest gimmick or commercial **slathered** across the media. One can only **infer** by watching this media frenzy that we are a nation **steeped** in team spirit.

Fans begin each season wondering who the next **prodigy** will be. They fill sports bars on Monday nights listening to coaches trying to **exonerate** their players of any wrongdoing as they go through the typical **litany** of the pros and cons of the various strategic plays attempted in the earlier games. It's as if they're trying to **vindicate** themselves of the choices they've made and divert the attention away from their mistakes.

I often get **nostalgic** listening to them. They remind me of the days I played and coached ball. Sometimes I wish I could turn back the clock and play ball again. But, because that's not possible I'll just have to be content with my view from the big-screen TV.

How would you sign the following sentences?

1. This **fervor** of excitement has **spawned** a whole new line of products.

   _____

2. Fans begin each season wondering who the next **prodigy** will be.

   _____

3. Coaches sometimes try to **exonerate** their players of any wrongdoing.

   _____

4. Teams today are very **ubiquitous** due to the amount of publicity that they get.

   _____

5. She tried to **vindicate** herself after being shut out for the third game in a row.

   _____

Selection 17.3: Contemporary Music

Have you been paying attention to the lyrics of some of the music hitting the airways today? While some of the songs have **ominous** messages **encrypted** in them, others have such a **sonorous** quality that you wonder how they ever made it on to the airwaves. I'm not sure what **compels** some of the artists to come up with the lyrics that they do, but it seems from time to time that the same morbid message keeps cropping up in songs.

I've often wondered what **redemptive** qualities a song has that makes a point of **denouncing** all of the values that most of us cherish. It's as if the lyrics are **anchored** in messages that promote anger and destruction through the use of **acerbic** words. Frequently, listeners get so caught up in the beat that they aren't even **cognizant** of what they're hearing. On the surface what appears to be an innocent piece of music is actually a **scurrilous** piece of prose designed to make **disparaging** remarks about basic beliefs.

257

CHAPTER 17
....
Additional
Vocabulary-Building
Activities I

The **scenarios** described in the songs often don't **mesh** with the realities of daily living. Rather, they become an **oration** supporting violence, greed, and wrongdoing. I realize that it is the songwriter's **prerogative** to write what he or she wants, but at the same time I think we should be more **stringent** about what can and can't be played on public airways.

How would you sign the following sentences?

1. Some songs today have **ominous** messages **encrypted** in them.

    _____

2. Some contemporary artists use **acerbic** lyrics to get their point across.

    _____

3. It is a songwriter's **prerogative** to write what he or she wants.

    _____

4. I think we should be more **stringent** on what is aired across public airways.

    _____

5. Sometimes the **scenarios** described in songs are in direct opposition to real-life experiences.

    _____

Selection 17.4: Problems at the Mall

Recently my Deaf friend told me about a problem they had at the mall. Let me tell you what happened. It seems for the past couple of years they've been having their silent dinner at the food court at the mall. People from all over the community would come, eat, sit and visit, and just have a good time. Basically, they were being very **nonintrusive**; in part they were giving sign language students a forum to **enhance** their skills.

Well, last month the security guard at the mall **confronted** them and told them they couldn't meet there any more. At first they were **devastated**; then they got **disgruntled**. The manager told the guard to tell them that they were taking up too many seats and that they'd have to find another place for their silent dinner. One of the members tried to explain that there were plenty of seats and that they were mall customers just like everyone else. The security guard wouldn't hear of it. He basically told them they'd have to leave.

The situation started to **intensify** when my friend told the guard they were being **discriminated** against and that he couldn't keep Deaf people out of the mall. He went on to tell him that they couldn't be **coerced** to leave. The conversation reached an **impasse** when the manager couldn't be contacted for comment. Word of what happened spread throughout the state, and next month more Deaf people plan to attend the dinner. The mayor's office has been contacted for help, but phone calls haven't been returned. In our **egalitarian** society, it doesn't seem legal that they can be banned from having their dinners at the mall.

How would you sign the following sentences?

1. They were being very **nonintrusive;** they were just sitting there minding their own business.

    _____

2. The conversation reached an **impasse** when the manager couldn't be contacted.

    _____

258

PART III
....
Multiple-Meaning
Words, Idioms, and
Vocabulary Building

3. They felt they were being **coerced** into leaving.

_____

4. At first they were **devastated**, then they became **disgruntled**.

_____

5. In our **egalitarian** society, it doesn't seem legal that they can be banned from the mall.

_____

Selection 17.5: The United Nations

The United Nations has been in existence for as long as I can remember. They have a wonderful **infrastructure** and serve as peacekeepers for member countries throughout the world. They function as **mediators** when global problems arise and **impose** sanctions on countries that they **deem** are not following humane practices toward their fellow countrymen.

Through the years the UN has been responsible for sending billions of dollars in food and aid to wartorn countries. Their aid **transcends** all boundaries. Their goal is to make others more comfortable and prevent the masses from dying from disease or starvation. The organization is **undeterred** by leaders of countries who **rebuff** their efforts and try to **admonish** them from trying to come into their so-called domains.

It's too bad today there aren't more organizations like the United Nations. If there were, perhaps more wars could be **averted**, there would be less human suffering, and the world would be a more humane place to live.

How would you sign the following sentences?

1. The United Nations has wonderful **infrastructure.**

_____

2. One of the functions of the UN is to **impose** sanctions on countries that present a threat to other countries.

_____

3. Their aid **transcends** all boundaries.

_____

4. The organization is **undeterred** by leaders of countries who try to **rebuff** their efforts.

_____

5. If there were more organizations like the UN, perhaps more wars could be **averted.**

_____

CHAPTER 18

Additional Vocabulary-Building Activities II

Selection 18.1: The Pillar of the Community

In every community there are certain individuals who stand out as **pillars** of the community. What earns them this **acclaim**? Is it the amount of money they **amass** over the course of a lifetime, the charitable acts they perform, or a combination of both? Regardless of how we define this unique group of individuals, they all seem to share one common characteristic. They are all **dynamic** individuals who make a **significant** contribution to society.

Bev is one of those **sterling** individuals. She is a professional woman who volunteers on several community projects, cares for her ailing mother, and is a **prominent** fund raiser. She is a **contemporary** woman unruffled by the **frenzy** of daily living, committed to making her community and the world a better place for those who will follow in her footsteps.

Her willingness to support others **spans** more than three decades. She has **spearheaded** several fundraisers to help women whose families have been **splintered** by alcoholism, divorce, and abuse. In addition, she has been a **champion** for those needing extended treatment for cancer and AIDS. With the **advent** of her support group, those otherwise facing social isolation and **stigmatization** have found acceptance and encouragement.

Bev continues to serve as an **inspiration** to others in her community. She is indeed a pillar of strength and an **incredibly** kind and caring individual.

How would you sign the following sentences?

1. Bev is a true **pillar** of the community; she gives far more than she takes.

2. She is a **dynamic** individual who has made a **significant** contribution to society.

3. Her involvement with the community **spans** more than three decades.

4. She has **spearheaded** several fundraisers for causes she believes in.

5. She has helped women whose families have been **splintered** by alcoholism and abuse.

259

Selection 18.2: The Plight of Immigrants

One of the **stark** realities of the plight of immigrants lies in the fact that many of them are **exploited** by the dominant culture. Faced with poor living conditions and substandard wages, many of them **succumb** to a life of misery and pain. Why do so many continue to **emigrate** from their countries if the lifestyle that awaits them is one of **servitude** and low wages? Perhaps it's because the conditions in their countries are **abhorrent**, and they fear for their lives if they don't escape.

In a new country, they frequently lack health insurance while **enduring** difficult jobs. Faced with the barrier of communication, they find themselves trapped with no tools to climb the socioeconomic ladder. Oftentimes, **stereotyped** by the larger majority, they struggle to avoid the **discrimination** often experienced by those who are different. Caught between a rock and a hard place, they must quickly adapt to their new surroundings in order to survive.

There are many reasons people continue to emigrate to this country. Some continue to come to establish a better lifestyle for their children. Access to a free public education is an **incentive** for many, making all of the sacrifices worth it. Escaping the **tyranny** of current dictatorships prompts others to leave, while others welcome hard work as a **respite** for having no opportunity to work at all.

Regardless of why they continue to come, many feel it is each and every country's moral and social responsibility to ensure that once they arrive on **domestic** shores that they are treated with the same **decorum** of dignity and respect central to the rights of all humans.

How would you sign the following sentences?

1. One of the **stark** realities of life is the **exploitation** of immigrants.

2. Many of them **succumb** to a life of misery and pain.

3. They are frequently **stereotyped** and **discriminated** against by the larger majority.

4. Many of them are escaping the **tyranny** of their former governments when they emigrate from their countries.

5. When they land, they should be treated with the same amount of **decorum** as others.

Selection 18.3: Developing Higher-Level Cognitive Strategies

With today's emphasis placed on high-stakes testing, many classrooms are focusing on rote memorization and failing to encourage the development of higher-level **cognitive** strategies. What is involved in this level of thinking? What types of activities do you find in classrooms that **embrace** a philosophy of teaching cognitive and **metacognitive** strategies to children?

If one examines Bloom's taxonomy, one quickly discovers that cognitive strategies are at the top of the **hierarchy.** Classrooms that focus on developing higher-order thinking skills are committed to helping students **transform** information into a strong conceptual framework whereby they draw **inferences** and critically examine information.

Within these classrooms students **engage** in thought-provoking activities, including responding to open-ended questions, entering debates, analyzing the reasons for their decisions, and thinking outside of the box. They learn to examine their thinking while developing strategies for solving problems.

In turn, these students can apply their newly **acquired** strategies to related problems, thus solving them **efficiently** and effectively. When faced with new **dilemmas**, they do not shy away from challenges but rather embrace them with a newfound eagerness to try to solve them.

Thinking skills can be traced to the early works of Socrates and Aristotle. Ever since the **advent** of time, humankind has tried to solve some of the mysteries of the world. By providing today's **emergent** learners with an exposure to critical thinking skills activities, the foundation is being laid for tomorrow's great analytical thinkers.

How would you sign the following sentences?

1. It is important today to introduce **cognitive** strategies into the curriculum.

_____

2. Many classrooms embed activities into the curriculum that promote cognition and **metacognition.**

_____

3. Critical thinking skills are at the top of the **hierarchy** in Bloom's taxonomy.

_____

4. Students need to be able to **transform** information into a strong conceptual framework.

_____

5. When students become **efficient** at developing their ability to think critically, they have developed higher-level cognitive strategies.

_____

Selection 18.4: Relationships

There are an abundance of contemporary books and articles on the market today that focus on forming and maintaining relationships. The topic has **intrigued** psychologists for years and given them **fodder** for numerous articles as they examine and describe the way individuals relate to each other. One topic that has particularly **piqued** their interest is how different people respond during times of conflict. They have recorded numerous arguments on tape depicting the dynamics that occur when two or more individuals disagree. These heated debates have been captured, and the spontaneous interactions have been analyzed for patterns of behavior. Some of the more common behaviors include matching anger with anger, walking away from the situation altogether, or clamming up.

In general, they have observed some people **feigning apathy** when being bombarded with **caustic** remarks, while others become **livid** and match their opponent with equally sarcastic and biting comments.

Recently, a renowned author wrote an article describing how it can be a positive attribute to maintain your **equanimity** even during times of stress. However, he also stated that the most **taciturn** individuals can become very vocal if pushed to the limit on a topic for which they have a passion.

262

PART III
....
Multiple-Meaning
Words, Idioms, and
Vocabulary Building

How would you sign the following sentences?

1. The topic has **intrigued** psychologists for years and given them **fodder** for several articles.

   _____

2. One topic that has **piqued** their interest is how people interact during disagreements.

   _____

3. Some people **feign apathy** when being bombarded with **caustic** remarks.

   _____

4. It is a good idea to maintain your **equanimity** in the face of adversity.

   _____

5. The most **taciturn** people can become vocal if pushed too much.

   _____

Selection 18.5: The Essay

All of us at one time or another have had to write an essay. Usually this assignment is given in an English composition class where you have to create the standard five-paragraph exposition, complete with an introduction, conclusion, and three paragraphs in between.

I remember the time a friend of mine shared his essay with me. It was a story about the characteristics of **bellicose** people. He emphasized how **erratic** their behavior can be and how they can be **perfidious** people. He further described them as advocating **sedition**, drawing unsuspecting individuals into their lairs and persuading them to participate in **belligerent** activities.

He resorted to using **hyperboles** in his paper to make some of his points. He really wanted to emphasize the **egregious** qualities exhibited in these types of people. What he had to say was **germane** to the topic he had selected. As I read it, I remember developing a great **animus** toward them. It was hard for me to **fathom** how anyone could have such a belligerent **disposition.**

It's been several years since I read that essay but some of his descriptive language made an impression on me. He definitely had a way with words and could capture his audience's attention, even if he was writing about topics that some would find hard to stomach.

How would you sign the following sentences?

1. My friend wrote his essay about the characteristics of **bellicose** people.

   _____

2. He resorted to using **hyperboles** in his paper to emphasize his points.

   _____

3. What he wrote was **germane** to the topic.

   _____

4. I developed a great **animus** to the people described in his essay.

   _____

5. He talked at length about the **egregious** qualities that they exhibited.

   _____

Additional Vocabulary-Building Activities III

Selection 19.1: Washington, DC

Washington, DC, is considered a **megalopolis** due to the dense population of people who reside within that geographic area. The inhabitants of the area represent diverse cultural and ethnic backgrounds that espouse different **dogmas,** religious beliefs, and practices. Without a doubt, the city represents a **diverse** group of individuals who contribute to the fabric of the United States.

The city is full of an **eclectic** group of art galleries, featuring **abstract, austere,** and **esoteric** paintings and sculptures designed to provide residents as well as visitors with an array of options to choose from. The **intricate** designs have prompted several viewers to **covet** several of the pieces displayed in both the museums and the galleries.

In addition to the cultural offerings of the city, there is also an abundance of restaurants with **tantalizing** dishes prepared to satisfy any appetite. With food choices arranged **aesthetically** on plates, diners have the option of selecting everything from Indian fare to Greek cuisine with everything in between. Prices vary from moderate to expensive, depending of the type of atmosphere and the location of the restaurant.

It goes without saying that this important city is also the nation's capital. From this vibrant political hub speeches are delivered, legislation is passed, mandates are established, and life-altering decisions are made. It is truly a Mecca for political activity. Because Washington can be such an exciting place to visit, it is best to go in the spring or fall when the days are warm and you can go for extended walks while taking in all that the city has to offer.

How would you sign the following sentences?

1. Washington is considered a **megalopolis** due to its dense population.

   _____

2. Different cultural groups frequently espouse different **dogmas** and traditions.

   _____

3. Some of the art work was very **esoteric;** I could look at it for hours.

   _____

4. The **tantalizing** dishes satisfied my palate.

   _____

5. The food was **aesthetically** arranged on the table.

   _____

Selection 19.2: Raising the Barn

When reading historical accounts of the early settlers who put down their roots in rural America, one is frequently reminded of the **benevolence** exhibited by mankind. There are numerous stories of families in **dire** need of supplies and shelter and of the assistance they received. Countless stories have been told of how the neighbors would come together, and within a very short time they would raise a barn.

The early settlers were very **pragmatic** people, exhibiting good common sense by separating out their **intrinsic** needs from their **extrinsic** desires. Their homes were not **ornate** but, rather, were designed to protect them against the **ominous** weather that could develop quickly and without warning.

Several poignant memoirs have been written about the **affinity** displayed among family members and friends during the early days on the frontier. Reading the **chronicles** describing the hardships these **intrepid** men and women endured provides readers with new insights into what life on the prairie was really like. One can only imagine that is must have taken a **tenacious** and hardy group of people who were willing to make great sacrifices so that new towns and communities could be established.

How would you sign the following sentences?

1. Several **poignant** memoirs have been written about the early pioneers.

   _____

2. They had so protect themselves against **ominous** weather that could develop at any time.

   _____

3. Many of the early settlers were in **dire** need of food and shelter.

   _____

4. Reading the **chronicles** provides one with new insights into these **intrepid** men and women.

   _____

5. The early settlers were very **pragmatic** people.

   _____

 ### Selection 19.3: The Forces of Nature

Meteorologists spend a lifetime studying weather patterns and predicting storms that can **intensify** at a moment's notice, wreaking **havoc** on area inhabitants and causing destruction that can take years, if not a lifetime, to repair. Modern technology has made it possible to **detect** severe weather patterns and make earlier predictions of **impending** violent weather, thus saving lives. However, little can be done to change the course of Mother Nature and the damage that can be left in her wake.

Volcanoes that have been **dormant** for years can suddenly erupt, covering the landscape with molten lava and ash. **Formidable** storms frequently develop in the form of tornadoes when masses of cold and warm weather collide. Varying in intensity, these funnels can cut a wide path of destruction, leaving hundreds hurt and homeless.

In recent years hurricanes and **tsunamis** have become extremely deadly in nature. When total communities are **eradicated** by **fatal** mudslides and flood waters, residents have been forced to flee their homes and these **dire** conditions in order to survive. Once the storms **subside**, they return to the area to find total

265

CHAPTER 19
....
Additional
Vocabulary-Building
Activities III

devastation with all of their **sentimental** belongings destroyed or washed away. While some return with the hope of rebuilding again, others are **adamant** about relocating, salvaging what they can, and beginning a new life.

How would you sign the following sentences?

1. Storms can **intensify** at a moments notice and wreak **havoc** on a community.

   _____

2. New technology has made it easier for meteorologists to predict **impending** violent storms.

   _____

3. Volcanoes that have been **dormant** for years can erupt, covering the landscape with molten lava and ash.

   _____

4. With **fatal** mudslides **eradicating** total communities residents have been forced to flee their homes.

   _____

5. Once the storms **subside**, residents return to find total **devastation** with all of their **sentimental** belongings destroyed.

   _____

Selection 19.4: The Bibliophile

Rich is a **bibliophile**. He has a **voracious** appetite for learning and devours everything he can on a wide array of subjects. He has collected a multitude of books. Having read and studied over ten different languages, he is **fluent** in Spanish, French, German, Italian, and Russian.

It is easy for him to **assimilate** new information, so learning languages is not difficult for him.

His interest in learning is not limited to languages; he collects books on history and **savors** both biographies and autobiographies. He loves to read historical prose that focuses on the **pragmatic** lives of the early pioneers and the forming of the constitution. He will collect several volumes and then delve into them until his interest in a subject is satisfied.

Rich also enjoys studying calculus, physics, and trigonometry. While in college, he devised some **esoteric** theories that were understood by only his major professors. The rest of us were left in the dust. His ability to apply these theories to reality has allowed him to **improvise** on more than one occasion when he needed something that was not readily available.

He is truly a **renaissance** man who enjoys collecting and **perusing** books at his leisure and garnering as much information from them as he can. He has a **propensity** for learning and because of that will probably remain one of the most **versatile** individuals around.

How would you sign the following sentences?

1. Rich is a **bibliophile;** he lives in the library among the stacks of books.

   _____

2. He will **delve** into several volumes until his interest in a subject is satisfied.

   _____

3. While in college, he devised some **esoteric** theories only understood by his professors.

_____

4. He has a **propensity** for learning, spending hours with his nose in a book.

_____

5. He is probably one of the most **versatile** individuals around.

_____

Additional Vocabulary-Building Activities IV

Selection 20.1: Careers in the Field of Science

The field of science is very broad, affording those who choose to major in it a wide variety of job opportunities upon graduating from their respective programs. It is **evident** to those who **avail** themselves of science that the field is vast and the careers endless.

With global warming gaining national attention, **geologists** as well as **meteorologists** have joined forces with physical scientists to try to determine the causes that are responsible for contributing to this **phenomenon.** Recently, scientists **convened** in Washington to discuss the **toxic** effect global warming could have on society. **Oceanographers** were invited to join in the discussion to share their insights into how we could harness energy found in the sea, thus eliminating some of the **potential** culprits contributing to the problem.

Other areas of science gaining global attention today lie within the field of biomedicine. Some of the **beneficiaries** of this branch of science are those who have lost limbs or the use of limbs due to accidents or disease. Sophisticated **prosthetic** devices have made the lives of so many individuals so much better. By **simplifying** their lives, prosthetics have enabled people to regain their sense of independence. Prior to the development of these devices, the **prognosis** for these patients was less than satisfactory. Today, due to the advances in technology, many are leading independent lives not previously thought possible.

How would you sign the following sentences?

1. It is **evident** to all of those who **avail** themselves of careers in science that numerous job opportunities await them.

    _____

2. **Oceanographers** as well as **meteorologists** are joining forces to confront the problem of global warming.

    _____

3. It is feared that global warming could have a **toxic** effect on the environment.

    _____

4. New advances in biomedicine have aided in the development of new **prosthetic** devices.

    _____

5. In the past, the **prognosis** for these individuals was less than satisfactory.

    _____

268

PART III
....
Multiple-Meaning
Words, Idioms, and
Vocabulary Building

Selection 20.2: The New Power Plant

For the past ten months, the city council has been engaged in heated debates with the community over the proposed new power plant. City leaders had no idea the topic would create such **discord** among local residents. Although they recognized that some people might feel **adamant** against the decision to build it, they thought there would be more **harmony** among the majority of area residents.

At each of the recent meetings, a number of **dogmatic** individuals **dominated** the conversation, trying to persuade area residents why they should vote against the proposed plant. They explained that the new plant would not be **compatible** with the existing system and that it would create more headaches for them down the road than they realized.

They brought in **prestigious** leaders from **adjacent** communities to address the topic, believing that their **status** in their communities would lend **credence** to the debate. Emphasizing that the new plant would not be **durable** enough to withstand the forces of nature, they **literally** outlined what the future would hold. They went to great lengths to describe why they were **skeptical** and why they thought the civic leaders would be wise to reconsider the proposal.

The **astute** city council members responded by presenting them with pages of **tedious** facts and statistics. In the end both sides were ready for a **respite** from the discussion. The vote will take place at the next meeting. It is **anticipated** that a large crowd will converge on the meeting and will depart either **exceedingly** happy or **distraught**.

How would you sign the following sentences?

1. City leaders had no idea the proposal would create such **discord** among community members.

   _____

2. Each side was **adamant** about its beliefs and views on the topic.

   _____

3. A number of **dogmatic** individuals **dominated** the conversation, making it difficult to focus on the facts.

   _____

4. They brought in **prestigious** leaders from **adjacent** counties.

   _____

5. The **astute** city council members presented them with **tedious** facts and figures.

   _____

 ## Selection 20.3: The Gathering

Annually, Thanksgiving is spent at my grandmother's estate in upper New York state where she has lived for her entire life. My **agile** grandmother is now in her early eighties but still very much the **matriarch** of the family. Every year she invites all of the family as well as selected friends to attend the gathering at her estate.

She is a very **gregarious** person and has always had a **zest** for life. Through the years those who know her have tried to **emulate** many of her positive **attributes**. Without a doubt, her **charisma** is felt by those who have been fortunate enough to get to know her through the years. Not only is she **amiable**, but she looks for ways to connect her guests with one another while emphasizing their unique and noteworthy contributions.

269

CHAPTER 20
....
Additional
Vocabulary-Building
Activities IV

PART I

PART II

PART III

PART IV

Last year poets, artists, and musicians were invited to the estate. While some of her guests appeared to be a bit **eccentric**, they all seemed to enjoy the company of the others. I was **intrigued** to see how even the most **bizarre** characters seemed to enjoy the **banter** of those around them. It's always been fun just to remain on the **periphery** and observe the actions of others.

I don't know how many more years my grandmother will be able to host this event. I just know that she has always been the **epitome** of the perfect hostess, and when these events cease I will experience a great sense of loss. Through the years, I feel I have been fortunate to rub shoulders with some of the most **erudite** people of our time, and for that I will always cherish the gatherings.

How would you sign the following sentences?

1. My **agile** 80-year-old grandmother is still the **matriarch** of the family.

   _____

2. She is a very **gregarious** person who has a **zest** for life.

   _____

3. Without a doubt, she has a certain **charisma** about her that is admired by many.

   _____

4. Some of her guests appear to be a bit **eccentric**, exhibiting **bizarre** behaviors.

   _____

5. I like to stand on the **periphery** and listen to the **banter** of the group.

   _____

Selection 20.4: The National Agenda

Did you know that there is a national agenda to improve the education of deaf children throughout the United States? A group of important stakeholders have developed an agenda designed to address the **vital** educational needs of these students. They are taking very **prudent** steps to ensure the changes they are recommending are anchored in evidence-based practice.

After months of evaluations, discussions, and sifting through **data**, they have **corroborated** their findings and have now established a new set of **criteria** for use in restructuring current programs. If these recommendations are adopted, it will **signify** a new direction for the field to take.

Upon first glance, many of their recommendations appear to be **feasible**. They are **pragmatic** in nature and are designed to hold all educators **accountable** for their instruction and **assessments** that they are using on a daily basis. The **philosophy** behind the recommended changes is that more critical thinking skills strategies and activities should be integrated into the curriculum. This would shift the **onus** of learning onto the student and provide for a more student-centered classroom learning environment.

Emphasis would continue to be placed on literacy, but strategies for transferability would become a **pivotal** part of each objective and classroom learning activity. If instructors are taught to **diverge** from their current **dispositions** regarding classroom instruction and embrace this new **pedagogy**, it is believed that students' achievement will skyrocket, and they will escape the learning **plateau** where they have been **stymied** for so many years.

How would you sign the following sentences?

1. They are taking very **prudent** steps as recommendations are developed.

   _____

2. They have **corroborated** their findings and have established a new set of **criteria.**

   _____

3. Many of their recommendations appear to be **feasible.**

   _____

4. This would shift the **onus** of learning onto the student.

   _____

5. The stakeholders are hoping the classroom teachers will embrace this new **pedagogy.**

   _____

Selections for Interpreting and Transliterating

Leisure and Employment

Selection 1.1: Baking Bread

Do you like to bake bread? I do. Let me give you a simple recipe to make a perfect loaf of white bread that is delicious every time. To make this loaf of bread you will need the following ingredients: $5\frac{3}{4}$ to $6\frac{1}{4}$ cups of flour, one package of active dry yeast, $2\frac{1}{4}$ cups of milk, 2 tablespoons of sugar, 1 tablespoon of butter, and $1\frac{1}{2}$ teaspoons of salt.

You begin by getting a large mixing bowl. In this bowl combine $2\frac{1}{2}$ cups of the flour and the yeast and set it aside. Next, get a medium pan. In the saucepan heat and stir the milk, adding the sugar, butter, and salt until it becomes warm and the butter almost melts.

Then you are ready to add the milk mixture to the flour mixture. When you do this, beat it with an electric mixer on low for about thirty seconds. Then turn your dough out on a floured surface, and knead in enough of the remaining flour to make a moderately stiff dough.

Keep in mind that kneading is important. If you have never kneaded bread, it is simple. Push down on your dough with the heels of your hands, curving your fingers over the dough. Continue pushing the dough down until it becomes elastic. When it's not too sticky and will hold its shape, place it in a bowl and let it rise. After it has doubled in size, punch it down and shape into a loaf. Put it in a pan and let it rise. When it has doubled in size (this usually requires thirty minutes to an hour), it's ready to bake.

Bake your bread in a 375-degree oven for about forty minutes. When you take it out of the oven, immediately remove it from the pan and let it cool.

Warm bread is delicious with any meal; it's especially good on cold winter days when you're eating soup or stew.

Selection 1.2: Applying for a Job

Finding a job in a competitive market can be challenging for even the most qualified individuals. Today many computer-savvy folks have designed websites that help promote their skills. On these websites they may list their resumes, jobs they have held, and even a photo of who they are. While some of these are done with the help of a web designer, others are done by the individual with just the basic information displayed.

Whether you design a website or represent yourself only in person, there are certain tips that you should follow if you want to secure a job. First, find out as much about the employer as possible. Maybe you know a friend who works for the company. Try to determine exactly what the company is looking for.

Second, read the advertisement carefully. Do you have the skills it is looking for? If you don't have all of the skills, do you at least have part of them? Can you modify your resume to show your strengths, so the person reading your informa-

273

CHAPTER 1
....
Leisure and
Employment

PART I

PART II

PART III

PART IV

tion will see that you can meet some of the requirements? Remember, you want to highlight your strengths, not draw attention to your shortcomings.

Third, drop off, mail, or e-mail your application, resume, and a letter requesting an interview. In your letter be specific about what job you are applying for. Express your interest in working for the company or agency. Be sure to include all phone numbers and email addresses where you can be reached.

If you are contacted for an interview, arrive fifteen minutes before it is scheduled to begin. Remember to dress appropriately. First impressions are made during the first five minutes. Interviewers will form an opinion of you before you even open your mouth to speak. Once the interview begins, listen attentively and ask questions at appropriate times. Make sure those in the room can see your interest in their organization.

A day or two after the interview, send a follow-up letter thanking the individual for taking time to meet with you. Interviewing for a job is a learning experience. You should be able to walk away from each interview and mentally assess the things you did well and the things you might want to improve upon before the next time. You might be the perfect candidate for the job. However, if you are not hired, you will at least have the satisfaction of knowing that you put your best foot forward.

Selection 1.3: Traveling to Europe

How many of you have ever traveled to Europe, either alone or with a group? If you have visited some of the European countries, you'll be able to relate to what I'm going to say. Those of you who have traveled extensively probably have a number of stories that you, too, could share with the group.

When traveling abroad, you can go individually, as couples, or as part of a travel group. Sometimes special tours are organized for Deaf people. If you go on one of these trips, there is usually an interpreter or interpreters available 24/7. This makes it nice for visiting museums, art galleries, and other points of interest.

Before you can leave the United States, you must obtain a passport. Depending on where you live you will be able to get your passport from several different places. In some small towns you can go to the courthouse and take care of everything right there. In larger cities you might have to stop at two or three locations in order to secure the picture and all of the necessary paperwork. Whenever you decide to take a trip abroad, it is always wise to find out what you'll need well in advance of the trip so you have ample time to gather what you need.

When you arrive at your destination, you might want to convert some of your U.S. dollars to the currency used in that country. Then, as you purchase your souvenirs you won't have to worry if merchants will accept U.S. dollars.

When traveling throughout other countries, it can be fun to sample the local cuisine by eating in restaurants that cater more to the locals than to the tourists. These restaurants tend to serve more authentic food that is typically found in the area. Be careful to ask how spicy some of dishes are before you order so you'll be able to eat your selection.

Be sensitive to local customs. Educate yourself to the required protocol prior to attending an event or frequenting an establishment. If you know that the restaurant expects you to sit on the floor and eat your food from community bowls and you're not comfortable with that, don't attend. A polite decline will save everyone from embarrassment or a stressful situation in the long run.

Plan your trip well in advance. Prioritize where you want to go and what you want to see. Be realistic about your time constraints. Traveling can be an experience you will treasure for a lifetime if you do your homework before you go. If you approach it with an open mind and you are eager for an adventure, you are sure to have a good time.

Selection 1.4: Going Hunting

Hunting can be a very popular sport among both men and women. While some folks in the North hunt pheasant and quail, those in the South and West may hunt deer. Those who hunt birds frequently go out in the field with one or two dogs or sometimes even a pack of them. The dogs sit quietly at their masters' feet waiting for the command to go and retrieve the bird.

The hunters stand waiting for the flock of birds to fly overhead, aim, and fire. If they are lucky enough to get a bird or birds, they command the dog or dogs to retrieve them. At that point, the dogs run through the field or into the water to retrieve the birds and then bring them back to their owners.

Deer hunting is very different than bird hunting. Deer hunting can be done by just walking through the woods and tracking a deer or going to a hunting camp where one scouts the deer. In either event, the goal is to kill a deer, thus providing meat for weeks and months to come.

One popular way to hunt deer is to use a deer stand. A deer stand is usually constructed in the trees and allows the hunter to climb up where he or she has an aerial view of the ground. Then as deer run or walk by, the hunter can get the deer in his or her sight, aim, and shoot without being seen. If hunters are lucky enough to get a deer, they climb down from the deer stand and retrieve their prize.

Some hunters spend hours in a deer stand in search of the perfect buck. Some are lucky and within hours have spotted their prize; others wait hours in the cold to no avail. After a few or several hours, they can become cold and disappointed and return home. While some may think hunting is a cruel sport, most of those who participate are very humane and help keep the animal population under control, thus reducing the number of animals that starve to death because of limited food resources.

Selection 1.5: Waiting Tables Can Be Hard Work

Waiting tables can be extremely hard work. You're on your feet eight or ten hours a day, hustling back and forth to the kitchen, bringing orders to anywhere from one person to large groups of people. Keeping orders straight and balancing plates, trays of glasses, and desserts can be challenging to say the least. But this is not the worst part.

When families arrive with children who are unruly, it can become a nightmare. Frequently when children are tired or very hungry, they scream, cry, or run around. When parents try to console them, glasses may get tipped over, food may be thrown on the floor, ketchup can get squirted over everything, and the table ends up in total disarray.

Families are not the only ones who present a challenge for a waiter or waitress. Sometimes customers become very rude and abusive. They don't like the way their food is cooked, they may feel what they got is not what they ordered, and send the server back and forth to the kitchen numerous times to try and get it right. That alone is bad enough, but when their attitude is obnoxious, it makes it very difficult for the person trying to serve them.

Oftentimes servers balance two heavy trays at one time. With both arms full from wrists to shoulders, they weave in and out of customers who are on their way to their tables or to go to the restroom. Stopping to answer questions along the way, they never seem to lose their balance or upset their trays.

Parties require special skills from servers. In order to do a good job, the waiter or waitress wants to make sure that all of the orders arrive hot and at the same time. He or she tries very hard to keep up with all of the refills so the guests at the table will appreciate the service, want to schedule their next party at the restaurant, and perhaps ask that he or she be their server. When servers do an excellent job like this, although it is very hard work, the tips can be generous, offsetting the demands of the job.

275

CHAPTER 1

Leisure and
Employment

PART I

PART II

PART III

PART IV

Selection 1.6: Working as a Parking Lot Attendant at Disney World

I'll never forget the story my friend Katie told me about the summer she worked as a parking lot attendant at Disney World. She and her best friend had been looking for a summer job that wouldn't be too difficult and one that they could do together. So when they saw the ad in the paper that Disney World was hiring parking attendants, they decided that would be an easy job that wouldn't require too much skill, so they decided they should apply.

Luckily for both of them they were both hired. They knew it would be an easy job. What they hadn't counted on was how boring it would be. Day after day as the cars pulled into the amusement park, they would tell the people where to park. Their jobs consisted mainly of saying "go to your left" or "go to your right and park in the first available spot." One day out of sheer boredom they came up with an idea. They thought it would be great fun to tell all of the white cars that came into the park to park in one specific lot.

So sure enough—all morning long as the cars filed into the amusement park they would tell all of the red, blue, and green cars, you get the picture, to go to Lot A on their left and all of the white cars to go to Lot B on their right. They continued to direct all of the cars this way until lunchtime. By two o'clock Lot B was filled to capacity with all white cars. I mean it was solid white. There wasn't one car that was a different color in that lot.

Late in the afternoon the tired park goers returned to the parking lots, ready to head home for the day. Now stop and imagine what they found when they went to find their cars. Instead of looking for a white car here and there among the others, they found row after row of white cars. You can imagine they weren't happy. They were hot, tired, and this wasn't funny. You guessed it! Several of the people complained to the management.

Later that day, Katie and her friend were called into the office. They were told never to do that again. They were also warned that if they did, they would be fired. Disney did not want unhappy customers. Needless to say, they didn't do it again. But, I have often laughed when I think of her telling that story. I'm glad I wasn't at Disney that summer, and I'm especially glad I didn't have a white car, but it's fun to imagine what that parking lot must have looked like.

Life Experiences I

Selection 2.1: Rescue from the Third Floor

Tracinda, her husband, and their 1-month-old son live on the third floor of an apartment building in New York. He works nights and she works days—that way they can take care of their son and don't have to put him in daycare at such a young age. It cuts down on the time they have together as a couple, but they both agreed that this is a good arrangement.

Recently, a tragic event happened. It was a cold, stormy night and Felix had gone to work. The weatherman had predicted an electrical storm, but by ten o'clock it seemed that the only thing that was going on was that the cold wind was going to continue to blow and that the electrical storm probably wouldn't materialize.

Tracinda finally got the baby to go to sleep, put him down, and thought she'd catch a couple hours of sleep before he woke again for his next feeding. She had only been asleep for about an hour when she woke up to the smell of smoke in their apartment. She ran to the window, looked out, and realized the building was engulfed in flames. It didn't take her long to realize that the only way out of the apartment was through the window. The floors below her were filled with smoke and flames.

In a state of panic, she grabbed the baby, ran to the window, and started shouting for help. She knew if someone didn't come and help her soon, they would both be lost in the flames and smoke. As the smoke filled the apartment, she held her son close to the window for air. Fortunately, firefighters arrived, and they were both rescued. After they were both treated for smoke inhalation, they were released from the hospital.

Later, when interviewed by the media, Tracinda talked about how lucky they were to get out alive—some of her neighbors hadn't been so lucky. She got teary eyed when she talked about losing friends and everything they owned. She said for them it could have been so much worse; she just felt lucky to have her son and still be alive.

Selection 2.2: Getting Stuck in the Mud

It had been raining cats and dogs all day long, and the ground was saturated with moisture. The sky was a leaden gray, and there was no sign of the rain stopping anytime soon. Puddles of various sizes were everywhere, and the ground made a squishing sound every time you had to walk on it. What's more, mud was starting to collect around sidewalks and curbs where the rain had washed the dirt from barren flower gardens.

Around one in the afternoon Jeanne had to head out toward her daughter's school. She had promised she'd be there by one-thirty to sign a book to Harley's class. As she started out, she knew she was in for a rough time. Visibility was reduced and the traffic was moving at a snail's pace. As she crept along with the other cars, she noticed a car accident ahead. Apparently a car had hit the retaining wall and had done a 360, taking out three other cars as it spun in a circle. Cars were backed up at a standstill waiting to get on the entrance ramp to the freeway. It didn't bode well.

277

CHAPTER 2
....
Life Experiences I

PART I

PART II

PART III

PART IV

Jeanne decided she would turn her car around and head in the other direction so she could arrive at the school on time. Just as she started to turn, her car slid to the right and ended up in the median. It scared her at first, but once she got her composure back, she tried backing up and getting out of her predicament. Once she backed up, her wheels got stuck in the mud. She tried to go forward but to no avail. The more she tried to move, the deeper her car got stuck in the mud.

Finally, she pulled out her Blackberry and called a friend for help. About thirty minutes later the tow truck arrived and pulled Jeanne from the median. She was so embarrassed and realized the folly of her actions. She vowed never again to take a short cut through the median.

Selection 2.3: Drive-Through Flu Shots

Have you ever had a flu shot? Do you plan to get one in the future? Many people swear by them. They think they help keep them healthy during the cold and flu season. It used to be that the only places you could get a flu shot were the doctor's office, health center, or a clinic. Doctors made a special effort to make sure the elderly got theirs first.

A new trend has taken over in this country. It involves drive-through flu shots. Set up like a fast-food drive-through, individuals can remain in their cars, roll down their windows, hold out their arms, and medical personnel will give them their shots without their ever having to leave the comfort of their own vehicles. Recently, a group of educational interpreters experienced this new trend.

One afternoon before classes started they decided to get in their cars and drive to the designated location. They got in line behind several other vehicles and inched along as they waited their turns to roll down their windows, hold out their arms, and get their vaccinations. At the end of the line, healthcare workers provide clipboards with information that the recipients of the flu shots are required to fill out. All of this takes place in a large circular fashion. You drive up, circle the building, receive your shot, and complete your paperwork and then exit where you came in.

The day the students went, they said that they had to wait in line for approximately ten minutes to get their flu shots. As the cars inched forward, they queued up and got ready. They feel it is a wonderful, fast, new way to receive flu shots with very little inconvenience to the patient.

Selection 2.4: Displays at the Grocery Store

Marvin works at the grocery store. He's worked there for about fifteen years now. He started out as a bag boy, moved up to checker, and now he's the assistant manager in charge of setting up displays. Every week he designs new displays that reflect the specials of the week. Sometimes he sets up seasonal displays, and other times they are promotional in nature for new products.

Last week he put together an elaborate display of baby food. Gerber was doing a promotional sale where moms could buy three boxes of cereal and get two free. Marv was asked to build a display at the end of the aisle that would draw attention to the cereal. What he created was a display about six feet tall from top to bottom. It was circular in design and featured all of the different boxes of cereal. He started with five pieces of plywood cut in perfectly round circles, each one cut a little smaller so he could build a tiered display.

At the base he placed over a hundred boxes of cereal on the wood with all of the box fronts facing outward. Each box was placed about two inches away from the box next to it. Then, he made a second row before adding the next piece of wood. He continued with the display until he reached the very top layer. At the very top there was room for between six and eight boxes. All total it resembled a giant wedding cake with over a thousand boxes of cereal, and although it took several hours to assemble, the finished product was a real eye catcher.

278

PART IV
....
Selections for
Interpreting and
Transliterating

Shortly after Marv finished he was ready to begin work on another display. Just as he was getting ready to head down the soap aisle to start the next display, something caught his eye. He stopped to look just as a woman with a baby in her cart turned too sharply down the baby food aisle and collided with Marv's display. Hundreds of boxes of cereal fell helter-skelter onto the floor. All he could do was look in awe as the woman stood embarrassed turning bright red before the chaos on the floor.

 Selection 2.5: Getting Stuck in a Dressing Room

My friend Rosie is crazy. She can't go anywhere without something funny happening. She's just one of those people. You know how some people have good luck, some people have bad luck, and then there are some people who are just funny. Rosie has these experiences that other people probably have, but the way she tells the story you can't help but laugh.

Recently, she was telling a group of us about shopping for new clothes. Part of the reason this is funny is that Rosie hates to shop for clothes. She just does. She'd rather work out in her garden and have mud up to her elbows than go in a store shopping for something to wear. Maybe it's because she was planning a trip to her high school reunion or maybe it's because it had been raining so much lately that she couldn't work outside that she decided to get out of the house and go shopping.

Whatever the reason, her shopping experience was typically Rosie. It started out with her trying on pants. She told us that she had found the cutest pair of pants in just her size. She's rather a small woman, and sometimes it's hard for her to find clothes. These pants were black with small sunglasses embroidered in all different colors all over them front and back. They looked to be the perfect size but she decided she better try them on.

When she went to go into the dressing room, the male attendant gave her a number—you know, for how many items she had—and sent her into the dressing room. This dressing room was one large room with a hall down the middle and several dressing rooms on both sides. She went into the fourth or fifth room and put on the pants. They fit perfectly and she was so excited. She went to take them off, and that's when her problems started.

She couldn't get them unfastened. She tried and tried, and she couldn't get the metal clasp to release. At first she thought she'd just buy the pants, wear them home, and figure it out once she got there. Then she had second thoughts. What if she had to go to the bathroom before she made it home? That would never do. She couldn't ask the attendant for help—the guy would think she was crazy, and she knew she'd be embarrassed to have some kid helping her out. What was she going to do?

Then she heard two women talking in another dressing room close to her. She decided they were her best bet. She went over to their room, knocked on the door, and said "excuse me." One of the women opened the door. Rosie explained her dilemma. At first the woman tried doing just what Rosie had done but had no luck. Finally, she told her, "I'm going to have to unzip the pants." Rosie said that was fine. By then she was desperate. Finally, the woman got them unfastened. Rosie was so grateful; she thanked the woman profusely and went back to her dressing room.

Once there, she took off the pants and put her own back on. She was so relieved. When she told us the story, we asked her if she went ahead and bought the pants. She said she did—that she knew her husband could fix the metal clasp so it wouldn't happen again. It was just funny to us—you see, one time Rosie went into a dressing room, tried on a dress that was too small, and almost had to buy it because she couldn't get it off. It took two of us to help her get out of it. She is just crazy.

CHAPTER 3

Games and Sports

 Selection 3.1: Flying Kites

March is a great month to fly kites. There is usually just enough of a breeze to lift any kite high into the sky, making it fun to watch as it soars and glides through the air. Kids of all ages seem to enjoy kite flying, and the twins Jeremy and Josh are no exception. One brisk March afternoon their mom came into the playroom to see if they'd like to go out and fly kites.

"Jeremy, Josh, do you two want to go outside and fly your kites?" She asked.

"Oh yes, Mommy, that would be fun! Can we go now?"

"Let me get your kites while you two put your jackets on. Then we'll go to the park where you can fly your kites and play on the playground."

The boys got their jackets while Mom rounded up the kites. They all hopped in the van and drove to the park. It was a perfect day to fly kites. Mom helped each of the boys get their kites in the air. Then, she stood back and watched them run.

"Look, Mom!" Jeremy cried. "Mine is going higher and higher—I think it will reach the top of the sky!"

"Look at mine, Mom!" Josh called out. "Mine is going higher than Jeremy's. I think it will hit the moon!"

The boys ran and played until Josh's kite got stuck in the tree. All of them tried to pull it loose but to no avail. Finally Mom decided that it was a lost cause.

Josh started to cry, "But Mommy, that's my favorite kite—Daddy gave it to me for helping him clean the garage."

"It's ok, Josh, I know where Daddy bought it and we'll get another one just like it. Think how happy you've made the tree by giving him your kite to make his branches look pretty. You've shared your kite with the big oak tree."

With that Josh stopped crying. The boys played in the park for a while, then they all hopped in the van, headed toward the house, stopped at the store, picked up a new kite, and went home. By the time they got back the boys were very tired from running in the park.

Selection 3.2: Slalom on the Ski Slopes

One of the most popular events of the Deaf Winter Olympics is the slalom ski competition. Competitors come from all over the world: France, Germany, Switzerland, even China and Japan. Some of the most outstanding skiers are from the Norwegian countries. These are some of the strongest athletes in the world. They train for months getting adapted to the cold temperatures and thin air that they must endure as they traverse the slopes.

In order to reach the top of the slope, all of the skiers must ride the ski lifts or gondolas to the top of the mountain. The lifts swing freely in the air as the chairs glide up the mountain fastened to a steel cable. Once the skiers arrive at the top, they get off and get ready to go down the slope.

A slalom course is designed with poles that have flags on them, making it easy for the skiers to see at strategic places all down the slope. They are set up in a pattern that forces the skiers to weave in and out of them as they travel down the hill.

There can be as many as twenty-five sets of poles in descending order, all designed to challenge the skills of the skier.

The goal of the competition is to weave in and out through the course without knocking down any of the poles in record time. The winner is the athlete who successfully makes it to the bottom of the hill in the fastest time without falling or knocking over numerous poles. For each pole that is knocked down, points are deducted from the total score.

There are many skilled Deaf athletes who compete in this sport. Skiers from the United States usually come from the Northeast or the Northwest. They have grown up on the slopes and feel very much at home in high altitudes with temperatures that often drop below zero. Skiers from the Scandinavian countries have a definite advantage over the Americans, as it stays colder longer in these countries than it does in the United States.

Although the competition is hearty and the languages signed are different, all of the athletes enjoy the fellowship off the slopes of getting to know their competitors, learning a little about their culture, and sharing with them personal experiences of growing up Deaf.

 ### Selection 3.3: Team Sports

Are you athletic? Do you like to get involved by either playing or watching team sports? There are so many to pick from—for example, football, basketball, volleyball, soccer, and hockey. Football and basketball are two of my favorites. While both are very popular and are both fun to play and watch, they are very different.

Football requires two teams of eleven players each and is played on a field marked with hard lines. You need a quarterback, some running backs, and a few good linemen. The object of the game is to score a touchdown on your opponent's goal. Football players wear protective padding, helmets, face guards, and shoes with cleats. There are four quarters in a football game, and the games are either played outside or in an athletic dome.

Basketball, on the other hand, is played indoors on a court and requires two teams of five players each. Unlike football, you need a center, point guards, and forwards. The game begins with a jump, and each team tries to tap the ball into their teammates' hands. Like football, the goal is to score points, but this time by dropping the ball into the opponent's basket. Basketball players do not require the protective gear that football players wear. Instead they don shorts, tank tops, and tennis shoes. Both sports require players to be physically fit as they spend the majority of their time running up and down the field or court.

Selection 3.4: Children's Games

There are five children's games that my mom tells me they played when she was a child. They are leap frog; duck, duck, goose; hide and seek; red rover; and tug of war.

Leapfrog can be played by two or more people, but most of the time two or three will engage in this game. One child will squat down and put his or her hands on the ground. The second child will jump over the first, squat down, and wait for the second child to jump over him or her. This alternates back and forth until both or several children get tired of hopping.

Duck, duck, goose is a popular game. All of the children sit in a circle facing inward. One child runs around the outside of the circle tapping each child on the head saying "duck, duck." When the child finds a person that he wants to chase him, he will tap the child on the head and yell "goose!" At that point the tagged child will chase the first person around the outside of the circle, trying to catch him. If the first person is caught, he goes into the middle of the circle. If the goose cannot run fast enough to tag the child, the goose must go into the circle, and the game starts over again.

Hide and seek has been a popular children's game for years. The first rule is to establish home base. One person is it. She hides her eyes and counts to one hundred. All of the children hide. Then the child who hid her eyes tries to find them. As children are discovered, they run to home base to be "home free." If the person who is "it" tags one of them on the way back to home base, the person who was tagged becomes "it," and the game starts over again.

Red rover used to be played by elementary-aged children. It begins with two team captains picking their teams. Once both teams have been assembled, the children join hands or arms and make horizontal lines facing each other. Then the fun begins. The first team chants, "Red Rover, Red Rover, send (at this point a child's name is selected) right over." With this being said, the child runs from one side to the other and tries to break through the lines. If he is successful, he picks one child from the side and takes her back to his team to become part of the line. If he cannot break through, he must remain on the other team's side. The game continues until all of the players are gone from one side, or until both groups become tired or run out of time. My mom claims she played and enjoyed all of these games.

Topics for Classroom Lectures and Discussions

Selection 4.1: Classrooms Yesterday and Today

Students spend the bulk of their day in classrooms. And the classroom is the one environment over which the individual teacher maintains a large measure of control. In Boston these days, the world's largest public works project is burying six lanes of Interstate 93 right through the heart of downtown. Bostonians call it the Big Dig. They've uncovered lots of historical artifacts in this work, including parts of a school from the seventeenth century.

Imagine a moment in the future, a very long time from now. Our culture is buried deep beneath the ruins of time. An archaeologist many eons advanced uncovers a perfectly preserved home of the early twenty-first century. The first room he dusts off is an adolescent's bedroom. What does he find?

There's a computer. Next to it, an Ethernet connector that leads to the Internet—at 500 kilobytes per second. On top of it, mobile phones, with worldwide coverage, nights and weekends free. There is a radio AM and FM with CD player. Next to that an MP3 player with 500 songs (but not much Mozart). On the desk a connector for the digital camcorder. Just around the corner is a television, cable-ready with 120 channels.

Is this a typical find? Will he find more rooms like this in the neighborhood? What conclusions will he draw from his collection of artifacts?

Now imagine the same archeologist digs down the road a few miles and uncovers a school. Its cornerstone indicates it was built in 2004. He unearths a classroom, perhaps one that housed the occupant of the bedroom of someone living in the 2000s. What communication technologies does he find there? A chalkboard. A whiteboard. A lectern. Chairs. Perhaps he finds an Ethernet drop but nothing's connected to it. What conclusions will the archeologist draw from this collection of artifacts? What will he conclude when he compares them with the list from the bedroom?

Glance into a school classroom now. Or look carefully through your own. What information technologies are in evidence? How are the classrooms, and the people in it, connected with the world of facts and people and ideas outside? In many classrooms, students are asked to check their laptops and PalmPilots—their information technologies—at the door.

No matter what the age, our classrooms are not unfriendly places. For the most part, they are orderly and clean, which is more than you can say for the student's bedroom. Yet, it's the rare classroom in the United States where each student can, from his or her desk, turn to the Internet and find out the size of the middle class in Iraq or read Act II of *Hamlet* or call up a map of central Asia. Nor can the teacher. But most of those students, at home, could do that in an instant.

Think back to the classroom of twenty years ago, shortly before the current generation of high school students was born. How does it compare with today's classroom? What went on back then? How different is it from what happens in the

283

CHAPTER 4
....
Topics for Classroom
Lectures and
Discussions

classroom today? How much have our classrooms changed as a result of the infor-mation revolution? Would a teacher from 1986, if transported into your classroom today, be able to get the students through the morning curriculum and down to the lunchroom?

Look at Winslow Homer's painting *The Country School* of 1871. Would the teacher pictured there know what to do in a modern classroom? How long would she survive with today's second grade? And Homer's kids—what would they think of that twenty-first century bedroom? Would they know what to do?

In the world outside of school, there's been a revolution in how we collect, store, work with, and access information. Information of all kinds, from bare facts to fully embellished works of art, from personal calendars to institutional stock trades, from scholarly research to *The Simpsons*—it's done online now.

(*Source:* From Lengel, James G., & Kathlene Lengel, *Integrating Technology: A Practical Guide.* Pub-lished by Allyn and Bacon, Boston, MA. Copyright © 2006 by Pearson Education. Reprinted with permission of the publisher.)

Selection 4.2: Terrain and Temperature

If you travel extensively throughout the United States, you may frequently find that you are in awe of the diverse landscape that nature provides for us. In the West we are amazed by the majesty of the Rocky Mountains with their rugged peaks and clear lakes. The wildlife that inhabits the area provides us with a vari-ety of birds and animals to view as we hike through the aspen and pine trees that line the numerous winding paths.

Depending on the time of year that you visit, you might be greeted with a snowstorm or a warm spring shower. In the fall, the aspen leaves turn a vibrant shade of red and gold, alerting the traveler that winter will soon arrive, and blan-kets of snow will cover the slopes making way for the eager snow skiers.

Traveling either south or west from the mountains, the terrain flattens out as one enters the gateway to the desert. Here, land formations vary significantly from place to place. Surrounded by rock formations and cacti, the Painted Desert pro-vides a colorful backdrop for the seasoned hiker. Unlike the tree-filled peaks and verdant valleys in the mountains, the desert traveler is able to view a vast panorama where trees are sparse and the eye can see for miles. Animal inhabitants that reside in this area include reptiles and snakes that frequently prefer a warmer climate filled with hot sunny days and cool dry nights.

Selection 4.3: Banking Services

Since the 1900s, banking services have changed dramatically throughout the country. In the early days of banking, one went to the bank to get a loan, deposit or withdraw money from checking or savings accounts, and get checks. Today that has all changed.

With the advent of technology we no longer have to pay most bills by check. Instead, we can set up our banking online. By using the Internet we can log into our bank account and set up the names of the businesses we want to send monthly payments to, for example, your apartment or house payment, car, electric bill, insurance, and any credit cards that you might have.

Almost all banks are set up the same way. You enter the name of the person or business you want your check to go to, the mailing address, and your account number. It takes a few minutes the first time to get it set up, but once it's in the computer, you can just click on bill pay, bring up the payee, and then type in the amount. It is a very fast process.

When this service was first being promoted, Bank of America had an ad on TV. It went something like this: The camera zoomed in on a woman running her bath water. She went from the bathroom to the computer where she sat down, entered the amounts she wanted to pay, clicked on pay bills, and was finished in

284

PART IV
....
Selections for
Interpreting and
Transliterating

the time her tub was full. They used this to demonstrate how fast and efficient banking online could be.

Most banks today are set up where you can electronically transfer money from savings into checking or from checking into secondary checking accounts. By hitting the transfer function, you can easily move money from one account to another without driving to the bank and doing it in person.

Another feature of banking that was not available in the early 1900s is the ATM machine. In the early days ATMs were nonexistent. In order to get money out of your account you either had to go into the bank or find a business that would let you write a check for more than the amount of your purchase. Even then many businesses would only let you write a check for ten dollars over the amount that you spent.

Check cards, ATM machines, and the ease of online banking have tremendously reduced the amount of paper that goes through the system. Today when you write a check for something, many businesses run it through an electronic machine, deduct the amount from your account, and give your check back to you as a receipt. This cuts down on their paper trail to the bank as well.

When you look at the advances in the banking industry over the past twenty-five years, it is amazing to see how much the entire system has changed. It makes one wonder what changes will take place over the next twenty years. It should be fun to watch.

Selection 4.4: Teaching Tolerance to Young Children

Across the nation many schools are incorporating character education into their curriculum. Topics such as honesty, fairness, and respect are woven into lessons with the hope that today's children will embrace these values. One of the topics that is frequently included in character education programs is tolerance. Tolerance focuses on teaching students to recognize and accept the differences of others and to see those differences in a good light.

When some teachers approach this topic, they look at individuals with disabilities. By sharing poems and stories about people like Helen Keller, they try to teach children that we are all unique individuals and that we are all different in appearance as well as in what we like and dislike. These teachers emphasize what we all have in common while stressing differences that we can appreciate.

One teacher started her lesson by reading a story to her students about a mom who had a very young daughter. The two of them were waiting for a cab to take them home. When the cab pulled up, the man driving was an African American. The child wanted to know why his skin was darker than theirs. The mom modeled a very good answer. She told her daughter that people are like flowers in the garden of life and how boring flower beds would look if all of the flowers were the same color. She added that the different colors added beauty to the flowerbed, just like people with their different-colored skin added beauty to the world. The cab driver was impressed with the mother's story and said he would have to tell his daughter the same thing when she got old enough to ask questions.

By approaching differences in such a positive way through character education, teachers are hoping that children will become more tolerant from a very early age. By having open discussions and modeling positive behaviors, it is hoped that future generations will appreciate human differences rather than being fearful of them.

Selection 4.5: Live Versus Automated Phone Customer Service

Over the years, one of the major concerns businesses have had is with consumer satisfaction. The majority of all businesses depend on how satisfied their customers are, and outstanding customer service is the driving force that keeps customers coming back to the same businesses. Today many businesses have switched to

285

CHAPTER 4
....
Topics for Classroom
Lectures and
Discussions

automated phone systems to help route customer calls. Although these systems are designed to save money, many customers are not fond of them.

When consumers call businesses with a complaint, question, or concern, human nature tells them they should talk to a "real, live person." Frequently, when they begin to hear the litany provided by the automated phone system, they become frustrated with the process. Some systems are designed to route you through several choices before you even have the option of selecting the "O" to talk with an operator. These consumers feel that if customer service comes first, they should be allowed to talk with a live person much earlier in the conversation.

One way to improve such systems would be to let customers talk with a live person immediately when they place a call. With this option, consumers could go directly to the operator and avoid all of the choices that might or might not apply to their situation. Companies frequently don't understand the frustration that these automated services cause.

Consumers have been known to dial a number, listen to see if they want the information presented in English or Spanish, click on their language preference, and listen to a series of five or more choices. At the end of the selection, the person may be given an additional choice if none of the previous ones relate to what he or she needs. Once the person clicks on the last choice, he or she might still have to listen to an additional series of choices before ever getting the desired information. This can be very time consuming when you're in a hurry.

Although automated phone systems may be cheaper to operate than employing a full staff of operators who are equipped to answer questions, in the long run, businesses may find their sales increasing with better customer service. New companies starting out should be especially sensitive to having a live receptionist to provide quick and accurate information for questioning or concerned consumers.

Class Requirements and Activities

Selection 5.1: Writing a Research Paper

Any English teacher will tell you that there are specific steps you must take before you can write a research paper. First, you've got to pick a topic. Make sure that it's broad enough so you'll be able to find a number of journal articles about it. Then you should have sufficient documentation when you get ready to write. The topic should be something that is of interest to you. Otherwise, you'll get bored, and writing it will become a drudgery for you long before you're finished.

Once you've picked an interesting topic, make an outline of the important points you want to cover. This will help you focus on those articles that will support your main ideas. Depending on the length of the paper, you might only have five or six main ideas. Jot these down and head to your computer or to the library to see what you can find. Many libraries are set up so that you can do an electronic search. By typing in key phrases, you should be able to pull up a list of related information. Sometimes, abstracts can be accessed on the computer, while other times, full text articles can be found.

You can gather your research in a number of ways. You can bookmark your articles and read them at a later date, you can save the information on a jump drive, you can burn information onto a CD, or you can take notes on critical information to use later.

Once you have gathered all of your information, you are ready to write your paper. Frequently, an outline comes in handy here. Begin with your thesis, and in your opening paragraph be sure to refer to your supporting points. These points will become additional subheadings and paragraphs later. As you make each point, draw from your research to support your major tenets. Be sure to cite your research properly, giving full credit to any author's work whose ideas you are including. You do not want to risk plagiarizing anyone. In this respect it is better to overdocument instead of risking no documentation.

Once you have included all of your supporting paragraphs, you will want to write a conclusion. This paragraph should tie together all of the information you've included in the body of your paper. It should also refer back to your opening paragraph and your thesis statement.

The last thing you should include in your paper is a list of references. Be sure to include, author, date, title, journal, page numbers, etc., so the reader can go back to the main source if he or she wants additional information. You should always have another person proofread your paper for mistakes before you submit it. Today with spell and grammar check on the computer, papers should be submitted virtually error free.

Selection 5.2: Working with Students Who Need Speech Therapy

This semester we will be working with children in the public schools who need speech therapy. Because we will be going into the public schools, there are a few

287

CHAPTER 5
Class Requirements
and Activities

PART I

PART II

PART III

PART IV

points I want to remind you of. First, we always adhere to the rules established by the schools. We are entering the public school environment, and while there we must adhere to their guidelines. Every time you arrive at and depart from the school, remember to stop at the office and sign in or out.

While working in the schools, it is important that you dress professionally and comfortably. You will be working with young children. Sometimes you will be sitting on chairs, while other times you might find yourself on the floor with youngsters. Wear slacks or long skirts. Jeans are not permitted. Little ones can be very messy, and from time to time you will find little handprints, remnants of snacks, and washable paint on your clothes. I would recommend that you not wear clothing that will have to be dry cleaned or you will find you have an expensive bill by the end of the semester.

You will be providing therapy for the same child for the entire semester. When you meet the child for the first time, it is important that you take time to get to know him or her. Find out what types of activities the child likes. You will be establishing your goals based on the child's IEP. It is critical that you access the teacher's curriculum and his or her lesson plans. Feel free to look at those lesson plans so you know what books the child is reading, what sounds they're working on, and what the goals and objectives are for this child.

It will be your job to develop functional goals for the child. Keep in mind that although you will be working on individual speech sounds, functional language is our top priority. We want to ensure that the children we are working with have conversational skills that are readily understandable by other children and adults. You will be able to identify two or three major functional goals for the child. Under each of these goals you can list your objectives and then your activities.

Be sure to add an assessment component to your functional goals. It is critical that you collect baseline data on the child and that you have specific benchmarks and dates whereby you can measure your success. If you achieve one of your functional goals prior to the end of the semester, you can work on maintenance and spend most of your time working on another goal.

Selection 5.3: Comparing and Contrasting

Comparing and contrasting are such natural habits that we sometimes forget how important they are in our lives. From infancy we notice similarities. The dog is like the cat. Both are warm, have tails, and run. We also notice differences. The dog is different from the cat. One barks, one meows. One wags its tail in pleasure, the other in anger. When we point out similarities between things, we are comparing them. When we point out differences, we are contrasting.

We learn by comparing and contrasting the new and unfamiliar with the old and the familiar. We see a citron for the first time. What is it like? Well, we notice that it bears some similarity to a lemon. It is pale yellow and has a rind. On the other hand, we notice that the citron is larger and more acrid than the lemon.

Observation is the key. The more careful and detailed the observations, the more effectively the reader can see similarities and differences in the subject under discussion. Writers employ two basic organizational techniques when they compare or contrast. Sometimes they deal with, say, two people, point by point. They look at their heights first, then their ages, their occupations, and so on.

At other times it will be better to describe the first person completely and then move on to the second and finally emphasize similarities and differences in a summary. The choice of technique is just another decision writers habitually make.

Travel presents rich opportunities for comparison and contrast. James Michener and Mary Taylor give us incisive and balanced views of places they have traveled to. But many of the writers are seeing places for the first time and are writing for people who haven't been there are all. In these cases, they often shed light on the unfamiliar by setting it against the familiar.

Thomas Smith writes about a soccer game to illustrate contrast he has found in Central America. Mary Manning uses the theater to highlight the contrast

288

PART IV
....
Selections for
Interpreting and
Transliterating

between Belfast and her ordinary world. And John Updike compares the rich and poor in Venezuela to explain a system of class distinctions that might startle the typical American.

We see something of the world through seasoned travel writers. And in this way we can compare strange places with our own. The places that you have traveled may be near or far away, real or imaginary, but you can make any place interesting to your reader by singling out those details that struck you most forcefully or that remain most vividly before your mind's eye. These details can center on sights, smells, incidents, or people. Whatever they are, you can use them to engage the interests of your audience. In this way you can use comparisons and contrasts to highlight the unfamiliar by setting it against the familiar.

Selection 5.4: Down Home Days

Today and tomorrow in Madison, Florida, is what was formerly called "Down Home Days." I heard this year they've changed the name to "Four Freedoms Celebration," I think. The reason they changed the name is because Madison is known for the Four Freedoms Monument that stands in the town square.

If you're familiar with small country towns, most of them have a square downtown—you know, within the little communities. Madison is a very small town. I think it has three stoplights, two grocery stores, and two drugstores, and to do any clothes shopping you have to go somewhere else. It's kind of quaint.

Well, every year they have a Down Home Days celebration. It starts on Friday evening with the local dance studio in town bringing in some of their local students to perform on the main street in town. I always say this is for them to generate interest in the dance recital that is held later in the spring. There is only one dance studio in town, and children from 3 years of age through high school seniors take ballet, tap, and jazz lessons there.

Then on Saturday the day's events start with a fun run, which is a mile, I think, and then a 5K race. This is followed by a parade, and anyone who wants to be in the parade, I think, can join. Last year when I watched the parade, I got real tickled because everything from tow trucks to people's cars were in the parade. I think if you sign up you can be part of it. But when the parade takes place, a lot of the people in town come and watch it. A lot of the bands from the surrounding counties are invited and come and march. So between the floats, cars, bands, and horses, the parade lasts for about an hour. Oh, and I forgot the Shriners. They come with their little go-carts and make figure eights on the street. I enjoy them, but I don't enjoy the firetrucks and the ambulances when they sound their sirens.

In addition to the races and the parade, on Saturday a lot of the people frequent the many booths that are set up. On the square in town there is a gazebo in the center. It is like a park—you know, a city block square—so the vendors usually come in and set their booths up all outside so you can walk around the block and frequent the booths. You see everything there from some very nice woodwork to jewelry. Sometimes you'll see pottery, and that is on the high end too. You know, some of the woodwork that comes in is actual furniture like things for outdoors like benches, swings, or rocking chairs. Some of the pottery and jewelry is just phenomenal.

Then on the low end, sprinkled in with the expensive jewelry and furniture, are the booths that I refer to as the flea market fare. These vendors sell things like clothespin dolls, plastic flowers, inexpensive toys for children, and various and sundry items.

One year a couple brought in small propane tanks for gas that they had decorated to look like various farm animals. They had pigs, cows, roosters, and I can't remember all of the others. I don't know what possessed them, but they were selling them for over $50. I thought, oh my goodness, I can't afford this, not that I would want one, though. Sometimes you see some very nice things, some crafts you'd want to buy at very reasonable prices. Sometimes you don't see anything you'd want to buy, and you say this was fun, but no thank you.

Usually there are a variety of different kinds of food. They sell shark on a stick, chicken, and hamburgers. Many of your local groups or organizations will use this as a fundraiser to generate income. So you can buy a whole variety of things to eat. Many of the local churches set up food booths, as do clubs from the high school and the community college.

One of my favorite booths is run by the basketball coach at the local college. He uses the money to host a summer basketball clinic for underprivileged youth. They always serve chicken, and it is some of the best you've ever tasted. He is such a neat man—he stands about 6'8" and is so good with kids. After I finish my chicken from his booth, I usually get a funnel cake. Those are so good, but only if you eat them while they're warm.

After most folks finish eating, they stay in town for the afternoon events. These consist of a frog-jumping contest and a dog show. Last year was the first time I went to the frog-jumping contest. The local vet in town is one of the judges, and it really was fun to watch. These little kids come with frogs they have caught. They would set the frog down and then the judge only measures the first jump. Wherever the frog jumps when the child gets it to hop is what the judge measures.

In the evening the weekend events usually conclude with a street dance. I have never been to the street dance. My children have gone, and they say it's okay. I can hear the music from my house if I have my windows open. The dance usually concludes by eleven at night and the people head for home.

Down Home Days is a typical event that is hosted in many small communities. It is just a fun time for people to get out, see their neighbors, and socialize. From the parade to the dance it provides a good time for adults and children of all ages.

Selection 5.5: Graduating from Gallaudet

When Luis graduated from the Western Pennsylvania School for the Deaf, he was accepted at Gallaudet as a preparatory student. Because he was weak in English and reading, he needed some work in enhancing his skills before he could enter the freshman class. After a year of steady improvement, he was ready to begin his core classes.

As a freshman, he enrolled in English 1101 and 1102, Algebra, Biology, and literature courses. He registered for twelve hours a semester and had to work hard to maintain his 3.0 GPA. Oftentimes his roommate would ask him if he wanted to play basketball, and he would tell him that he had to go for tutoring instead.

At the end of his freshman year, he had successfully completed all of his courses and signed up for sophomore-level courses. He was still undecided about his major, and he continued to take core courses. Every semester he had room for an elective, and his advisor suggested he take courses from fields that he might eventually be interested in majoring in. He especially enjoyed courses in computer technology and art.

By the time he was a junior, he knew he'd have to declare a major. Although he loved his art courses and his computer courses, he felt that there wouldn't be jobs for him when he graduated. After thinking long and hard, he decided that he would major in education. He knew that there was a national shortage of teachers and felt he could teach either at a school for the deaf or in an inclusive program somewhere in the country. Knowing that there is a particular shortage of male elementary education teachers, he decided that this would be the perfect major. Not only would he have job security, but he felt he would be an excellent role model for deaf children and could possibly provide them with the needed foundation in reading and language arts so they would not need remediation as they got older.

Having made this decision, he spent his junior year taking education courses. He formed his philosophy of education, learned about classroom management, learned how to teach reading and math to elementary students, and even had the opportunity to participate in several practica.

By the time he was a senior, he was ready to student teach. He looked forward to the spring semester when he would go to the Western Maryland School for the Deaf and work with third-grade students. He felt he was well prepared to enter the classroom. Although he felt a twinge of anxiety, his excitement about becoming a teacher made him eager to begin.

CHAPTER 6

Life Experiences II

Selection 6.1: Bailey, Hudson, and Taz

Bailey, Hudson, and Taz are three dogs. Bailey is small and is a Bichon Frise. He is seven years old, all white and rather portly—or at least that's how the vet refers to him. He should only weigh about sixteen pounds or less, but currently he is topping the scale at twenty. Bailey was adopted after he had lived in three other homes. He feels quite at home, sleeping on the top of the back of the sofa and on the bed at night. His owner has had him for three years now, and he's become a very loving sidekick who's devoted and always by his owner's side. Bailey was originally purchased at a pet store and was very expensive. Because he is AKC registered, he sold for almost $600.

Hudson the XIV is also AKC registered and sold for $350. He's a Golden Retriever and only a puppy. At three months of age, he's awkward when he runs; he's still trying to master where he should go to the bathroom and is a bit rambuncous. He loves to chew on plastic two-liter bottles, the kind Coke and Pepsi come in, and feels that he should never be left alone. With a dark golden coat he's sure to turn into a beauty. His paws are large, and the vet estimates that he'll easily weigh a hundred pounds when he's full grown. He loves remote controls and cell phones, and his owner has to be sure to keep both items out of his reach.

Taz is the mutt of the group. He looks like a miniature Old English sheepdog with a long tail. Taz was adopted from the Humane Society for a donation. He is five years old, has long black and white fur, and the sweetest face you'll ever see. When he was much younger, he was hit by a car and suffered ulnar nerve damage to his right front leg. Today he has no feeling in that leg. Walking with a limp, he's a bit awkward but manages to get around fine. His owner protects his injured leg by putting a slipper sock (for toddlers) on his paw when he's out walking. This prevents the paw from getting nicked or further damaged.

Taz is a pretty laid back kind of dog. We say that he's very low maintenance. His only bad habit is that he loves to let out a long, loud howl and let you know when he wants to go outside. He, too, likes to sleep on the bed with his mistress and takes up a lot of space. Of all the dogs, I think I like him best!

Selection 6.2: Daisies, Brownies, and Girl Scouts

Depending on where a little girl grows up, she may be drawn into the world of Girl Scouts. The Girl Scout organization was founded by Juliette Gordon Lowe, and today if you travel to Savannah, Georgia, you will still find the headquarters for this organization.

Scouting became popular in the 1940s, and many young and older women today can tell you stories of their scouting activities. While some found themselves in troops where they earned cooking and sewing badges, other had leaders who were more comfortable in the outdoors and led the girls in activities that would earn them merit badges in crafts and outdoor activities. In the past, these girls usually started as Brownies in elementary school, gradually earned their wings, and became Girl Scouts as they got older.

Today girls of all ages can embark on an adventure with scouting. Depending on their ages, they might join the organization as a Daisy, a Brownie, or a Girl Scout. Kindergartners, ages 5 and 6, who want to get involved in scouting activities begin as Daisies. These little girls usually wear blue uniforms and divide their time between learning how to play games, do community service, and build friendships.

By the time they enter second or third grade and are 6, 7, or 8 years old, they have entered the ranks of Brownies. Brownies traditionally wear brown uniforms and continue to do service projects while enjoying arts and crafts and activities where they can make new friends and earn badges. Even at their young ages they become eligible to sell Girl Scout cookies, go on camping trips, and engage in other fun activities.

Between the ages of 8 and 11 they become Junior Girl Scouts. Then, once they are in sixth grade they become Girl Scouts. The world of scouting has become a hub of bustling activity. By the time these young women reach high school, they have the opportunity to become involved in a variety of service projects and activities. While some of these girls implement projects on their local and state levels, others become involved at the national level.

Within the scouting organization there are honors to be earned, scholarships to be awarded, and opportunities for girls to develop to their full potential. While some girls begin as Daisies and exit the organization at the Brownie level, others continue through high school and earn high awards as Senior Girl Scouts. The program affords all girls at all different levels a number of worthwhile opportunities.

 Selection 6.3: The Soup Bowls

Margaret turned to her mother and said, "You know, the annual Fill-a-Bowl Luncheon will be held in three weeks. Do you want to go again this year?"

"Yes," she replied. "We always have such a good time, and the money goes to such a good cause."

Jackie entered the room and caught the tail end of the conversation.

"What are the two of you talking about?" she asked.

Margaret was the first to speak up. "We were just talking about the annual Fill-a-Bowl Luncheon. Annually potters in the area make soup bowls and donate to our local soup kitchen. You know we have many potters in the area, and there are always a huge variety of bowls. Most of them are really pretty."

Her mom interrupted and spoke up. "Do you remember the year the potter made one and put a green glaze on it with a bunch of black squiggles? It looked like grass crawling with caterpillars."

Margaret started to laugh, "Yes, and you bought it and gave it to Chris. Anyway, anyone who wants to support the soup kitchen can buy a ticket for $20. When the doors open to the kitchen, all the people go in, pick the bowls they want, and then the cooks fill them with soup. At the end of the luncheon you can go into the kitchen and wash your bowl and take it home."

"What a great idea!" said Jackie. "I'd like to get a ticket when you get yours and go with you this year. What a great way to support an organization that does so much for others. When do the tickets go on sale?"

Margaret answered, "According to the paper they will be available tomorrow. You can buy them at the kitchen or at several of the church offices. I'll be happy to pick one up for you when I get ours. Come into the kitchen with me and I'll show you some of the bowls we've gotten over the past several years. Like I said, some of them are very pretty, and some are quite simple, yet unique. If you arrive at the kitchen early the day of the event, you get toward the front of the line and there's a better selection. The bowls are set up on long tables, and you just walk up and down until you find the one that you want. Then you take it into the kitchen to be filled."

"I can't wait to go. What a great way to do a fundraiser. Thanks a lot for including me."

Selection 6.4: First Immigration Wave: Mid-1800s to Early 1900s

A European potato blight in the 1840s began the immigration era, after Ireland and other areas, such as some provinces of Germany, were devastated by famine, resulting in about 1.4 million people immigrating to the United States. For example, the population in Ireland was estimated to be 8.5 million in 1845; by 1851 its population was reduced to 6.5 million. The loss of 1 million Irish people is attributed to starvation and resulting disease, and another million immigrated to America. An immigration of such magnitude had never been experienced before. Even during its founding years, only 850,000 immigrants entered between the American Revolution and the 1840s.

Another major cause for the drastic loss of lives among immigrants to the United States during the mid-1800s was the very poor sanitation conditions endured on the ships, which often led to epidemics and death on board. The normal mortality was 10 percent for steerage passengers of early ships, with 17,000 Irish immigrants dying during 1847, the peak of the famine period, and another 20,000 dying soon after arriving in the United States.

During this immigration era, around 2.6 million Europeans arrived in the 1850s, with some reduction of numbers during the U.S. Civil War and continuation of the large number of immigrants during the 1860s, which brought over 2 million newcomers, with numbers doubling during the 1880s to over 4.7 million arrivals. The 1800s marked a milestone in the history of U.S. immigration: "For the first time, more than a million immigrants . . . were from central—as opposed to northern—Europe," with large numbers of Jews, Italians, and various Slavic groups. In most instances, men came first, and millions of women followed some time later, bringing their children with them or sending the earning-age children before the rest of the family came. Grandparents were most often left behind, primarily due to two reasons: Older adults had more difficulty coping with the strenuous traveling conditions, and age was viewed as a handicapping condition by immigration officers. In most instances, men, who were often illiterate, could not provide sufficiently detailed information to prepare their families for the difficulties of the voyage. Women did not know exactly what to pack, what items to sell or leave behind, or what to expect during debarkation at Ellis Island. Most European peasants were fatalistic, and the immigration journey was a confused process and more dependent on luck than it should have been.

The 1890s brought some economic depression, reducing the number of immigrants to 3.6 million, with the following decade (1901 to 1910) experiencing an immigration peak of 8 million, in part because of the introduction of faster ships, reducing the voyage time from months to weeks and days. The steamers could also maintain regular schedules independent of inclemency of the weather, such as unfavorable winds. Steamers also provided dining facilities, and medical inspections and vaccinations were required at the port of embarkation in Europe. Even though steerage sanitation was still in need of improvement, the mortality rate decreased tremendously and almost disappeared.

(*Source:* From Gonzalez, Virginia, *English-as-a-Second Language [ESL] Teaching and Learning.* Published by Allyn and Bacon, Boston, MA. Copyright © 2006 by Pearson Education. Reprinted by permission of the publisher.)

Selection 6.5: The Smooth

I want to tell you about this situation I had in Alamosa, Colorado. I studied for my masters degree in a place called Adams State College in Alamosa, Colorado. Alamosa is about eighteen miles north of the New Mexico border in the San Luis Valley, and many of the local people there have been native to that region for a long time. They were typically referred to as the Mexican American population, but they were a combination of the local Indians of that area and some of the Mexicans who had moved into that territory. And, they had their own particular speech patterns and their own particular behaviors.

This happened one Saturday morning. I went into a local Shell station to get some gasoline, and a friend of mine who was going to the college came in and said, "Hey Bob, you'll never guess what just happened to me." I said, "What happened?" He said, "You know I got me my new 1955 Ford Crown Vic." What he had bought was a used 1955 Ford Crown Victoria, a very fancy Ford for that time, and he was very proud of it.

He said, "I was driving my Crown Vic down to Antonito, and on the way down there don't you know I had a flat." I said, "I'm sorry to hear that." "When I bought the car, I should have looked and there was no spare," he said, "So what I did, I got out and I hitched a ride back to Jimmy's Shell Station, and when I got back, I said, 'Hey, Jimmy, you'll never guess what happened to me, man. I had a flat tire and I don't have a spare tire in the trunk.' And, I said, 'Can you lend me a spare?'"

"So he's a good man, he lent me one, and then I had to go back on the highway and hitch another ride with the spare tire and a rim, and I had to take both the spare tire and rim back to my car, and when I got back, man, it was not my day. While I was gone, somebody had jacked up my car and stole two more tires and rims. And I said, What am I'm going to do? So I put that tire and rim that Jimmy had lent me on and I hitched back into town. And I said, 'Jimmy, you'll never guess what happened to me. While I was here getting a tire and rim, somebody jacked up my car and stole two more tires and rims.' He is a really good guy. He hunted around out back and he got me two more tires and rims. And, I had to find someone now who would give me a ride carrying these tires and rims. When I got back to my car, thank heavens no one had messed with my 55 Ford Crown Vic while I was gone this time. So I started putting the tires and rims on and just as I was about to finish putting the tires and rims on I almost got run over by a smooth."

I said, "What?" And he said, "I almost got run over by a smooth, you know a smooth, a thing that smooths the road."

Potpourri I

Selection 7.1: Cruise Lines Keep Adding New Attractions

Have you ever taken a cruise? You know, you can go on a cruise almost anywhere in the world today and spend as little as a few hundred dollars or as much as many thousands of dollars. It all depends on where you live, where you want to go, what time of the year you want to go, and how long you want to be gone.

People who live in Florida can get on a cruise ship and go to the Bahamas for three days or so for under $400. People living in northern California can go to Alaska for a week and spend between $1,200 and $1,500. Recently, I had friends who decided to take a cruise to Europe. They were content to take the time to sail across the ocean and then take trains to travel through the various countries that they wanted to see.

In the past, it seemed like only adults went on cruises. Today more and more families are taking to the seas. Annually, more than a million children under the age of 18 now go on cruises. In order to accommodate all of these children, cruise ships are starting to add amenities specifically designed to attract this population. Video arcades, spa treatments for teenagers, basketball courts, teen nightclubs, and onboard water parks are only a few of the new attractions that have been added. Some cruise lines actually offer programs for children by age groups, breaking them down into activities for children ages 3 to 5, 6 to 8, 9 to 11, 12 to 14, and 15 to 17.

In one year alone, over twelve million passengers sailed on cruises worldwide. In order to accommodate all of these passengers, new ships are being built on a regular basis. Many people are drawn to this type of vacation because once you pay for it, all of your meals and your room is covered. By traveling to unique ports people of all ages are able to experience enriching cultural experiences. Although a cruise might not be for everyone, it certainly has become a draw for a large number of people.

Selection 7.2: Music: Originals and Remakes

Some songs strike the fancy of recording artists as being so good that they want to take the music and put their own stamp of individuality on them. When this happens, an original song may be remade and referred to as a remake. There are pros and cons of both types of music.

For some fans, there is no song like the original one. Recorded by a favorite artist in a particular way, the listener gets used to hearing the beat, singing along, and sometimes fantasizing that he or she is the one performing the song. When listeners hear the title and know that it is going to be played on the radio, they perk up and get their vocal cords ready so they can belt out the tune. Frequently, they are disappointed when the music they hear isn't what they expected.

Some remakes are a welcome addition to the music industry. These songs take old, sometimes outdated, melodies and put a new twist on them. When this happens, the more contemporary crowd is drawn to the music—sometimes totally unaware that it is a remake of a previous song. It is only after these songs hit the top of the charts and are played on a variety of stations that someone may make a comment that the song is a remake.

296

PART IV
....
Selections for
Interpreting and
Transliterating

Are you a music listener? Do you usually prefer original recordings or remakes? Does it matter to you? Does it depend of what kind of music it is? What do you think? Which type do you prefer?

Selection 7.3: Award Winners

Most students are probably aware of the numerous awards shows on television, such as the Oscars, the Grammies, and the MTV Awards. This activity is an opportunity for students to acknowledge the positive qualities that they recognize in their classmates. It completes the sequence of activities on names by having each award named for the student who receives it. You can also record this activity and play it at a parent meeting or school assembly.

Procedure

1. Divide the class into small groups.
2. Give each group the names of five other students in the class to acknowledge at the awards ceremony.
3. Ask the students when they get the names not to let anyone know whose acknowledgments they are going to do. A surprise will make it more fun.
4. Instruct each group to take the names one at a time. Consider the things about the person that you like, admire, and appreciate—those things that make the person special.
5. Now that they have a list of qualities and contributions for which to acknowledge the person, direct each group of students to think of a way of summarizing in the form of a special award what that person has done for the group. For example, there might be a person who gets the *thoughtfulness award* for always being kind to people, helping people who are having problems, and so on. Or there might be a *good humor award* for a person who lightens up heavy situations and is always good for a laugh.
6. Hand out copies of the Awards Certificate Worksheet and have the students complete one certificate for each of the names they received. The award is named after the student who will receive it, and the person's special attribute is filled in on the line provided. Encourage students to decorate each certificate with colors and designs that make it personal to the recipient.
7. When all the groups are finished, they are to bring their awards to the awards ceremony (class circle). You, as master of ceremonies, will call on each group to make its awards. If students want to, they can pretend they are Oscar presenters and call for "The envelope please." That might add to the fun. Be sure that each group does a good job of explaining and displaying the award and letting the winner feel the full sincerity of the acknowledgment.
   You may want to discuss how to receive compliments graciously.
8. Close with a discussion using questions such as:

   What award did you receive at the awards ceremony?
   How did it feel to receive this compliment?
   Do you ever acknowledge yourself for these good qualities? If you don't, take the time to do that now.

Students can list people in their lives who deserve to be acknowledged for the things they have done for the students in the past month. The students could then be encouraged to make awards for these people, or in some other creative way acknowledge these people for their contributions.

Selection 7.4: Coffee Pots Versus Single-Serving Containers

Phil is like millions of other people who start their day with a cup of coffee. Sometimes he drinks two or three cups of his favorite roast before he gets going. When

297

CHAPTER 7
....
Potpourri I

PART I

PART II

PART III

PART IV

he has time, he brews a full pot and takes a travel mug with him in the car to enjoy on his way to work. Other times, when he's in a hurry, he pulls through one of the drive-through vendors and purchases a cup on the way. Rarely does he miss a morning without his favorite brew.

In the past, he, like most other folks, has relied on the traditional twelve-cup coffee pot to brew his coffee. Traditionally, these coffee pots were placed on the stove, heated until you could see the coffee perk or bubble up in the glass knob in the top of the lid. Then, at the designated time, you would remove the pot from the stove and enjoy it. More recently, the pot on the stove has been replaced by the electric coffeemaker.

These pots are designed to have your coffee ready in five minutes or less. You add the coffee, water, plug it in, turn it on, and you're ready to go. Many of the fancier models are designed with a timer to turn on at a designated time in the morning so when you get up, your coffee is waiting for you. Although these pots are designed to brew one to twelve cups you cannot take them with you, and if you're called out or have to leave in a hurry, the pot stays where you were, and the coffee is often discarded at the end of the day.

Soon these coffee pots may be a thing of the past as a new invention has become readily available in many of the stores where many of us shop. Brought to us by coffee makers, their latest big idea is to think small. As a result, they have developed what they refer to as single-serving coffee containers. Unlike travel mugs or hot plates, these diminutive coffee pots provide a self-contained coffee brewing system that has been installed in a new brand of coffeemakers to produce a single cup of steaming java. The inventors of this system feel these single-serving pots will replace the larger pots. Now coffee lovers will be able to brew and drink individual fresh cups of coffee, rather than frequenting the pot that has gotten strong or stale by staying warm all day. Furthermore, they feel this will eliminate the need to throw the leftover coffee down the drain at the end of the day.

This new product like many others will have to compete with the standard coffeemaker that has found its way into so many homes. Whether it will succeed at replacing the standard fare will depend in part on marketability as well as how well the consumers take to the new product.

Selection 7.5: Car Colors

What color is your car? Are you driving the same color car that's the most popular color among American drivers? How do you know if the color you picked is what most people prefer? Recently, a study was conducted to determine the preferred car color of Americans, and guess what they found out?

Twenty-five percent of the people surveyed preferred silver/gray cars. They felt this was a very dignified color, and it made them feel professional, elegant, or sophisticated when they drove their car. For men, it alluded a sense of business that told passengers that this is a man who knows what he's doing. It didn't matter if it was a BMW or a Mazda; those who selected this color felt it was the subtlest of the colors while conveying a message of being in control of the situation.

White was the second color of choice. Sixteen percent of the people surveyed preferred this color. Unlike gray, this color was selected because it was thought to be cool for folks living in the South during the summer; it didn't show dirt easily, and was a standard color found on most lots. Those selecting white cars also commented that they didn't "stand out" on the highways and weren't usually noticed by state troopers.

The third color of choice was natural or beige. Selected by 14 percent of the people this ran a close third. Like white, this is viewed as a cool color and hides dirt relatively well. Interesting enough, this color is thought to be the color of choice for older people. While it was more commonly found on car lots in the past, today those who want a car in this color frequently have to special order it.

Thirteen percent of the people drive red cars. Sometimes when you're traveling on the major highways or even in large cities, it seems as if more people drive red cars than the 13 percent who responded to the survey. Many sports cars are red. You see a number of Mazdas, Corvettes, and Jaguars. It also seems that there are more convertibles that are red than any other color.

Blue at 12 percent, black at 11 percent, green with 5 percent, and other at 3 percent completed the survey. Now that you know the colors of choice, what do you think of the car that you're driving? Is it a popular color? Did you buy your car for the color or for another reason? Sometimes, color is not the primary reason people select a car.

Life Experiences III

Selection 8.1: Tim's Trip to the Kennel

Tim and his wife Sondra have been married for two years. During that time, they have acquired a dog named Bandit. Bandit is a bit of a mutt—he's about 3 years old, brown and white, weighs about sixty pounds, and is a real lovable fellow. Needless to say, both Tim and Sondra have grown quite fond of him.

Because Tim's family lives halfway across the country from them, they frequently have to board Bandit before they can go out of town. Sondra typically takes Bandit to the kennel to be boarded. They charge her $25 a day to keep him and because they're usually not gone for more than five or six days, at best, it costs them around $125 to board the dog.

Last Christmas, Sondra had many last-minute errands to do, so she asked Tim if he would take Bandit to the kennel. He was more than happy to oblige. When he went to drop the dog off, the girl asked him the following questions: "Would you like us to give Bandit treats twice a day? Would you like us to give him play time three times a day? Would you like to have him groomed while he's here?" The list included about five different options.

Because Tim had never brought the dog before, he assumed that all of these additional services were free. So, naturally, he agreed to all of them. What pet owner wouldn't want his dog to have treats and be played with three times a day? Of course, he would want the dog to have a bath before he came back home and all of the other services too. Why not?

After agreeing to everything, he left the dog and Tim and Sondra went on their trip to see his family. After several days, they returned home. When Tim went to pick Bandit up, he was shocked when he was presented with a bill for over $325.00. What could he do but pay it? When he returned home, he showed the bill to his wife. She about died! "I have never paid that much money to board the dog! Have their prices gone up that much?" It was only then that she realized all of the services Tim had agreed to.

Since that time Tim has learned to say "No" when he takes the dog to the kennel. He has also learned not to make assumptions but to ask questions. Think how pampered the dog must have felt the one time his owner agreed to everything.

Selection 8.2: The Traffic Stop

It was a beautiful spring day—just warm enough to make Sanguita want to put the top down on her convertible. The sky was a deep blue and there wasn't a cloud in it. She hopped in her car and headed down I-95. Cranking the volume up on the radio, she was jamming as she pointed her car in the direction of the beach. It was a perfect day to relax, catch a few rays, and just "veg out."

She'd been driving for less than an hour when she noticed the trooper parked on the side of the road. She didn't give it much thought at first. Surely she hadn't been speeding or doing anything wrong—or had she? Then, without warning he pulled out. She saw the lights and realized she was the one he was following. As

300

PART IV
....
Selections for
Interpreting and
Transliterating

she pulled over to the side of the road, a million thoughts started racing through her mind. As the officer approached her car, she put down her window.

He said good morning to her and asked if he could see her license, vehicle registration, and proof of insurance. Sanguita opened her billfold, pulled out her license, and then rummaged through the glove box for the registration and proof of insurance. The officer looked over everything she had given him and then asked her if she realized that she had no brake lights and that her right turn signal light didn't work either.

Sanguita explained to the officer that she was clueless, that she never saw her car from the back while she was driving it, and that no one had ever told her that her brake lights didn't work. After explaining how dangerous it was to be driving without brake lights, the officer issued her a warning and gave her thirty days to get her car repaired. She promised she'd get it fixed and drove off toward the beach breathing a huge sigh of relief.

Tomorrow she'd schedule an appointment at the shop and get her car fixed. What could have happened to short out the brake lights? Who knows, but she'd deal with that hassle tomorrow—today she was going to catch some rays.

Selection 8.3: The Bridal Show

Have you or someone you know attended a bridal show? I went to my first one last Sunday, and I want to share my experience with you. Before attending, my daughter and I registered for the bridal show online. We were under the impression that by registering in advance we would be admitted for half price. So we paid our ten dollars by debit card and printed off the receipt.

When we arrived, we were told that we needed to pay an additional fifteen dollars to get in the door, five dollars for my daughter and ten dollars for me. That was ok, but we both were kind of caught off guard thinking that we had already paid the admissions fee.

Once inside, it was a sight to see. There were tables set up throughout the grand ballroom. Tables were set up all along the walls, and then rows of tables were set up throughout the room. There was plenty of room to walk up and down the aisles and stop at all of the tables. Now, let me explain about the tables. Some of them had vendors from catering services, some were photographers, others specialized in wedding attire, and of course there were the ones that focused on the honeymoon.

Because my daughter has already selected her dress, our concern was to focus on a caterer and find someone who could provide music for the reception. The first table we stopped at had a variety of food for you to taste. This included small sandwiches, cheese dips and seafood dips, crackers, meatballs, and an array of sweet treats. We tasted the various samples and then looked over the brochure. I think we were both surprised to find that for light hors d'oeuvres the cost was $29.00 per person. Obviously, this was not the caterer for us.

The next caterer seemed more reasonable. She had a chocolate fountain, a watermelon she had cut and turned into a fresh fruit basket, some small sandwiches, and various dips you could sample with chips or crackers. She did not have a price sheet but said she would work with her clients make it affordable. We took her card with the idea that we could contact her at a later date.

Our next two stops were the two tables with the wedding cakes. Both had cakes you could sample and books displaying pictures of cakes they had made for various special occasions. One was very pretty, but when we tasted it, we were very disappointed. Not only did it lack flavor, but it was very dry and not something we would want to serve to our guests. The second one was a little moister but again, lacking in flavor. We decided that neither of these bakers would work for us.

301

CHAPTER 8

Life Experiences III

PART I

PART II

PART III

PART IV

We saw many tables with DJs promoting their services and other tables with photographers. Because we want a string quartet and not a DJ, we avoided those tables. Some of the photographers had beautiful pictures on display, but all of them were more expensive than the photographer we had made an appointment to see the following week, so we didn't take any of their brochures.

After stopping at all of the various tables, sampling a couple of the chocolate fountains and tasting some punch, we decided it was time to leave. It was a fun afternoon and gave us a chance to see what is popular with many of the brides planning weddings this year.

Selection 8.4: The Blizzard

Have you ever been in a blizzard? If you have, you know that they're not much fun. Two years ago, my sister and I got caught in one driving from California back to Colorado. We were around Salt Lake when it started to snow. It was snowing so hard you couldn't see an inch in front of you to drive. I guess that's why they called it a white out. It was horrible. We had to pull the car off the road because we couldn't see to go any farther.

Once the snow let up a little, we found a room in a hotel because we knew we had to get off the road. The snow was piling up quickly, and we still couldn't see more than a foot in front of us. The hotel we found had one room left. We snatched it up, feeling lucky to be in out of the cold with a place to sleep.

During the night, the snow continued to come down. I guess it must have been around two in the morning when the power went out. Suddenly everything was just pitch black. We couldn't see a thing. We thought, well, if this is the worst thing that happens, we'll be okay. In the morning we'll be on our way.

By the next morning, not only was there no power in the hotel, but the pipes had frozen as well, and there was no water. We thought, oh well, we'll just get out of here and shower the next day when we arrive home. We checked out, and that's when our real problems began. During the night the wind had knocked over an electrical pole and the power lines were on our car. What's more, the car was buried in over eighteen inches of snow. There was no way the electric company could get in and remove the power lines until the snowplows made it into the parking lot.

Because the major highways were still closed, the hotel parking lot wasn't on the top of the list for the snowplows. We had no choice but to hurry back in the hotel and book our room for another night. After getting over our disappointment of not being able to leave, we decided to make the best of it. We walked a couple of blocks down the street where there was a restaurant with power and ordered breakfast. Once our tummies were full, we sat and just looked out at the winter wonderland.

Branches of trees were covered with inches of snow, power lines had about an inch of snow still on the tops of them. Everywhere you looked it was white. After spending three more days stuck in the snow, we were finally able to get in our car and drive home. That is a storm that I'll never forget.

Selection 8.5: Trying Out for the Dance Line

My friend Susie went to a public school in a small town in Arkansas. She was the only deaf student in the entire high school. However, she had a ton of hearing friends, and they all liked to hang out together. At the end of their sophomore year all of Susie's friends decided they should try out for the dance line. The girls selected for the squad performed at football games both at home and away and some basketball games. All of Susie's friends told her she should try out with them. They told her they'd help her learn the routines so she could compete.

With some apprehension, Susie agreed that she would try out. All of the girls had to sign up in advance. Long before the actual tryouts, senior girls on the team met with the ones wanting to try out to help the girls learn the routines that they would be judged on. For about a month, three times a week, all of the girls would meet in the gym after school. The senior girls would put on the music and teach them the steps.

Every day at practice Susie would stand between her friends and look to them to see when it was time to kick, when they should turn around, jump, and go down on the floor in a split. Her friends got a CD of the music, and every day they would practice at home turning the music up loud enough so Susie could feel the vibrations.

Finally, the day of tryouts arrived. Each of the girls was given a number to pin on her shirt. Then they were called in groups of six to perform the routines for the judges. Friends were not allowed to compete in the same group. When Susie's group was called, the six girls all stood in a straight line with Susie in the middle. The judges started the music, and they all performed the routines. Twenty minutes later, they were finished and the next group was called in.

After all of the girls were done, the judges called all of them back in the gym. They told them that they would vote and that the results would be posted after school two days later. It was really tough to wait. The day the results were posted, Susie wasn't sure she wanted to know. But, finally she mustered enough courage to inch her way forward and look at the list. Boy, was she shocked to see that she made it!

Interpreting: Preparation and into the Classroom

Selection 9.1: Immersion Weekends for Interpreters

Have you ever gone to an immersion weekend to help improve your signing, interpreting, or transliterating skills? There are several different types of weekends that fall under this umbrella, but most of them are designed to help improve an interpreter's skills. Let me tell you about the one I recently attended. It was scheduled for a Friday, Saturday, and Sunday.

It started on Friday evening and went from six until nine at night. There were about twenty-four of us who attended, and the opening general session was held with all of us together in one room listening to three different speakers. The topic that evening focused on mouth movements that are used in ASL. It really was an informative talk, and all of us left that evening eager to come back the next day and try out our new skills.

On Saturday morning we arrived at eight for coffee and muffins. By eight-thirty, we were divided into three groups, and all of the groups were hard at work. Group one focused on transliterating, group two on interpreting, and group three worked on receptive skills. There were about eight of us in each group working with one of the three instructors. We worked all through the morning until twelve and then we stopped for lunch.

After lunch, the three groups rotated. Those who had been working on interpreting went to the session on transliterating. The transliteraters went to the class on building receptive skills, and the people who had been working on their receptive skills went to the interpreting class. We spent the entire afternoon working on a different skill. By the time the afternoon ended, we were worn out. It was a good feeling of tired. We all felt we had learned a lot but we were exhausted.

Sunday morning we returned again at eight in the morning. By eight-thirty we were hard at work again. The group that had not yet had the opportunity to work on receptive skills went there. The group that hadn't had the chance to practice interpreting skills went there, and the remaining group worked on transliterating. By twelve o'clock we all stopped working in our individual groups and came back together.

At that time, we ate lunch, reflected on what we had learned, and completed an evaluation of the weekend. All of us who attended agreed that it was a marvelous learning experience. The presenters were awesome! Their constructive criticism was very helpful, and they made us feel like one day we would be able to join the ranks of other professionally certified interpreters. When someone asked me if I'd go back again, I told them I'd do it in a New York second. It was great! I just wish we could do this once a month. Then I know my skills would really take off. If you ever have a chance to do a weekend like this, take advantage of it. You'll be so glad you did. I know I was, and I'd go back next week if there was another one.

304

PART IV
....
Selections for
Interpreting and
Transliterating

Selection 9.2: What Is Expected of the Educational Interpreter in Elementary and Middle School Settings?

The elementary and middle school years pose many interesting challenges for educational interpreters. Just as preschool- and primary-aged students present everchanging development, so do pre- and early-adolescent students present a changing profile that varies both within the individual and between individuals at any given period. The educational interpreter who has an appreciation for the changing profile that characterizes this age group is probably an interpreter who is experienced with this particular age group. Interpreters who have no experience, either personally or professionally, with third, fourth, fifth, sixth, seventh, and even some eighth graders, will probably learn early in their work with this age group that a critical part of the changing profile involves the development of social competence.

A growing body of literature attests to the recognition that a child's social competence from 8 to 12 or 13 years of age is defined by relationships. Several categories of relationships can be found in the educational setting: peer relationships that exist between and among students who are deaf, hearing, and hard of hearing; teacher–student relationships; teacher–interpreter relationships; teacher–student–interpreter relationships; and the broader category of relationships that exist within educational communities.

Interpreters in the middle and upper elementary school grades must be sensitive to and knowledgeable of the dynamics involved in each of these relationships. Tanya Gallagher addressed language competence and its effect on peer relationships during these changing years. She described two kinds of peer friendships: *friendships of popularity* that occur when one is liked or accepted by one's peers, and *close friendships or chumships* that occur when mutual needs for intimacy are met.

The first friendship, friendship of popularity, is evidenced in group behavior. Students in the elementary and middle-school age group are likely to want to dress *like*, look *like*, and have things just *like* their peers whom they perceive as popular. Being different, especially different enough to have an interpreter, may challenge the student's sense of self-esteem and impact negatively on the student's relationships with peers.

I recall three different stories of young deaf girls who, each at about the fourth to fifth grade, experienced emotional struggles over their differences. In the first story, the mother of a very bright, attractive, and financially advantaged girl was devastated when her deaf daughter told her and her father that they could no longer sign to her when they went out to dinner—because, as she indicated, she wanted to pretend to be hearing. In the second story, the mother of a very popular deaf girl was worried when her daughter was feeling left out because her two best friends since first grade had become very talkative on the telephone in the afternoons. Her daughter wanted to become hearing so she, too, could talk on the telephone. In the third story, the mother of a very capable young girl who moved comfortably between sign language and spoken language indicated that her compliant and sweet daughter was becoming defiant and resistant, both at home and at school. There were indications that the daughter was becoming increasingly rude and inconsiderate to her interpreter, a woman she had previously adored.

An educational interpreter who recognizes the need for the deaf or hard of hearing student to be acclimated in the larger group probably experiments to find the most appropriate avenue for interpreting social exchanges. As the interpreter gains familiarity with different communication behaviors in the classroom, especially those behaviors that constitute "side conversations, the interpreter should become more proficient in representing the different communication behaviors—even the slang, sarcasm, and slander that are common to these side conversations. Certainly, a hands-off role is most appropriate for intimate communication behaviors or when social exchanges involving the deaf student are successful without the interpreter."

(*Source:* From Seal, Brenda, *Best Practices in Educational Interpreting*, pp. 81–82. Published by Allyn and Bacon, Boston, MA. Copyright © 2004 by Pearson Education. Reprinted by permission of the publisher.)

305

CHAPTER 9
....
Interpreting:
Preparation and into
the Classroom

PART I

PART II

PART III

PART IV

Selection 9.3: Interpreting Math Problems

Throughout the United States today over 80 percent of the full-time working interpreters are employed by the public schools. While working in this setting, they are responsible for facilitating communication in a variety of classes. Even those at the kindergarten and elementary levels find they are responsible for interpreting math, reading, social studies, science, and health classes.

At the middle and high school levels, interpreters find themselves in classes where Biology, Chemistry, Algebra, English Literature, as well as World History are common. During the day the interpreters usually change classes along with the students, thus providing the students with access to the curriculum.

Of all of the subjects that must be interpreted, mathematics can be one of the most challenging. Although standard computation problems can usually be set up with ease, computations found within word problems can be a bit tricky. From elementary school on through high school, students are faced with word problems. These require planning on the part of the interpreter to make sure the student is presented with a clear picture.

Take the following problems: Number one, Joel buys 18 marbles. Two marbles are in each package. How many packages does he buy? Number two, a land turtle has 27 pieces of tomato. It eats 3 pieces a day. How many days will the tomatoes last? Number three, Suzie plays the piano 7 times during each play. How many times will she play the piano in all 4 plays? Number four, Ann has 8 pair of slacks. Each pair has 4 pockets. How many pockets are on all of the slacks? Number five, there are 587 adults and 723 students at the graduation ceremony. Everyone has a chair. What is the least number of chairs at the ceremony?

By the time students enter middle school, many of them are working on pre-algebra skills. At this time the word problems change, and one problem may be related to another, requiring the student to compute the correct answer for the previous problem so accurate numbers can be plugged into the subsequent problem.

Think about these problems. Number one, Mr. Smith wants to fence in his garden using rope. How much rope will he need for his garden that is 20 feet wide and 40 feet long? Number two, Mr. Jones' garden is square. All of its sides have the same length. How much rope will he need to close in his square garden when each side is 20 feet long? Number three, Janice has 50 feet of rope to close in her garden. Her garden is 10 feet wide. How long is her garden? Number four, suppose you want to rope off a garden that has 5 sides. Each side is 8 feet long. How much rope will you need to close in the garden?

Having a basic understanding of math concepts is critical for interpreters. Taking time to visualize problems is also important. When interpreters take time to do both, they help facilitate clear communication, thus enabling the student to gain full access to the curriculum.

Selection 9.4: The Solar System

Do you know what a solar system is? A solar system is made up of a sun and everything within reach of its gravity. Nothing stands still in a solar system; everything moves. Our solar system is part of the Milky Way galaxy. The Earth is only one of the eight planets in our solar system. Mercury, the smallest planet, is also the closest to the sun and travels the fastest. It moves at about 107,000 miles per hour. Many people were taught that our solar system had nine planets, but Pluto, the planet furthest away, was recently determined not to be a planet after all.

Venus is the second-closest planet to the sun. It is so hot that lead, tin, and zinc would melt easily on it if they were placed there. Venus has a very rocky crust that looks like a chocolate bar that has gotten warm. Venus is about the same size as the Earth. However, it differs from the Earth because there is no water on the surface of this planet.

Our planet, the Earth, is the third from the sun. The Earth is made up of several layers. The inner core is solid and is made of nickel and iron. The outer core

306

PART IV
....
Selections for
Interpreting and
Transliterating

is made of the same elements, but it is liquid. The core is the hottest part of the Earth with the temperature almost as hot as the surface of the sun. The next layer is the mantle, which is made of molten rock. The outside layer is called the outer crust. It is what we stand on. If you compare the Earth to a basketball, the outside layer of the Earth would be as thin as a hair.

The planet that is the fourth from the sun is Mars. One of the first things that pops into people's minds about the planet Mars when they're asked is that it's red. Scientists studying Mars tell us that there are dust storms on Mars and that's why it is covered with a red haze.

All eight of the planets in our solar system orbit or move in an elliptical path around the sun. Each complete orbit around the sun is called one revolution. The sun's gravity is what holds the solar system together. There are many things we know about some of the planets today, and a lot things that we don't yet understand about the solar system. One thing we do know is that each planet has its own unique characteristics separating it from all of the others.

Selection 9.5: Time Zones

Do you all know what time zones are? Have you ever wondered why time zones were put on maps and why we follow them today? Let's talk about how and why time zones were established. First of all, we need to look back in time before people traveled great distances to look at how people knew what time it was.

For thousands of years, people would use the sun to tell time. When the sun came up in the morning, farmers and gatherers would know it was time to get up and start their day. When the sun was directly overhead, people knew it was noon, and then when the sun would set, work for the day would generally cease, and people would gather indoors for the evening meal and later retire.

For years, each community set its own time by the sun, and because the Earth rotates during the day, the sun is not overhead in all places at the same time. Therefore, when it was noon in one place, it might be ten or eleven in the morning in one town and one or two o'clock in the afternoon in yet another location.

Once the first transcontinental railroad was finished, it allowed people to travel from coast to coast. At that time, it became important to establish a timetable that everyone could follow so they would know when the train would arrive and when it would leave. Attention was given to where the sun was in the sky in different parts of the country.

In 1884 the first timetable was developed; the world was divided into time zones based on locations on the map. Starting with the prime meridian at Greenwich, England, it was decided that the time zones would be laid out along every 15 degrees of longitude and that each time zone would be one hour different for every 15 degrees. Since that time, the time zone map has been modified to make it more practical. Today, many time zone boundaries follow state or national boundaries. You can always use a map to find out what time it is in different locations of the world.

Keep in mind that the time east of you is always later than it is in your time zone, and the time west of you is always earlier. Within the United States, time zones are referred to by location. In the East, there is the Eastern Standard time zone; in the central part of the country is the Central Standard time zone, and the Mountain and Pacific time zones occur in the Midwest and West.

When you look in the phone book today, you can usually find a map of the United States that shows the different time zones. That can be very helpful if you are planning to call someone early in the morning or late at night. By finding the state and the city, you will know exactly what time it is.

CHAPTER 10

Topics Related to Deafness

Selection 10.1: TTYs

TTYs, also known as teletypewriters, once played a vital role for communicating within the Deaf community. From the early days of the huge TTY machines that were often covered with tablecloths when they weren't in use to the small portable TTYs that could be used with pay phones, they provided a link to members of the Deaf community.

From the early days Deaf people could identify their friends by their typing styles, how they said hello, and how they signed off at the end of a conversation. When the original machines came out, they vibrated too much and were so noisy that people living in some apartment buildings on floors beneath Deaf people could feel the ceiling shake when they typed on them.

Those using the machines for frequent communication quickly developed a group of abbreviations that could be used to expedite conversations. GA was the standard signal used for "go ahead," and SK was the standard indicator for ending a conversation. By using the GA, one person could let the other person know that he was done with what he wanted to say, and it was the other person's turn to respond. This helped slower typists out. The person on the other end of the line wouldn't interrupt while the slower typist was trying to get his or her thoughts out. By waiting until the GA was typed at the end of the thought, it meant that you still had the floor.

During the conversation, if you had to look for information, or if someone came to your door and you needed to leave for a minute, you could type HD for hold. It was always polite to type HD several times if you needed to be away for more than several seconds. In this way you could type HD and add "still looking" or let the person know you hadn't hung up on them.

Stop Keying or SK was always used to signal the end of the conversation. After both parties were done talking, someone would say something like "Okay time for me to stop—see you tomorrow SK." Then the person on the other end would also type SK, indicating she was finished with the conversation too. Once in a while, one of the people would remember one more thing he or she wanted to add and would type it and then add their SK. While some individuals ended with just SK, others would type it two or three times.

Today many of the TTYs have been replaced with VPs, Blackberrys, Sidekicks, and other handheld devices. While once TTYs were very popular, today they are quickly becoming a machine of the past, foreign to the younger Deaf generation. With more and more technological advances, it will be fun to see what the handheld devices will be replaced with during the next thirty years.

Selection 10.2: Teaching Deaf Studies in Inclusive Classrooms

Have you ever stopped to think about the impact an educational setting can have on your cultural development? Where you lived, where you went to school, what your cultural background is, what the cultural background of the majority of students was where you attended school, and how you fit in with your peers

308

PART IV
....
Selections for
Interpreting and
Transliterating

all contributed to your cultural perspective of who you are and how you fit in that environment.

If you attended a school where you were part of the majority culture, you assimilated a number of the values of that group without even questioning what you were doing. This subliminal unwritten curriculum influenced your development as you prepared to function as an independent, successful, contributing member of society. However, if you attended a school where you were part of a minority culture, you might not have received information on your culture's rich heritage. This can be particularly true when deaf students are included in general education classes.

I'm sure all of you are aware that over 80 percent of students who are deaf or hard of hearing receive part if not all of their education in public schools alongside their hearing peers. Unlike students who attend residential schools where they have the opportunity to develop a sense of Deaf community and Deaf identity, those enrolled in inclusive settings may find they are the only student with a hearing loss in their grade level, and sometimes the only student who is deaf within the entire school. As a result, these students can grow up feeling like they are the only deaf or hard of hearing student in the world.

What can be done to help these students develop a positive identity that includes being deaf or hard of hearing? Teachers can begin by integrating Deaf studies across the curriculum. Beginning in kindergarten, teachers can incorporate some of the basics for interacting with Deaf people when units on sound awareness are taught. In first-grade social studies, Deafness and communication can be stressed when the topic of family life is taught. Throughout the K-6 curriculum, teachers can integrate lessons on deafness, including sensitivity activities, providing basic information about ASL as a language, and including Deaf history and organizations and recreational activities that have been established for Deaf or hard of hearing individuals.

By providing students with information on Deaf studies, it is hoped that each student will begin to shape his or her own unique identity, whether it be within the hearing or the Deaf community. The goal of all education should be to help students when they leave school feel to satisfied with whom they have become. By teaching Deaf studies, it is hoped that hearing students will broaden their perspectives on life and that deaf and hard of hearing students will find their place in society.

Selection 10.3: Video Conferencing Technology

Video conferencing technology has opened the doors for Deaf people by providing easy access to communication. The days of the TTY message relay are going by the wayside as more and more Deaf consumers take advantage of video relay interpreting known as VRI.

When using this technology, consumers as well as interpreters use web cameras to capture the signing. Videophones, PCs, and televisions equipped with web cams are all used to connect one person with another. Depending on the speed of your Internet connection and the type of camera you have, one-to-one conversations can take place.

Deaf students are now finding that they can chat with their friends or contact their advisors and instructors when they have questions for them. Dialing over the Internet, they can make connections with anyone who has compatible equipment. Video conferencing is not limited to one location. When the equipment is set up, you can call all across the United States, or into other countries.

Hearing people as well as Deaf people are taking advantage of video conferencing. James, who lives in Georgia, can use it to call his mom who lives in Wales to let her see how fast her grandson is growing. Dan can call his dad from California and show him the engagement ring he recently bought for his fiancée in Montana.

Furthermore, this equipment is being used in interpreting programs to connect college students with deaf high school students around the country. Erin, Alana, Kelly, and Abby, who are interpreting students in Valdosta, can now connect with deaf students in residential schools in Delaware and Oklahoma and provide tutoring for them. Once connected, the deaf student appears on the tutor's computer screen, the tutor appears on the student's screen at the residential school, and the tutoring process begins.

Videoconferencing has brought communication to a new level. By using videophones, signing can be seen clearly, and deaf individuals can connect with their friends and family and talk with them whenever they want.

Selection 10.4: Deaf, Deaf World

During Deaf Awareness Week have you ever gotten to experience "Deaf, Deaf World"? I'm not sure that's the actual name of it, but let me tell you about an event I attended last spring. I was taking an ASL class, and my teacher told me that we were required to attend this event. He told us when we got there and entered the room that we wouldn't be able to use our voices. He said we needed to experience what it was like to communicate without using our voices to make our needs known.

I wasn't sure what to expect when I entered the room. There were lots of people who were already there when I got there. All around the room against the walls tables were set up with signs over them telling you what they were. There was a bank, a VR office, a school, a hospital, as well as other offices. One area was set up like a classroom where you could learn about Deaf culture, and I think get some instruction in basic sign language. I never made it over there.

I remember once I walked in the door there was a table to my left that had a big bowl on it. Inside the bowl were colored disks that looked like poker chips. Every once in a while the lights would flash and there would be some message signed. Some people got really frustrated because they didn't have any idea what they were supposed to do when the lights flashed. Some students would write questions down on paper because they couldn't communicate even when they were using gestures.

It really was an awesome experience! Deaf people sat behind the tables, and they were very patient with the hearing people who would approach their areas. After it was over, one of my fellow classmates said she had made a big mistake while she was in the room. She said every time she didn't understand something, she meant to sign that she didn't know but instead signed that she didn't care. She didn't realize it until later that night. Then she was so embarrassed. She said she wanted to go back and tell all of the people that she was sorry.

Many of my classmates said they'd go again next year. They said they felt all instructors should require their students to go. They thought it was a really worthwhile experience. I don't think I've done it justice here, but if you ever have the chance, you should go and experience it. You'll be happy that you did.

Selection 10.5: Living with Deaf People

I want to tell you some of my experiences living with a couple of women when I first started teaching school. I started teaching back in 1970 at the School for the Deaf in Colorado. During that time, training programs frequently didn't teach any classes in sign language. I was a graduate of one of those programs. Then these programs would send students who had no previous experience with the language or oftentimes with the Deaf population to schools for the deaf to student teach.

When I entered the residential school for the first time to do my student teaching, I was 20 years old and was placed at the high school level teaching high

310

PART IV
....
Selections for
Interpreting and
Transliterating

school seniors, many whom were my age. I remember walking into the classroom, seeing all of them sign, and saying to my supervising teacher, "Oh my gosh! I don't know the language. What am I going to do?" And her response was, "Well, either you'll get it or you won't." I think she probably took pity on me.

Now, there was a Deaf woman who taught science at the school. She told me that she owned a house, rented rooms, and asked if I would like to rent a room and live there. She said another Deaf woman who worked at the bank also rented from her, and I was more than welcome to do the same. I agreed, and that's when I moved in. This was probably one of the best experiences I've ever had.

It was during the time before captioned TV, before most people had TTY machines, back in the days when the Deaf Club was very popular and most students went to residential schools—back in the days when we really had the facilities for Deaf people that are not as prominent in today's times as they once were.

Well, I became their interpreter 24/7. I tell my students frequently that while I learned to sign, my roommates were very patient. The three of us would go out to eat at restaurants. After about the second or third time of asking them what they wanted, I'd be too embarrassed to ask them again. So, I would guess and order what I thought they wanted. Then when the server brought the order, and it wasn't at all what they had asked for, I'd tell them that she must have misunderstood me. I never wanted to admit that I hadn't understood what they had asked for.

One time, while living with them, I locked myself out of the house. It was early in the morning and I still had my pajamas on. I forget what I had gone out to do, and the door locked behind me. I stood out there for what seemed like an eternity pounding on their window with a shovel handle trying to get their attention so they would let me back in. Finally, one of them saw one of the dogs barking. She didn't hear the dog, she saw it because I was making such a racket that she looked out, saw me, and let me back in. I'm sure I was quite a spectacle for all of the neighbors.

I also recall the time, probably my very first experience, when they had a party and I was the only hearing person there. It was definitely being in the minority. I was a little slower to catch the jokes. Everyone would laugh, and I would have to sit on the side and process a little bit longer before I finally got it. This was a marvelous experience—we lived together for about a year before I went back to work on my master's. It's an experience that I'll always cherish. I learned a great deal—I would always recommend to anyone regardless how many classes that you've had that you get out and socialize in the Deaf community, because this is truly where you learn the language.

We can teach you the grammar, syntax, and the rules of the language in the classroom, but until you really get a chance to use it in a conversational sense, it doesn't really become your own—I don't think. So don't ever hesitate to enter new groups, go to new places, and use the skills that you have. Mine certainly developed by having the opportunity to talk with native users and have them be patient enough to work with me as I started to learn the language.

Potpourri II

Selection 11.1: Homes of the Rich and Famous

Have you ever looked at books or watched programs that feature homes of the rich and famous? They go beyond what most of us can imagine or envision. Usually their homes have between fifteen and twenty thousand square feet or more and countless bedrooms and bathrooms. Depending on where they are located, they may house multiple fireplaces or swimming pools both indoors and out.

One of my favorite celebrity homes has a semicircle of glass that surrounds the back of the house. Thousands of rectangular glass panes create a wall of glass that allows the resident to look out at the expanse of the ocean. Extending floor to ceiling, the entire height of three stories, it is a sight to see. Regardless of where you're sitting or standing in the back of the house, you have an exquisite view of the water.

This particular home features a magnificent entryway flanked with large plants located on each side of the front door. Approximately ten feet into the entryway is a large fountain with water that cascades down into a marble font filled with alabaster shells. Upholstered benches form a semicircle around the fountain, providing visitors a place to sit and wait to be formally received.

A spiral staircase winds its way up to the second floor. Once you arrive on the second floor, the hall is lined with paintings. Created by the masters, they grace the wall with their beauty. Under the paintings are a series of tables that provide support for a variety of sculpted pieces and pottery brought back from all over the world. In essence, it is a small art gallery.

One wing of the second floor is full of bedrooms. Each of the twenty bedrooms has its own bathroom. Each of the bedroom doors, at eye level, has a little brass plaque that identifies the name of the room. This assists guests in finding their rooms when they spend the night. Ten of the bedrooms are on one side of the hall and ten on the other.

There are numerous fireplaces throughout the house. While some are located in some of the bedrooms, the most expansive one is placed between the living room and the dining room. Opening into both rooms, it is made of stone, and the mantle is massive. Although the ones in the bedrooms are electric and very realistic, the one that opens into the dining and living rooms burns wood and requires a great deal of work. A large pile of logs is set beside the fireplace, and on a cold evening the stack rapidly diminishes.

Although I could talk for hours about this house, I can't imagine living in a home that is so massive. Even if I could afford it, I'm afraid I'd get lost just trying to find my way into the kitchen.

Selection 11.2: Candidates for Governor Spout Platforms

Within any political party, two or more candidates can vie for the backing of their party so they can compete against the contender from the opposite party. It doesn't matter if the candidate is a Democrat or a Republican; before you can compete for

312

PART IV
....
Selections for
Interpreting and
Transliterating

any office or elected government position you must first win the election within your own party before you can go further.

The primaries are usually held in the summer well in advance of the November elections, and candidates are cautioned to avoid harsh negative attacks on their intraparty opponents that will make it hard to unite after the election is over. The goal is to win the party nomination without giving too much fodder to the other party prior to the primaries.

Last year two men were in the runoffs for the Democratic nomination for the governor's race in Florida, Davis Nelson and Graham Smith. Not too long after each declared his candidacy, the two men agreed to meet to defend their platforms and garner support for their campaigns. A debate was scheduled and was held in the Exhibition Hall in Gainesville. The media provided coverage of the event, so those who were interested could listen to their views.

Nelson began the debate by stressing that he was campaigning on his values. He continued to say that he felt it was time to put the interests of children first and that tax dollars must be allocated for education to protect the future of this country. He went on to say that healthcare issues and underemployment had to be addressed.

When Smith had his turn at the podium, he stressed that although education seemed to be a top priority, it was time to examine family values and put money into parenting classes, thus reducing the number of children who arrive at school presenting discipline problems for the teachers. Listening to Smith's bold stand that government should intervene in family values, the audience became silent. He went on to stress that more funding needed to be poured into programs for senior citizens and programs that offer assistance for those who are unemployed and underemployed.

Although several barbs were exchanged throughout the one-hour exchange, at the end of the debate both men shook hands and were very congenial when they left the stage. Smith and Nelson will have other opportunities to address additional issues in future debates.

 ### Selection 11.3: Airports

Have you ever flown out of a large airport? I am always fascinated at the design of many of the modern ones. They can accommodate multiple runways, a vast array of terminals, shops, restaurants, and a variety of places for the travelers to relax while waiting for connecting flights.

The shops have everything from books and bath needs to clothing and snacks. For those who need something more than a candy bar, restaurants are readily available. In today's larger airports you can find everything from fast food like McDonalds, Burger King, and Wendy's to those establishments that provide a full steak dinner.

The airport in Tampa, Florida, has gone a step further to accommodate its passengers. Located across from the International Mall, travelers can be bused to and from the mall as they wait for their connecting flights. This mall is huge and has hundreds of stores. It is shaped like a big "Y" with the more typical stores like Penney's and Sears on one wing and the more expensive stores like Coach and Saks Fifth Avenue on the other wing. For those travelers who have both time on their hands and money, it is a wonderful convenience. It is also helpful for those travelers who arrive in Tampa with lost luggage and are in need of a business suit for the next day.

Of all the airports I have traveled in and out of, I think the ones in Denver, Dallas, and Atlanta are the largest. When you drive into these airports, the parking lots are huge, and frequently you must ride a bus to get from the parking lot into the terminal.

Once inside, you usually have to ride an escalator up to the second floor and go through security. Those of you who have flown know what is involved there.

313

CHAPTER 11
....
Potpourri II

PART I

PART II

PART III

PART IV

As you weave back and forth through the line, you finally arrive at the security checkpoint where your bags, purses, and any other security items are scrutinized for dangerous items.

When going through this checkpoint, laptops must be removed from their carrying cases, belts and shoes must frequently be taken off, and usually change and keys must be removed from one's pockets. In the event that the sensor picks up any additional metal, you must stand with your feet shoulder length apart, with your arms extended, to be scanned with a wand.

Once this procedure is complete, you are free to put your shoes and belt back on and put the change back in your pocket. You can then put your laptop back in its carrying case and proceed to your gate.

In a large airport, several gates can originate from one hub, so from one central location you may have paths for gates going out in several different directions. Furthermore, in large airports such as Dallas, you are required to ride the train to the various terminals and then ride on the walking sidewalks to your gate. The train system is designed with a color-coded map that allows for ease at getting off at the appropriate gate.

The Atlanta airport differs from Dallas in the respect that all of the gates are in one building and you ride the train to the various destinations. Moving sidewalks are also available for those traveling short distances. I remember arriving in Atlanta one time with very little time to get to my connecting flight. As I hurried to get on the train to arrive at the next terminal, we waited for what seemed like a very long time for the train to start. Finally, the lights blinked and a voice came over the loudspeakers informing everyone that the train had broken down and that all travelers would have to use the moving sidewalks. I remember my panic as I raced along the sidewalk to my final destination.

Recently a colleague and I traveled to Colorado Springs and flew into their airport. Of all the airports I have flown in and out of, I think it is one of my favorites. Located in the middle of the prairie, it is not huge, but large enough to facilitate a number of flights.

As we entered the airport, we were struck by the beauty of the sculpture and the artwork. While walking through the terminal, we couldn't help but notice the paintings on the walls and the metal sculptures that were suspended from the ceiling by using fine steel cables. It was exquisite!

As in most airports, the gate areas have long expanses of windows, providing the traveler with a panoramic view of the surroundings. These windows line both sides of the gate area giving viewers the opportunity to not only see the local terrain but also to observe the planes as they land and take off from the airport.

Once on the plane you must store all of your carryon baggage under your seat or above in the bins lining the plane. Prior to take off, the stewardesses will close the bins so no suitcases will fall on the passengers when the plane both takes off and lands.

Deplaning passengers also ride trains or moving sidewalks as they search for the baggage claim area. There, large conveyer belts deposit bags on a revolving storage area until passengers can retrieve them. Once bags are retrieved, passengers exit the airport at the ground level.

Both flying and airports can be a lot of fun. Just sitting and watching people walk to and from their flights can be delightful—especially if you enjoy "people watching." Travelers are diverse and always provide you with a kaleidoscope of behaviors and forms of attire to observe.

Selection 11.4: Adult Day Care

I read an interesting article in the paper recently about the growing number of new facilities for adults, primarily for individuals who are suffering from both dementia and Alzheimer's disease. Who would have thought that today that we'd be setting up daycares for the adult population very similar to daycare centers for infants

314

PART IV
....
Selections for
Interpreting and
Transliterating

and the pre-K population that have been so popular for the past thirty years ever since the baby boomers went to work and started having children?

I think the sad commentary on adult daycare centers is not the fact that they're available or that they provide wonderful services, because they do, but because of the clientele that they serve. One of the things that I have always thought would be the hardest is to go through the aging process, have your body stay very physically fit, and have your mind start to deteriorate. Especially if you are aware of the fact that you're not able to function the way you once were able to. This, I think, is one of the saddest portraits of the graying segment of society, those senior citizens who, due to the aging process, are not able to continue functioning mentally at the capacity they once did.

Alzheimer's has really taken its toll on people. You know there's hardly a day that goes by that you don't hear a story on the news or read a story about someone who has some form of Alzheimer's or some new research that they're doing to try to slow the progression of it. How hard this must be for people who have loved ones who have this disease to sit back and watch them deteriorate to the point that they function like an infant again. I often think of some of the adults who I've known through the years who have been very physically active, who have been in good health who live to be sometimes 100 years old. Then their minds start to go, they can't remember things, and they can't communicate with others very well because those portions of their brains are just not functioning like they once did. This has got to be so frustrating for the individual and so traumatic. You know they are aware of what they want to express, and it just won't come out. You know with Alzheimer's the brain continues to deteriorate, and sometimes people with that disease become very violent or wander away.

And I think part of that must be tied into frustration. Think of the frustration of not being able to express yourself, not being able to communicate. That has to be very hard on the individual. I think it's marvelous that these centers have been set up today so that people do have a place for their loved ones to go where they'll receive very good care. Some of these facilities are set up with varying degrees of care—for those who can still live semi-independently, there are apartments where people can just check on them.

For those who have reached the stage where they need far more care and assistance, there are modified assisted living environments where they receive more services. So I think the adult daycare, where some people drop their parents off during the day and then pick them up at the end of the day and bring them home at night, when they can be there to watch them, is a good option. Others have to stay in a residential facility because they've reached the point at which people at home can't take care of them.

So, adult daycares serve a very useful function today, and they're located in so many cities and provide a quality of life that we previously didn't have. Maybe some of you have loved ones who have been receiving services in these facilities. If so, I hope you have found one that you're very happy with to help deal with this devastating disease.

PART I

CHAPTER 12

Potpourri III

Selection 12.1: Bike Across America

Do you like to ride a bike? Have you ever considered riding it for long distances? Some friends of mine are part of a bike club. Some of the members are hearing and some of them are Deaf, and they all sign. A few years ago one of the interpreters in our town, who loves to ride bikes, organized the group. The only requirements to join are that you've got to have a bike, and you've got to enjoy riding. The rest is up to you. When they first set up the club, their goal was to train for a forty-mile ride.

The first Saturday they got together, they all brought their calendars. They decided that they'd ride together, as a group, every other Saturday. One member of the group would be responsible for setting the course, making sure it included enough miles and that it wasn't too hilly. They decided they'd start with ten miles at first and gradually build up to forty. So, every other Saturday they met in front of the Student Center, got on their bikes, and set off on the course.

The first week they went from the Student Center and rode five miles north past the high school and Highway Patrol station. Once they hit five miles they turned around and came back. Two weeks later they rode eight miles east to the small town of Lee, then went ten miles south to Clifton, and then retraced their route. Some of the riders could only go part way, so they would either wait for the others to return and join the group again, or they would head back early.

After months of training, several of them were ready to try a weekend bike ride. They registered for the event, and when they showed up at the starting point they were amazed to see the number of bike riders. It was awesome! During the weekend they made so many good friends and made plans to ride again in a longer race during the summer. It was as if it had gotten in their blood and now they didn't want to give it up. What a positive thing to be hooked on!

If you think you'd enjoy doing this, you should check in your community and see if there's a bike club already set up. If so, you should go to one of the meetings and join. It's a wonderful way to make friends, a great way to get in shape, and it's neat to see different parts of the country. Some of the bike clubs join together with other clubs in different states and ride with them during their summer vacations. What a great way to get fit and build friendships as well as self-esteem!

Selection 12.2: Cat Lovers

There are some people in the world who just love animals. I mean all animals. Cats, dogs, pigs, hamsters, ferrets—you name it, and they will tell you they either have one for a pet or had one as a pet in the past. Then there are some people I know who just like cats, dogs, and fish. They've found a way to have their cats and dogs live together in the same house and get along fine. I tried that once, but it didn't work so well for me.

Then there are other groups of pet owners who either seem to be those who love cats or those who love dogs. These people usually have cats or dogs but not

316

PART IV
....
Selections for
Interpreting and
Transliterating

both and will tell you up front what they like and what they wouldn't have. My neighbor is like that. She is a dyed-in-the-wool cat lover!

I always refer to her cats as the "step cats." She lives in an old-fashioned farm house with about eight steps leading up to her huge front porch. It's really a neat old house. She has five cats. Wow! That's too many for me. But anyway—each of the cats seems to like a different step, and when you go and visit her, you have to walk in between them going up the steps because they refuse to move.

The cat that sits on the right side of the bottom step is all gray with a white star on her chest. I think she must be the oldest of the group because she never budges when she sees you coming. She just looks at you with at air of indifference like oh, it's you again. I imagine she was a beauty in her day, but now she's gained a little weight and her coat has lost some of its luster.

On the third step from the bottom in the middle of the step is a black and white cat. She calls him Tuxedo. He's young and feisty, and you'd better not get too close to him or he'll think you're playing with him. I've gotten scratched a time or two when I got too close, and he thought my leg was a play toy. I can tell you, that wasn't much fun.

On the next step are two of her cats, Eli and Lily. They're sister and brother, and both of them are afraid of their own shadows. Usually, when they see some-one coming they run for cover. You have to be careful when you approach them so they don't run toward you, causing you to trip. That's always been my fear that I'll jump, try to avoid them, and fall flat on my face.

Her fifth cat usually hangs out on the top step in the flower pot. My friend has two huge pots full of geraniums, and for some reason Rascal loves to curl up in the flower pot. He almost looks fake when he's sleeping and has been known to make more than one child jump when he or she got too close and tried to touch him. Like I said, she is really a cat lover. I think she'd be lost without her cats.

 ### Selection 12.3: The Hundredth Day of School

When you were in elementary school, did you celebrate the one hundredth day of school? This is a popular day among elementary-school children. Some teachers ask the students to bring in a hundred of anything to celebrate. Children have been known to bring in one hundred pennies, jelly beans, rubber bands, googley eyes, and paper clips. Sometimes teachers ask their students to write papers about what they've learned during the first one hundred days of school. Below are some papers from some first graders about what they learned during the first hundred days.

One child wrote, "Today is the hundredth day of first grade and we got new pencils. I got one with horses on it and it has a pink eraser. And I learned to not hit and push."

Another student put on his paper, "I learned to jump rope. I didn't know how to jump rope when I started school. So, if you come to the same school I will teach you how to jump rope because kindergartners don't know how."

An autistic child wrote: "I like to count to 100. I can count 1, 2, 3, 4, 5, 6, 7, 8, 9, 10, 100. I count the starts. What does 98 plus 2 equal? It's 100. Just e-mail and use the computers. Just go to school. I'm so happy." It said, "Dear Class I love 100. Love Daniel."

Here are two more: "Hi My name is Jennifer. I am 100 days smarter. I learned how to spell 'are' and how to spell 'what.' It is cool to be here and I like my teach-ers Ms. Megghan and Ms. Brandy. And I like clusters. It was on Wednesday I learned about Hawaii. I learned there are hump backed whales. And there are 8 islands in Hawaii and water turtles. I like my life a lot."

The last one wrote: "What I learned is time lines. I will show you what time lines are. They are stuff you do in the past."

Selection 12.4: The Money Pit

Our house gives new meaning to the movie *The Money Pit*. We bought this house about eighteen years ago, and it's been a work in progress ever since. Before I tell you everything that's wrong with it, let me explain why we bought it in the first place. We had moved into a very small town, and after renting for about two years, it was the only thing on the market that would meet our needs, sizewise, that is. You see, we have four children, and they were all living at home at the time.

The man who had owned the house before us was supposedly a builder and had taken the original structure and added onto it. Originally, the house was one story. It had a living room, kitchen, bathroom, and three bedrooms. When the previous owner had it, he decided he would expand the house. First, he added a laundry room, another bedroom with a bathroom attached, and a family room. But I guess that wasn't enough. Some time later he added an upstairs over the family room that had two more bedrooms with a bathroom in between them.

What started out as a frame house was then bricked in so it looked like it was all built at the same time. Well, when we bought the house we knew it needed some work. How much work it needed was a huge surprise to us. One of the first things we did after we bought the house was to remodel the family room. It had been done in the 1960s with dark paneling and orange shag carpet. My husband decided to remove the paneling and texture the walls. It was then that he discovered there was no sheetrock on the studs.

That was the first project—adding sheetrock that should have been there from the beginning. While he was adding sheetrock, he decided to put in overhead lights as there were none in that room. That's when he discovered the aluminum wire going into the electrical box. Needless to say, that was a fire hazard just waiting to happen. Through the years he's had to replace walls, wiring, and rotted wood from the staircase leading up to the second floor.

When he went to replace the toilet in one of the bathrooms, he discovered that the standard toilet he had bought as a replacement wouldn't fit because the man had used a substandard commode and then built the walls around it. In order to put in the new toilet, the walls had to be moved. Not only that, there is not one straight wall in the new part of the house. Obviously, the man couldn't measure, and while some of the walls from top to bottom are only off a quarter of an inch, others are off by almost an inch and a half.

We have both decided that once all of our remodeling projects are done, we will sell our "money pit" and move to something smaller and newer. I think my husband has grown tired of being a weekend plumber, carpenter, and electrician. If we had known what we were getting into, we probably would have pitched a tent somewhere and waited until another house became available. While some people spend their summer vacations painting and just doing general maintenance, we've spent ours correcting poor workmanship and hazardous conditions. Our only hope is that we can finish our projects within the next couple of years so we can relocate and start having our weekends to ourselves again.

Selection 12.5: My Dog

I want to tell you about a new dog we recently got. Before I tell you about him, let me tell you about a previous dog that we had. Several years back my husband and I moved from a farmhouse into town. We purchased a fairly large house that had five bedrooms. Two of the bedrooms were in the front of the house, one was in the back of the house, and two were upstairs in the back of the house. Because our bedroom was upstairs in the back of the house and my two youngest daughter's bedrooms were in the front of the house downstairs, I told my husband that we needed to get a dog. That way, if anyone tried to get into the house, the dog would bark, and we would hear him.

318

PART IV
....
Selections for
Interpreting and
Transliterating

So, I set out on a mission to find a dog. I had decided that instead of buying a dog or going to a pet store, it would be better if I looked at animal shelters and adopted a poor little dog that just didn't have a home. So, I looked, and I looked, and sure enough I found a dog in an animal shelter in Monticello, Florida. Actually, I had gone into an animal clinic to ask about getting a key to the shelter located behind it. And, while I was in the animal hospital I noticed this little dog that was in a cage, and I said, "What a cute little dog!" And the woman said to me, "Oh, he's up for adoption." I said, "Really?" She said, "He gets along really well for only having three legs."

Well, I looked at him; I have to tell you, this dog was a cross between a Yorkshire terrier and a poodle. And, with his long fur, I looked at him and said, "Oh, this is great—you don't even notice he's missing his back right leg." So I told the woman I would take the dog. She said he would have to stay and be neutered and that I could pick him up the following Friday.

When that Friday arrived, I took my four daughters, got in the van, and went and got the dog. I told them on the way that the dog only had three legs, but that he was a sweet little dog, and that with his long fur, no one would ever notice his missing back leg. We picked him up and brought him home. He got out of the van, and the first thing the men who were cleaning the street, the city workers, said was "Oh my gosh, what happened to his other leg?" Well, obviously my daughters never believed me after that.

We had this little dog—his name was Toto; he had been named that. I'm sure that the person who had previously had him thought he looked like the dog from the *Wizard of Oz*. We had Toto for about eleven years; he was 4 when we got him. Yes, that's about right—maybe we had him for about a couple of years longer. Anyway, by the time Christmas rolled around this past year Toto had lost his hearing, he had become blind, and of course he only had his three legs. He was really a special needs dog. And he had gotten to the point where he was just very, very old and was not doing well, so we had to have him put to sleep. That was very sad.

So, since Christmas time, I've been looking for another small dog. Well, the other day a woman from another college in Madison, Florida, e-mailed me and said, "There is someone who has a little dog that she needs to get rid of because she is allergic to it. Would you be interested in this dog?" And I said, "Yes, I would." She said, "It's a Bichon Frise, 5 years old, housebroken, and has had all of its shots." So I said, "Ok, give me the lady's number, and I'll go look at the dog."

So, I did; a couple of days later I went around the corner. This woman, I found out, lives very close to me. I got the little dog, and brought him home. I didn't realize that he was an AKC-registered little dog. This is actually his third home. He's a white fluffball and his name is Bailey. So we've now had Bailey for two days. Bailey seems to be a pretty friendly little guy and loves to sleep with someone at night, so he's sleeping with my daughter. He does have four legs. Now, he—I think—will be a pretty good companion. He weighs about fourteen pounds.

I have to tell you that my love of dogs goes way back. The first dog I had was when I first started teaching. And this little dog—well, he really wasn't so little—was an Old English sheepdog. Tugboat weighed 110 pounds. When he stood on his hind legs, his front paws would hit my shoulders, and we could look each other in the eye. He was a delightful dog—Tugboat was from a breeder who had bred the dogs that Disney used for *The Shaggy Dog*. And, he was sold for pet stock because he was bigger than a show dog for an Old English. So you can imagine that he was a pretty good-sized dog.

I have to admit I really am a dog lover, and I guess I always will be one. I don't know how many of you are. But, if you are, you can certainly appreciate what one goes through when one has to have a pet put to sleep, or one's pet dies. I think you automatically want to replace it. And, even when we replace a pet, special memories of the former one always stay with us.

CHAPTER 13

Life Experiences IV

Selection 13.1: A Walk in the Woods

Jeff loves to walk in the woods. It doesn't seem to matter to him what season it is, he just loves to get out and walk. He lives in the mountains, and there are so many different kinds of trees, including aspen and pine trees, that he never gets bored walking and looking. Aspen trees are some of his favorites. In the spring and summer their leaves are green, in the fall they turn from green to gold to orange, and then they fall off the trees in the winter. Jeff's told me that if you can catch it right in the fall, it looks like the hillside is almost on fire.

Not only does he enjoy the trees, but he's an avid bird watcher. He loves to look up in the trees and see how many different kinds of birds he can identify. Sometimes he takes his dog with him on his walk. Chief is a "real man's" dog. He's big, boisterous, and loves to chase birds. When he sees them on the ground, he barks and makes all of them scatter. Jeff thinks it's funny to watch them fly off in a hundred different directions.

One time when Jeff was by himself, he noticed a bird's nest that had fallen out of the tree. He scooped it up, took it home, and put it in an incubator he kept for chicken eggs. It wasn't very long before the baby birds hatched. Once they got old enough to fly and be independent, he set them free. Another time while he was out walking he spotted a beautiful bald eagle. You know, they have just been removed from the endangered species list. It was just regal! He stopped walking and watched it for some time before he continued on.

Another time he noticed some interesting tracks along the trail. He couldn't figure out what kind of an animal would leave tracks like what he was seeing. Just out of curiosity, he continued to follow the tracks. When he finally caught up with the animal, he felt foolish. It was just tracks from a dog that had part of one of its paws missing. He just knew he had come upon a unique animal.

Jeff's lucky. All around his house are mountain trails. While some of them wind around going up the mountain, others go straight up the side of the mountain. The mountains aren't real steep where he lives, so when you hit the various plateaus, you can walk for miles through valleys filled with wildflowers in the spring time. The panoramic view from these peaks is phenomenal. Sometimes in the winter he likes to go snowshoeing. Because that's such hard work he limits his walks to one or two miles.

I think he developed his love of walking while he was in college. He's always liked plants and found if he walked he could see a number of plants that are different shapes and sizes. He discovered that some of them seem to grow out of rocks while others can live in water and in cracks in the sidewalk. He has several books on plants and can tell you a lot about them. That's probably why he likes to walk so much. He really enjoys getting in touch with nature.

 Selection 13.2: Barbara the Pig

Julie, a friend of mine, used to go to the school for the deaf in our hometown. While she was enrolled in the school, her mom worked there as a tutor. Neither

320

PART IV
....
Selections for
Interpreting and
Transliterating

Julie nor her mom liked one of the houseparents. As you've probably guessed, the houseparent's name was Barbara. So when Julie and her mom decided to buy a pot-bellied pig, they decided to name her after Barbara. Barbara even had a sign name. It was a B close to the shoulder. Well, let me tell you about Barbara. She got into more stuff than a 2-year-old child.

One day when Julie and her mom were out shopping, they had left Barbara in the back yard. Somehow, the pig managed to get the back door open and got into the kitchen. She succeeded in opening all of the cupboard doors where the food was kept. Well, Barbara had a feast! She ate everything she could get her snout on. Can you imagine the mess that she made? Anyway, after she was very, very full, she waddled into the bedroom, somehow leaned against the door, and fell asleep.

When Julie and her mom got home, they found the mess. Yikes! Then they went looking for Barbara. When they tried to open the bedroom door, it wouldn't budge. She just weighed too much, and she refused to move. They tried and tried to encourage her to get up by calling her name and talking to her. But, it was to no avail. Finally Julie had to crawl in through the bedroom window, wait until Barbara was hungry again, and then she could get her up and get her out of the room. Wow! What a mess they had to clean up.

Another time they left her in the yard, and the UPS brought Julie's mom a new comforter. He saw the pig but thought if he put it on the top of the clotheslines, it would be fine. So, he balanced the package between the lines and left. Barbara was just too curious for her own good. She nudged the pole until it finally made the package drop. Then she tore it open and proceeded to chew holes in the new bedspread. When Julie's mom arrived home, she found a bedspread covered with holes about the size of apricots. Needless to say, she wasn't a happy camper. She called UPS, bawled them out, and asked them what they were thinking.

Through the years, Julie has told me many stories about Barbara the pot-bellied pig. I just love to listen to her talk about her. She has such beautiful ASL, and when she starts one of her stories, I always know it'll be entertaining. I've never had a desire to have a pet pig, and listening to her convinces me that I'll never want one. But, it sure is fun to hear her talk about the adventures she's had while owning a pig.

Selection 13.3: Violet's Tanning Experience

My friend Violet recently shared her experience about wanting to get a tan and how she got the look she was after. I knew that she was planning on going on a trip to Europe, but what I didn't know was that she wanted to have a tan before she left. You see, instead of flying to Europe, Violet and her friend Mary were taking a cruise to Europe and were planning to travel by train once they got there. The trip was being sponsored by Violet's alma mater, the Texas School for the Deaf, and from what she said, it sounded like it was going to be a lot of fun. So, before she went, she decided she needed a tan.

Violet knew she'd be wearing an evening dress for one of the banquets on the ship; she also had several swimsuits that were cut differently, and she didn't want to have any tan lines. At first she considered going to a tanning bed, but from everything she'd heard, she didn't think that was for her. She didn't want her skin to wrinkle, and she was afraid down the road of getting cancer. So, she opted for a spray tan.

She looked in the phone book and found what looked like the perfect place to go. She used her video phone, made her appointment, and showed up in plenty of time. After she paid her money and signed the form, the woman came to take her to one of the spray tanning rooms. The woman explained that she could take off all of her clothes if she wanted. She told her how to stand so the insides of her legs would get tan, and what to do when the spray started to hit her face. The woman told her she would turn on the machine and leave. When it was finished, she'd need to wait between twenty and thirty minutes for the tan to dry and then she could get dressed and leave.

Violet was a little concerned about removing all of her clothes. She had seen a special on TV in which some tanning salons had hidden cameras and took pictures of people in the nude. She didn't want to find pictures of herself on the Internet. After she searched the room for hidden cameras, she decided she'd keep on her underwear and she'd remove everything else. She got all ready, the woman turned on the machine and she left.

Violet followed the directions to a T. She held out her arms. She stood with her feet slightly apart with one foot about six inches further in front of her than the other one. She watched for the red light, because she knew that meant that the spray was about to hit her face. When she was all finished, she looked down at her feet and that's when the panic set in. She noticed her feet were all speckled. In a panic she opened the door and started out down the hall to find the woman. It was then that she realized she didn't have any clothes on.

She let out a holler and the woman came running. Once inside the room, the woman explained to her that she just needed to take the rag she had provided and smooth it out. Once Violet did that, the speckles disappeared. After the allotted twenty minutes, Violet put on her clothes and left. When she woke up the next day, she was pleasantly surprised to see what a nice even tan she had. She was really thrilled with the results and told all of her friends that she'd do it again. I wish you could have seen her tell the story. It was so much fun to watch. She is such a nut!

Selection 13.4: The Pizza Party

Mike and Cindy love pizza. It doesn't matter what kind. They'll eat cheese, pepperoni, sausage, onion; you name it, they'll eat it. One of their favorite kinds is pineapple and Canadian bacon. Because they're both health nuts they limit how often they eat it. But, once every two months or so they order a variety of pizzas, invite some of their closest friends, and they just sit around, eat pizza, watch movies, and have a good time.

Well, let me back up for a minute and tell you something else about Mike and Cindy before I go any further. About three months ago they rescued a dog that had been displaced after the last hurricane. It had been in a shelter, and both of them fell in love with him. He's just an overgrown mutt, but has an endearing personality. They brought him home, and he's been part of the family ever since. At first Rufus was pretty timid. He'd sleep on the floor, never got into anything, didn't play with toys, and pretty much just behaved like a well-trained dog. I'm telling you all of this because when I tell you what happened at the last pizza party, you'll appreciate knowing about the dog.

Let's see, it was about a month ago that I was invited to their house for the party. Usually, I can't go because I work the night shift most of the time and am never off the night of the parties, but last month I was lucky. It just so happened that I was off the night they were going to have it. I was excited because I like pizza too—especially barbequed pizza. That and the ones with grilled chicken on them—they're two of my favorites, and Cindy told me they'd order those if I was coming.

I got there a little late, and most of our other friends had already arrived and had started to eat. I went in, visited, and was just catching up on the latest news when Rufus came bounding out of the kitchen with a big piece of chicken pizza dangling from his mouth. He lay down on the carpet with all of the guests just like he thought he should. Cindy about died. There he was on her light tan carpet with a piece of pizza, tomato sauce and all, ready to hit the floor. She bolted for the dog and retrieved the pizza before he knew what happened. And don't you know it was the last piece of chicken pizza.

322

PART IV
....
Selections for
Interpreting and
Transliterating

Even though I didn't get my favorite kind of pizza that night, my friends had already eaten all of the barbeque before I arrived, it was well worth it just to see Rufus with that big piece of pizza hanging out of his mouth. I don't know what was funnier—seeing Rufus with the pizza or seeing Cindy run after him. Pretty funny!

Selection 13.5: The U-Turn

Have you every moved from one town to another and had to get used to where everything was located? If you have a good sense of direction, it's not too difficult. If you don't have a good sense of direction, it can be particularly challenging. Just getting from home to work, from home to the gym, class, the mall, or the grocery store can be an adventure.

About five years ago, my friend Tammy moved from a very small town of about 5,000 people to a very large city of over 500,000 people. In order to travel anywhere in the city, you usually had to cross over a bridge. I think the town where she lived had about seven or eight bridges, and, of course, if you got on the wrong bridge going the wrong direction, it could take you more than thirty minutes to find a place to turn around so you could get going in the right direction again.

When Tammy first moved to the city, she would call her mom crying if she got lost or got going on a bridge the wrong way. Then after a few months, the phone calls got to be less and less, and she started to navigate her way around town pretty well. She found which bridges took her to which parts of town and which ones to avoid during rush hour. She also asked her friends for directions for short cuts so if there was a major accident on the freeway she could take a detour and get where she needed to be without waiting for hours for the traffic jam to clear up.

Well, one night a friend of hers called her and told her she was sick. She asked her if she'd mind going to the store for her and bringing her some orange juice and some cold medicine. She had started running a fever, was chilled, and just really didn't want to go out. Tammy said she'd be happy to help. Her friend lived within ten miles of her, and she didn't even have to cross any of the bridges. Tammy already had her cow-print pajamas on, but she decided there was no reason to change. She had orange juice and cold medicine at her house, and she could just put them in a bag, drive them over, and come right back. After all, she didn't want to stay around her and risk getting a cold.

So she put the items in the bag and took off. When she got to the first light on Eisenhower, she couldn't remember if that was where she was supposed to turn left or if it was on Lincoln. Once she had passed Eisenhower, she realized that was where she should have turned. So at the next corner she decided to turn around and go back. Little did she know that there was a sign close to the ground that said No U-turn. As she made her U and was headed in the right direction, she noticed the flashing blue lights in her rear view mirror. She pulled over and got out of the car.

When the officer approached her and saw what she was wearing, he told her to get back in the car. I guess he thought her cow pajamas might be too distracting to the other drivers. Anyway, he gave her a ticket and told her to look for the signs in the future. She tried to explain to him that she was new in town but he wasn't very sympathetic. She took the ticket, made it to her friend's house, and then went home. Next time she'd be more careful about paying attention to the signs.

Life Experiences V

Selection 14.1: Driving on the Ice

I don't know how many of you have lived in climates where it snows or where the weather gets very cold and ice is a concern. If you've ever lived in the Midwest, umm, or even in the North, on the northeast coast, you've probably experienced what I'm going to talk about. Several years ago we lived in Pennsylvania in a town called Altoona. Altoona was an interesting town in that it was built around rail yards, and it had a big changing station for trains to come into, so many of the neighborhoods were built on triangles. Instead of having streets like in most cities that are parallel to each other and then perpendicular with a lot of streets running east and west or north and south, these streets would make a triangle. It was a very odd shape. For any of you who are from PA, you know what I'm talking about, but this is how Altoona was set up. Well, we lived in Altoona, and I worked at a college that was in Cresson. Cresson was a little small community up on Cresson Mountain. It was probably about thirty miles—well, between twenty-five and thirty miles from Altoona to Cresson—and I would drive up and down the mountain. The first year we lived there, we rented a house in Altoona while we looked for a house to buy in this small community on the mountain. Houses up there were hard to find because most people didn't move out once they moved in. During that year, I would drive up and down frequently. Well, one morning I was going up fairly early to work, and we had had an ice storm the night before. We had what's called black ice, and if any of you are familiar with this it means the roads are clear where you can see the asphalt, and the ice forms on top of it. You don't even know it's there necessarily because you can't see it. I was driving up the mountain when I hit a patch of ice, and my car probably spun around three times. I went from my side of the highway to the other side before I stopped. I'm sure I made three complete rotations. It was very, very frightening. Fortunately for me, no one was coming, no one was behind me, no one was going down the mountain, or I'm sure it would have been a very nasty accident. It was one of those things that not all pieces of the road have ice so you're not aware that it's there, and I just hit a patch and lost control of the car. It's kinda like when you hydroplane. You know you're stuck, and you can't get traction, so you just have to go with the flow of it.

Recently, one of our daughters moved to North Carolina, and this has been her first experience driving on both snow and ice. We cautioned her a while back, "You be careful because you will hit patches of black ice where you're driving. It's just fine and then all of a sudden you hit one of these pieces and you don't have control over your car. The best thing to do always is to drive slowly and give yourself plenty of space between cars. You know the same thing is true with ice—no, not ice, with snow. You can get stuck in the snow unlike ice where you can lose control and can end up just circling. With a car on the snow you can get your tires stuck in it and can't get any traction." This also happened to me when we lived in Pennsylvania. My husband went out and shoveled the driveway for me one morning. While I was backing out, I got too close to where he had shoveled this pile of snow. I got the back wheels stuck in it and couldn't get out. He had to come out and reshovel the driveway. He wasn't very happy with me. Part of this is just if you don't have a way to get traction on packed snow, it can be very much like ice. This is why so often in the Northeast or even in the Midwest you'll see people who put sand bags in their trunk to weigh down the back end of their car in the winter so if they get stuck the weight will help with traction, and it can also be useful if you do what I did. Sometimes when people get stuck they get out and put sand around their tires, which will give them enough traction to get out of the snow. So I caution any of you, if you've never had this experience, and you move to a location where snow and ice occur on a fairly routine basis in the wintertime, be careful when you get out and drive on it. It's very easy to navigate on those types of roads if you know what you're doing.

I grew up in Colorado, and we had lots of snow. Snow in Colorado is generally very different than snow in Pennsylvania. Snow in Colorado is very dry and powdery compared to snow in Pennsylvania, and that's why skiing out there in the winter is so good. In Pennsylvania, it's a much wetter snow, and then when the temperature drops, it can freeze and can become very icy. So quality of snow is different and can influence how much ice you'll end up with. So do be careful if you've never driven on it, but don't be afraid of trying it. People drive on it all the time and are quite successful.

Selection 14.2: The Cruise

Several months ago my husband and I were talking about places we'd like to go and things we'd like to do. He made the off-handed comment that he had no interest in going on a cruise. I asked him if he really meant it, and he said he did—to him it would just be like being in a mall with a whole lot of people, and it would just be something he wouldn't enjoy. I said to him that I had always wanted to go on one, at least just one time, just to experience it to see if it was something I'd like to do. My sister had asked me several years ago if my husband and I would be interested in going on a cruise with her and her husband to Alaska. I said before any of us ventured out on a cruise that long, one of us needed to try something shorter to see if we really liked the concept of a cruise. So, as my husband and I sat talking that day about his not wanting to go on a cruise, I said, "You know, I'd really like to do this. I think I'll call one of the girls"—you see we have four daughters.

I said, "Hmmm, I think I'll ask one of the girls if they'd like to go with me and plan a year from summer to go." I called the first daughter in Jacksonville. She's been on a cruise—I was trying to think if she's gone once or twice, but she's gone once and to Europe twice. So I called her and said, "You know, I'm really thinking of going on a cruise next summer and I was wondering if any of you girls would like to go." She said, "Definitely." She talked about how much fun she had had when she went and said to count her in.

I called another one of the girls and asked, "Would you like to go on a cruise? Your sister and I are going." Yes, she wanted to go too. Well, to make a long story short, all four of our daughters decided that they'd like to go. Then one of them said that we need to include our aunt who's from Mexico because she's such a delightful person that they thought she'd have fun with us. So we called her up, couldn't get her, but talked with her husband, and explained that we were planning an all-girl cruise a year from summer and did he think that she'd be interested in going. He said for sure that he thought she'd thoroughly enjoy it. There are a couple of other female family members that we're planning on inviting. All of us will start looking at our schedules, as this will take a little doing to coordinate this.

One of my daughters finishes up her master's next May, so it'll have to be after May. As soon as we can start to get an idea of months and weeks, we'll start our planning. One of the girls laughed and said she was going to go back to the gym so she could have a good figure to wear her bikini on this cruise. I think it

325

CHAPTER 14
···
Life Experiences V

PART I

PART II

PART III

PART IV

will be a fun time. My husband will get to spend some time with one of his brothers while all of us go on this adventure.

We've decided that we don't want to go and be gone very long, probably a three-night, four-day cruise. We found that you can now leave from Jacksonville, which will be nice because one of the girls will fly in from Charlotte to Jacksonville; one will fly up from Tampa to Jax, and we can drive down. That's where we'll plan to board the ship. My sister-in-law will fly in from Denver, so I think it'll be an exciting time. Never having been on a cruise ship myself, I'm looking forward to it. I enjoy traveling, and I think just to get to go and see what it's like will be lots of fun.

Someone has said that the food is phenomenal and that there's food available all day long. I guess I should go on a diet a couple of months before we go and shed a few pounds so if I put them on while we're on the boat it won't be a big deal. But I think it will be a great experience, and I'm looking forward to the mother–daughter time. How many of you have been on a cruise, and did you enjoy it? I hope so. I hope this will be a good investment of both time and money, and if not, I'll at least have a chance to see my children and that in itself will be fun.

Selection 14.3: Jan's Girls

Every mother will tell you that her child or children have unique characteristics that make each of them special in her eyes. If a mother has more than one child, she will go on at great lengths to describe the similarities and differences in the children. My friend Jan is no different. She has four grown daughters and is proud of each and every one of them. According to her, they are each beautiful and talented in their own ways.

Her oldest daughter is the tallest of the group, has brown hair, dark brown eyes, and a dancer's physique. According to Jan, she's gorgeous, very bright, quite artistic, and has a passion for dance. Second to her passion for dance is her love of the ocean and walking on the beach. She loves to spend her free time walking on the sand soaking up the warmth. Being a cat lover, she has two felines that she dotes on.

One is a long-haired cat that is rather rotund. Pushing between sixteen and eighteen pounds, she's a force to be reckoned with. She'll curl up in your lap and keep you warm during the cool, winter months. Her other feline is black and has patches of fur missing due to allergies. He is the less social of the two and generally retreats under the bed when visitors arrive.

When her oldest daughter was in college, she majored in dance and still dances today. One time she asked Jan if a group of the dancers could stay at their house so they could go to a dance concert in another town, not far from where Jan lived. Jan welcomed the dancers and their professor with open arms. At the end of the weekend, the girls left her a thank you note referring to her as Donna Reed. It was really cute and a weekend that Jan will always treasure.

Her second-oldest daughter is short like Jan and built very much like her. She's petite, has dark curly hair, very dark eyes, and is also a real beauty. She is also very artistic, but excels in math as well. Jan laughs that while her second daughter was in college, she used to bring home problems in calculus and trig that went way beyond where Jan's mathematical mind would go. However, being a good mom, Jan would smile and nod, pretending that she understood.

One time while in college, she invited a group of her friends home for the weekend. They were a delightful group of students from different countries and cultures. Jan said it was a real international weekend and that she sat around the table listening to the future leaders of our country. It is a fond memory she'll have for a long time.

Not only can Jan's second daugter solve complex engineering problems, but she has also developed a knack for drawing and painting and delights in putting

326

PART IV
....
Selections for
Interpreting and
Transliterating

her talents to work. She has created several pieces of art throughout the years that are treasured by her family members and her friends. Jan has several pieces that she has done for her throughout the years. Her sisters also have their own treasures that she has made for them.

The third daughter is somewhere in height between the first and the second. Unlike her older sisters, she has blonde hair and blue-gray eyes. She is also striking, and her personality is a lot like Jan's. She followed in her mother's footsteps and became a teacher, and the two of them can talk for hours about educational issues. She also has a very creative nature, and although she doesn't paint or draw like her sister, she has a knack for putting collages and picture frames together. She also has a knack for decorating and a good eye for what will go together.

All of the girls have a wonderful sense of humor, but the third daughter seems to find herself in more situations than the others that just make you want to laugh. Jan loves to hear her share stories about her friends, her teaching, and her new experiences as a newly married woman. She sees humor in most things and has a delightful way of sharing stories. Many people have commented that she is a bright spot, bringing smiles to almost anyone she talks to.

The fourth daughter is the shortest by far—topping the height chart at only four foot eleven. With red hair and bright blue eyes, she's stunning. A gymnast by training, she still has an athletic build, although she doesn't compete any more. Unlike her sisters, who joined Future Homemakers of America while they were in high school, she opted to join Future Farmers of America. During her junior and senior years of high school, she raised hogs and showed them during the livestock show.

A mixture of femininity and creativity, there isn't anything she can't do. Like her other sisters, she's very artistic, very independent, and knows what she wants out of life. She's definitely not a morning person, but by evening she comes alive and can delight you with her many stories. She's developed a real passion for cooking and loves to watch the cooking shows on TV and experiment with new dishes. Jan thoroughly enjoys having her around to cook.

I wish you could meet Jan and the four girls. When they all get together, they're all so different, but complement each other so well. Jan's husband learned years ago that once they get going, he can't get a word in edgewise. He's just excited today that he has a new son-in-law that he can sit and visit with. The man their daughter married is delightful and fits in perfectly with the other members of the family. Jan's husband especially enjoys having another man around to shoot the bull with.

Potpourri IV

Selection 15.1: Car Shows on MTV

How many of you have had the chance to see the new program—I think it's on MTV—where they take cars and remodel them for the person who has donated the car? Do you know what I'm talking about? I don't watch MTV—I don't watch TV much, for that matter, but one day I came home from work, and I thought I just need to unwind a little bit, so I turned on the TV. It had been left on this channel where they were doing this car. The car that I saw was a Cadillac that had been refurbished.

Apparently they've done trucks, they've done cars, and the Cadillac they were doing had been custom painted. They used a color of rose—it was a pinkish red that they had custom mixed. They had taken rims for the wheels and painted them. Inside they had done it over too. It had a TV in it, and it had a six- or eight-CD changer. The seats were all done in leather. It had all of these wonderful features.

But then the thing that really caught my eye was that apparently this girl who had this car was a real lover of shoes. She had every kind of shoes imaginable, and when the makeover people had gotten her car, they found in the trunk that she had just taken and thrown in all these different shoes. It was rather messy. So somehow they designed a shoe rack for her trunk with a sliding, um, like a sliding shelf that would come out that was all divided into little shoeboxes not with lids—just the rectangles where you could put all these shoes. She must have had fifteen pairs of shoes in these boxes they built for her, so when she opened the trunk, she could pull these out. The boxes were designed where she could slide them up and out so she could get to the pair of shoes that she wanted. You know, kind of like in your kitchen where some people have their food on sliding shelves where you can pull out the shelf and see what you have. Well, this is the way her shoes were done in her trunk.

So they gave her back her car, and she was so excited. I think the people who remodeled or refurbished it spent $20,000 on it. It was a pretty penny; it was an old Cadillac. Well, anyway I watched this; it was fascinating. At the end of the program she drives off in this. Then she shows it to her family, and everyone thought this was a pretty neat deal. You know, she just didn't want to part with her old Cadillac.

Well, one evening I was talking to my son on the phone, and I told him that I had happened to turn on the TV and I had seen this show. He knew exactly what I was talking about, and he said, "My friend Dave"—one of his friends—"they've accepted his car and during the summertime his car is going to be one of the ones they're going to do next. I'm not sure what they're going to do to it." It really is fascinating. One of these cars had three TVs put in the back seat where people could watch different shows on TV at the same time.

This has really been interesting to me. I don't spend that much time in my car, but I'm sure for some people who do, this is a big thing to do. I know today it's not uncommon to see cars with TVs and VCRs or CD players in them. Perhaps some of you have watched this show and are more knowledgeable than I am, so if you get a chance to see it, take the chance and watch it because it really is neat to see the before and after and see what they can do with a little bit of money. And if you have an old junky car or an old "beater" car, you might consider submitting your car to the MTV show.

Selection 15.2: Seasons of the Year

Have you ever noticed that some people really have a distinct preference for different seasons of the year? In some parts of the country, there are four distinct seasons: fall, winter, spring, and summer. In these locations, there is a definite change in temperature; there are changes to the trees, to the flowers, to the grass—the temperature changes dramatically from winter to summer. States such as Colorado, Nebraska, and Kansas all have four distinct seasons, as do the New England states.

In the fall, many of the leaves go from green to gold or red, if they're an aspen tree; in the winter those trees lose their leaves. In the spring, the leaves come back again and remain on the trees throughout the summer. Trees are one way we see a real change in the four seasons. Another big change you'll notice in states that have definite seasonal changes is in temperature. In the fall, the nights start to become cooler, in the forties or fifties at night, sometimes even high thirties where the daytime temperatures may stay in the low to mid seventies. Many people are very, very fond of fall weather because of the cool evenings and warm days. Then, as the season changes to winter, the temperature drops significantly. In these locations, snow usually becomes part of the routine for winter. Temperatures may drop to zero, ten below, even as low as thirty below and only climb in the daytime into the teens.

Snow generally starts to fall as early as October or early November, and snow may continue to fall up until the end of March. Occasionally, these states will see a snowstorm in April, but this is usually rare. Then spring arrives by April and lasts through May. By the time we're into June, the temperatures have started to get quite warm. June, July, and the middle part of August, you may see temperatures ranging anywhere from the eighties to one hundred depending on if a heat wave is sweeping through the country. The evening temperatures will drop down into the fifties or sixties. And then we go back into fall.

Many people are really affected by seasons in the year, by sunshine, by winter months compared to summer months. Some people are far more sunshine oriented, and some people love the snow and love to be out in the cold. It really varies. You know, in Seattle and in Oregon, because of the number of months that they have rain and cloudy skies and don't see sunshine a lot of time, they use mood lights there to help people get a sense of sunlight, like what we enjoy in the southern part of the country.

As you look around the country and think about relocating, pay attention to the type of climate an area has. Some people can't go from the South and move to the North because they don't get acclimated very well. On the flip side, some people who have lived in the North or the Northwest can't move to the South because the temperatures are so warm. So finding out the kind of person you are and the type of weather you like are critical to finding out how happy you're going to be in any one given area.

Selection 15.3: The Importance of a Good Manager

Motivation is everything. You can do the work of two people, but you can't be two people. Instead, you have to inspire the next guy down the line and get him to inspire his people. The natural tendency of most businesspeople is to promote from within in order to reward loyal employees. This is a great policy, but it has some

329

CHAPTER 15
....
Potpourri IV

PART I

PART II

PART III

PART IV

major flaws that must be considered in each case. Employees who perform labor and critical jobs are important, but managers are more important, because they directly influence many more people.

If you look closely at those firms that have been consistently profitable, you will see that their success comes from maintaining, developing, and keeping great managers. Managers are the folks who implement your policies and keep workers motivated. Just because you have a vacancy in your business, please do not think that you have to promote from within. Sure, you want to give your employees the first chance to move up, but the benefits must be weighted against the possibility of promoting an incompetent worker.

There is no law that says you must promote from within. Your question should be—Who is going to do the best job for your company? Longevity should also not be the primary criterion used to promote from within; rather, your goal should be to find the best person to be a manager in your company, whether that person comes from within your business or from outside. Some people are going to say that this policy is unfair to your workers; however, it's much more important to be fair to the entire business by attracting the best managers wherever they may be. The requisite skills of a great worker and the requisite skills of a great manager are not similar. However, you may have an employee who is better than anyone you can hire from the outside. Your job as manager of your business is to find the best person for the job. Managers are critical to your organization. Find managers from either inside or outside who will do the best job for you.

 ### Selection 15.4: Local Fast Food Chain Pushes Its New Image

Coming soon to a fast-food restaurant near you are adult meals featuring salad, bottled water, pedometer, and advice to walk more. A local fast-food chain announced Thursday the plans to develop "go active meals for grownups" at all 13,500 of its U.S. restaurants. These restaurants are trying to make their fare and their image seem healthier. A target of obesity lawsuits and a magnet for criticism that fast food is bad for you, our local fast-food chain also launched a marketing blitz to address health issues head on and tout new diet-conscious items at its outlets.

As part of its advertising, the company said in June it would roll out healthier choices in meals for kids nationwide such as the option to substitute apple slices and juice for fries and soft drinks. It will also distribute brochures telling customers how to modify their orders so they can consume lower fat calories and carbs, such as by skipping the cheese or a bun. The promotion has been employed at its New York region restaurants since January. Also new will be the low-fat salad dressing that has been tried out in a number of test markets throughout the country. The company said nutrition information comes in response to a call from the U.S. Department of Health and Human Services this year for the private sector to help fight obesity.

Our local fast-food chain is really trying to promote balanced eating and exercise and is committed to taking the lead role by educating its customers on this seriously important health issue. By introducing entrée salads, the chain has helped get the American people thinking on the right track while also helping to increase sales. It has been moving to add healthier choices to its restaurants worldwide, including adding salads in Europe this spring. If it wants to improve the health of the people by providing salads and bottled water, it could stop using partially hydrogenated oils in its fries, which contain fats that are a real promoter of health disease. They also can lower the fat content in their burgers, use low-fat cheese, and provide more baked goods instead of fried food.

Our local fast-food chain promised two years ago to provide a healthier type of cooking oil for its fries. However, at this point they have not found an appropriate replacement. Those who are truly health conscious continue to monitor the changes that are being made to the restaurant, picking and choosing what they eat to reflect a healthy lifestyle.

Selection 15.5: A Story About My Dad

My name is Robert, and I want to tell you a story that happened to me and some members of my family. It begins back in about 1947 when my father returned from World War II after having served in the infantry in Germany. I remember that day very, very well. A man who I had never met suddenly got out of a yellow cab in front of our house at 256 Tacoma Street in Denver, Colorado. When he came into the house, he grabbed my mother and hugged her and kissed her, and I had no idea who this man was who was coming between me and my mother.

Later, and very soon, I began to realize that this was my father, and like any young boy somewhere between 5, 8, or 9 years of age, I often asked him questions about his war experiences. I would ask him if he shot a gun, where he was, did he ever kill anyone. And I always got about the same answers. He said very little, and he would often say that war was very ugly and that he really didn't want to talk about it. But, I was a little guy, and I wanted to talk about it.

I asked him if he brought home any mementoes, because some of my friend's fathers had brought home things, things they had taken off of prisoners and weapons or artifacts from the countries that they were in, but my father brought home nothing, at least nothing that I was aware of. So I continued to ask him and continued to wonder what he did in the war.

I heard a few stories. One, I know that he was one time on patrol, and they captured some German prisoners. When they returned, he was asked to return some of those prisoners back to the front line some five, six, seven hundred yards away. Shortly after, while he was taking them back, the rest of his troop continued on and they were massacred in a crossfire. I also know he was hospitalized once with frozen feet, and ultimately returned to the United States for treatment and then returned back to war.

But I know very little else, because like I said before, he didn't want to talk about it, and only later could I begin to understand why. In fact, a few years ago Tom Brokaw wrote an elegant book, titled *The Greatest Generation*. Tom Brokaw had decided that those men and women, who were the ages of my mother and father, now in their eighties, some nineties, some late seventies, but mostly in their eighties, were the people who had lived through the Great Depression, gone off and saved the world from a madman named Hitler, fought a war, many of them dying, came back, and without asking for anything, put aside their weapons, and built this country into the great country that it is.

When they came back and went back to work, they asked for very little. These are great and strong people. And my father's unwillingness to talk about death and destruction is now understood by me for the very first time. I know now why we never had a gun in our house, a bullet in our house—even a BB gun for his son was not allowed in our house. Things that killed people were just not allowed. We didn't even talk about them. We didn't hunt, and we didn't fish. We didn't kill animals; for whatever reason, that was just not done.

I'm not quite certain what his values were before the war, but I am quite certain what they were after the war. So hopefully you have a picture of him, because I want to tell you another story about him.

Picture the man who was part of the wonderful generation of men and women who helped salvage this country and get it started again, who asked for virtually nothing, who were strong determined people, and who did not romanticize death and destruction in any way and refused to have his children romanticize it in any way. But I was a boy, and as I grew my fascination with what I didn't know grew with it. When he stopped answering my questions about guns and death, I just started looking around for other things to do.

I made slingshots, and I threw rocks, but we didn't have any guns. And then one day by accident, rummaging through something in our garage I found a bullet, a real bullet. This bullet fascinated me, so much so that I decided to do something with it that I probably shouldn't have; no, I know I shouldn't have.

I took that bullet out and wedged it between two wires in our fence. Not knowing how weapons worked, my assumption was that if I could point the bullet at the anthill and somehow get it to go off, it would go in that direction, not thinking very much about how guns and rifles have barrels to guide the bullet and the direction you want it to go. Well, at any rate I wedged the bullet into the fence and then went inside and found a book of matches. Then I went outside and one after another after another lit matches under the casing of the bullet until finally under heat the bullet exploded.

But it didn't go straight, it went into my arm. And suddenly, after the ringing in my ears stopped, I looked down and a huge amount of blood was dripping off the ends of my fingers, and my arm was numb. And I said to myself, uh oh, I've done something really bad and my dad is really, really going to be angry. But right away I noticed I was bleeding a lot and I had to do something.

So I ran inside and called my mother who was working about five blocks from where we lived, but the line was busy. We didn't have call waiting in those days. In fact, most of us still had party lines. Ask someone to explain that to you. At any rate I stood there bleeding and making these phone calls on the inside and then I realized what a mess I was making by the telephone stand, so I'd run back outside and stand for a minute, but I was bleeding a lot.

Then I'd run back inside and call and the phone was still busy, so I'd go back outside and each trip I would leave a fair amount of blood on the kitchen floor and the downstairs and out back. Then I would come back inside and make the phone call again. And, finally I didn't know what to do because the line remained busy.

So I called my aunt, my mother's sister who lived about fifteen minutes across town. I called her and said "Aunt Sheila" actually we called her Aunt Toots—"Aunt Toots, I've just shot myself and I can't find my mother, can't reach my mother on the phone, and I don't know what to do," and I hung up. Well, my aunt called my mother's line at work, and it was still busy.

So she frantically jumped in the car and started driving across town. I kept trying to call my mother, and finally the phone rang. Now weakened from the loss of blood, I said, "Mom, something bad has happened, and I've shot myself, and I'm bleeding bad, and I think I'm going to die." And I hung up. Well, my mother hung up and drove the few minutes from her office to the house and found me sitting sort of crumpled up by the side of the house and indeed in a fair amount of blood.

And she dragged me around to the side of the house and turned on the garden hose, trying to rinse the blood off so she could see what was going on. She couldn't get the bleeding stopped, so she stuck her finger in the hole. That's right, she stuck her finger in the hole. Then she grabbed me and dragged me across the street, where, had I only remembered, but I didn't, there was a doctor's office.

Dr. Curtis was an unusual man, also someone who had served in World War II. He had a cleft lip and palate, which made his speech kind of hard to understand, and he was gruff. It may be hard to understand now, but doctors during that time all smoked in their offices. They might put their cigarettes down to do something, take a drag, come back, and do some other things.

Well, when I came into the office, everyone moved aside. We went back to a little examining room, and he reached under my arm around my armpit and found the exact place to put pressure on it to stop the bleeding. And then he casually picked up a piece of vein and said, "Well, you cut this right in half—no wonder you're bleeding." Then proceeded to put a tourniquet on my arm and with no Novocain, because I really didn't need it, sewed my vein back together and my arm.

The bullet had gone in, hit a bone, and exited back out in about the same place it went in. I was fortunate that my mother came home and got me over to

332

PART IV
....
Selections for
Interpreting and
Transliterating

him in time because I had a substantial blood loss. But at any rate old Doctor Curtis put my arm back together, or at least the hole back together, patted me on the head, probably charged my mother ten dollars for all of it, sent us home, and said, "Give him some orange juice—he's a little low on blood."

When we got back home, the horror of it all started to be amplified. The phone book had accepted a lot of blood and had swelled to more than twice its size. There was blood all over in the kitchen and on the floor and out on the back steps. And finally, for the first time, my mother, who's normally a very together person, cried and yelled in anger at me, "What have you done? What have you done?"

I said to please not tell my father because the man who had preached all his life or at least all of my life not to have a gun in the house would be so upset, really disappointed, that I had not listened to him. But she said there is no way I cannot tell him about this. So, I waited the rest of the day for my father to come home. When he got home my mother greeted him at the door, and they had a long ten-minute conversation.

He came in, patted me on the head and said, "You know I don't think you want to be playing around with bullets and guns. They can hurt you and others." To this day I've never owned a weapon, and I've never fired another shot, except one time I went duck hunting and shot a shotgun. However, I inadvertently hit the decoys instead of the ducks and sank this man's expensive decoy. He never asked me to go hunting with him again.

In my family guns were a no-no, and they almost took my life. (Courtesy of Robert L. Johnston)

References

Baker, C., & Cokely, D. (1980). *American Sign Language: A teacher's resource text on grammar and culture*. Silver Spring, MD: T.J. Publishers.

Borden, B.B. (1996). *The art of interpreting*. Plymouth, MI: Hayden-McNeil Publishing.

Byrnes, J. P. (2001). *Cognitive development and learning in instructional contexts*. Boston: Allyn and Bacon.

Cokely, D., & Baker-Shenk, C. (1991). *American Sign Language: A student text, units 1-9*. Washington, DC: Gallaudet University Press.

Gonzalez, V., Yawkey, T., & Minaya-Rowe, L. (2006). *English-as-a-second language (ESL) teaching and learning*. Boston: Allyn and Bacon.

Humphries, T., & Padden, C. (2004). *Learning American Sign Language*. Boston: Allyn and Bacon.

Janaro, R., & Altshuler, T. (2006). *The art of being human*. Boston: Allyn and Bacon.

Jones, M. (2005). *Criminal justice pioneers in U.S. history*. Boston: Allyn and Bacon.

Kelly, J.E. (2001). *Transliteration: Show me the English*. Alexandria, VA: RID Press.

Lengel, J., & Lengel, K. (2006). *Integrating technology: A practical guide*. Boston: Allyn & Bacon.

Lentz, E.M., Mikos, K., & Smith, C. (1992). *Signing naturally: Student workbook level 2*. San Diego, CA: Dawn Sign Press.

Makkai, A., Boatner, M.T., & Gates, J.E. (2004). *A dictionary of American idioms*. (4th ed.). Hauppaugh, NY: Barron's Educational Series.

Markowicz, H. (1980). Some sociolinguistic considerations of American Sign Language. In W.C. Stokoe (Ed), *Sign and culture: A reader for students of American Sign Language*. Silver Spring, MD: Linstock Press.

McKechnie, J. (Ed.) (1993). *Webster's new universal unabridged dictionary*. New York: Simon & Schuster.

Mikos, K., Smith, C., & Lentz, E.M. (2001). *Signing naturally: Student workbook level 3*. San Diego, CA: Dawn Sign Press.

Mulderig, G.P., & Elsbree, L. (1990). *The health handbook* (12th ed.). Lexington, MA: Heath.

Nist, S., & Simpson, M. (2001). *Developing vocabulary for college thinking*. Boston: Allyn and Bacon.

Newell, W. (2006). *Giving directions in American Sign Language*. Personal communication.

Newell, W., Campbell, C., Holcomb, B., Holcomb, S. Caccamise, F., & Peterson, R. (in press). *ASL at work— level one*.

Padden, C. (1983). *Interaction of morphology and syntax in American Sign Language*. Unpublished doctoral dissertation, San Diego, CA: University of California.

Schein, J.D. (1984). *Speaking the language of sign*. New York: Doubleday.

Schein, J.D., & Stewart, D.A. (1995). *Language in motion: Exploring the nature of sign*. Washington, DC: Gallaudet University Press.

Scheetz, N. (1998). *Manual communication: Signs for everyday use*. Austin, TX: Pro-Ed.

....
References

Seal, B. (2002). *Best practices in educational interpreting*. Boston: Allyn and Bacon.

Smith, C., Lentz, E.M., & Mikos, K. (1988b). *Signing naturally: Teacher's curriculum guide level 1*. San Diego, CA: Dawn Sign Press.

Smith, C., Lentz, E.M., & Mikos, K. (1988a). *Signing naturally: Student workbook level 1*. San Diego, CA: Dawn Sign Press.

Strike, K.A., & Moss, P.A. (1997). *Ethics and college student life*. Boston: Allyn and Bacon.

Stokoe, W.C. (1980). *Sign and culture: A reader for students of American Sign Language*. Silver Spring, MD: Linstock Press.

Supalla, T., & Newport, E. (1978). How many seats in a chair? The derivation of nouns and verbs in American Sign Language. In P. Siple (Ed.), *Understanding language through sign language research* (pp. 91–132). New York: Academic Press.

Valli, C., & Lucas, C. (2000). *Linguistics of American Sign Language* (3rd ed.). Washington, DC: Gallaudet University Press.

Index